Cardiac Diagnostic Tests

A GUIDE FOR NURSES

SHARON VanRIPER, MS, RN, CCRN
Clinical Nurse Manager, Cardiology
University of Michigan Hospitals
Ann Arbor, Michigan

JOHN VanRIPER, BSN, RN
Community Service Coordinator
Ann Arbor Public Schools
Ann Arbor, Michigan

W.B. SAUNDERS COMPANY
A Division of Harcourt Brace & Company
Philadelphia   London   Toronto   Montreal   Sydney   Tokyo

161324

W. B. SAUNDERS COMPANY
A Division of Harcourt Brace & Company
The Curtis Center
Independence Square West
Philadelphia, Pennsylvania 19106

NOTICE

Cardiology is an ever-changing field. Standard safety precautions must be followed, but as new research and clinical experience broaden our knowledge, changes in treatment and drug therapy become necessary or appropriate. The editors of this work have carefully checked the generic and trade drug names and verified drug dosages to ensure that the dosage information in this work is accurate and in accord with the standards accepted at the time of publication. Readers are advised, however, to check the product information currently provided by the manufacturer of each drug to be administered to be certain that changes have not been made in the recommended dose or in the contraindications for administration. This is of particular importance in regard to new or infrequently used drugs. It is the responsibility of the treating physician, relying on experience and knowledge of the patient, to determine dosages and the best treatment for the patient. The editors cannot be responsible for misuse or misapplication of the material in this work.

The Publisher

Library of Congress Cataloging-in-Publication Data

VanRiper, Sharon.
   Cardiac diagnostic tests : a guide for nurses / Sharon Van Riper, John Van Riper.
     p.   cm.
   ISBN 0-7216-2493-6
    1. Heart—Diseases—Diagnosis. 2. Heart—Diseases—Nursing. I. Van Riper, John. II.
Title.
    [DNLM: 1. Heart Diseases—diagnosis—nurses' instruction. WG 141 V217c 1997]
   RC683.v29   1997
   616.1'2075—dc20
   DNLM/DLC   96–18816

CARDIAC DIAGNOSTIC TESTS   ISBN 0-7216-2493-6

Printed in the United States of America

Last digit is the print number: 9   8   7   6   5   4   3   2   1

This book is dedicated to many loving family members and friends who provided encouragement and inspiration, but most importantly it is dedicated to the two people who gave me such rich beginnings of love, support, and unflagging devotion; my parents.

svr

I dedicate this book to all of my friends and family but especially to my children, Eddie and Timmy. Through their eyes I am able, once again, to view the adventure that is life, experience the joy of new knowledge, and marvel at the wonders that are all around us. My world is much richer since they became a part of it.

jvr

FOREWORD

With health reform sweeping the nation and technologic advancement in diagnostic testing continuing to move forward at an ever increasing pace, the need for concise yet complete descriptions of our utilization of cardiovascular diagnostic tests is becoming increasingly important. In this book, the editors and authors present a detailed overview of the major diagnostic tests which are currently used in modern cardiovascular therapeutics. Descriptions of electrocardiography, echocardiography, thallium imaging, radionuclide ventriculography, magnetic resonance imaging, positron emission tomography, and computerized axial tomography are all reviewed in a clear yet concise way. In addition, the authors discuss the use of certain laboratory tests and invasive procedures, including cardiac catheterization and electrophysiologic testing. The chapters are beautifully prepared with a glossary of terms and definitions at the beginning and examples of patient education sheets and critical pathways at the end. The chapters focus on multidisciplinary interventions which will be helpful in preparing the patient for these tests, as well as pertinent nursing interventions during and after each procedure. With an increasing number of patients being cared for in the outpatient arena, a reference text such as this is especially helpful for nurses and other health care professionals involved in the care of patients in rapid turnaround environments where access to quick knowledge is especially important.

Cardiac Diagnostic Tests, A Guide for Nurses, will be a significant reference text for members of the health care team who deal with cardiac patients in a variety of settings. I enjoyed reading it very much and I know you will too.

Kim A. Eagle, M.D.

PREFACE

Technology in the diagnosis and treatment of cardiac disease has changed drastically in the past fifteen years. Diagnostic tests and therapeutic interventions have become very sophisticated, often requiring indepth specialty training to perform and interpret. However cardiovascular disease remains the leading cause of death in the United States and most of the western world. This book is written to help nurses and other direct patient care providers understand the various diagnostic tests, both invasive and noninvasive, that are used to develop a treatment plan for the patient with heart disease. Testing and diagnosis are the first steps, followed closely by interventions that are often very complex and expensive.

The purpose of this book is to describe each diagnostic test in detail. Patient instructions and specific preparations for each test are detailed. For diagnostic tests that require special monitoring or post-procedure care, nursing interventions are described. Several chapters are authored by nurse practitioners and have excellent tips for ordering tests and the appropriate care surrounding them. Nearly all the chapters have a critical pathway that describes the multidisciplinary care that might be given for a specific diagnosis.

A number of invasive therapeutic interventions including PTCA, stents, atherectomy, and intracardiac catheter ablation are also discussed. Pacemakers and implantable antiarrhythmia devices are described, including the newest third generation devices. Pertinent nursing considerations and patient education materials are also included.

A thorough review of current thrombolytic agents and the new antiplatelet drugs are covered in the introductory chapter, along with a review of each of the major forms of cardiac disease. The ECG chapter is a complete overview of basic rhythms as well as 12-lead interpretations. Each chapter has a glossary of terms that can be used as a quick reference.

It is my hope that this text will be used as a guide to prepare patients for diagnostic and therapeutic procedures, and to recover from them afterwards. I also hope that the nurses who use it will find useful descriptions and illustrations of why tests are used and how they are interpreted. Finally, I hope that, in a small way, I might be able to make the job of staff nursing just a little easier (by providing a quick reference guide) for the thousands of dedicated professionals who are struggling to make it all work in an environment that is constantly changing with dwindling resources. Keep up the great work!

No preface is complete without acknowledgment of those individuals who helped to make this book a reality. I would like to thank my editor, Barbara Nelson Cullen, Marie Pelcin, and Joan Sinclair from W.B. Saunders for their encouragement and assistance. I appreciate the support and encouragement of the book sales force at W.B. Saunders with whom I have worked for many years as they provided learning materials and references at so many nursing seminars. Finally, a very special thank you to Marty Tenney at Textbook Writers Associates, Inc. for her calm and efficient preparation of the final product.

In addition to each of the contributors, I would like to thank several colleagues who provided assistance in a variety of ways, especially Elizabeth Nolan, MS, RN, Cheri Davis, BSN, RN, and Wendy Rose, MA. I am grateful to several of the cardiologists at the University of Michigan who offered manuscript critiques, illustration materials, and overall advice, with a special mention to Drs. Sunil Das and Steven Werns. It is an inspiration to work with such a talented group of people, and I greatly appreciate your support and assistance.

SVR

CONTRIBUTORS

JULIE R. CLIFFORD, MS, RN
Acute Care Nurse Practitioner
University of Michigan Hospitals, Ann Arbor, MI
Cardiac Disease: An Introduction

COLLEEN M. CORTE, MS, RN
Doctoral Student
University of Michigan, Ann Arbor, MI
Echocardiography

MARGARET GILLIGAN, MS, RN, CRNA
Certified Nurse Anesthetist
St. Joseph Mercy Hospital, Ann Arbor, MI
Electrocardiography

EVA KLINE-ROGERS, MS, RN
Acute Care Nurse Practitioner
University of Michigan Hospitals, Ann Arbor, MI
Positron Emission Tomography

EVAN PADGITT, MS, RN, CNP
Primary Care Nurse Practitioner
David Winston, MD and Associates: Internal Medicine, Ann Arbor, MI
Nuclear Medicine Studies; Magnetic Resonance Imaging and Computerized Tomography

JUDITH HOGAN RADKE, MS, RN, CRNA
Certified Nurse Anesthetist
Houston, TX
Laboratory Tests

CATHERINE GAGE RICCIUTI, MS, RN, CCRN
Educational Nurse Specialist
University of Michigan Hospitals, Ann Arbor, MI
Laboratory Tests; Cardiac Catheterization; Critical Pathways

MARGARET RICKLEMANN, BSN, RN
Staff Nurse, Emergency Department
University of Michigan Hospitals, Ann Arbor, MI
Electrophysiology Studies

SHARON VANRIPER, MS, RN, CCRN
Clinical Nurse Manager
University of Michigan Hospitals, Ann Arbor, MI
Electrophysiology Studies; Critical Pathways

REVIEWERS

LINDA M. CELIA, MSN, RNC
Hahnemann University Hospital
Philadelphia, Pennsylvania

NANCY C. GROVE, RN, BSN, MED,
MSN, PhD
University of Pittsburgh, Johnstown
Johnstown, Pennsylvania

ANN M. GURKA, RN, MS, CCRN
Clinical Nurse Specialist
Cambridge Hospital
Cambridge, Massachusetts

M. CHARLENE LONG, RN, MS
University of Southern Florida
College of Nursing
Tampa, Florida

BARBARA J. MARTIN, RN, MS
Rush Presbyterian-St. Luke
Medical Center Chicago, Illinois

KELLY MCKNIGHT, RN, BN, MSc.
Instructor
Red River Community College
Winnipeg, Manitoba, Canada

MELINDA E. MERCER, MSN, RN,
CCRN, CS
Hahnemann University Hospital
Philadelphia, Pennsylvania

PATRICIA GONCE MORTON, RN, PhD
University of Maryland School of
Nursing Baltimore, Maryland

JACQUELIN S. NEATHERLIN, RN,
PhD, CNRN
Baylor University School of Nursing
Dallas, Texas

COLLEEN S. PFEIFFER, RN, MS, CCRN
William S. Middleton Memorial
Veterans Administration Hospital
Madison, Wisconsin

SARA M. SUMNER, RN, CCRN
President
Criticare, Inc.
Holmes, Pennsylvania

KAREN L. THEN, RN, BN, MN
Assistant Professor
Faculty of Nursing
University of Calgary
Calgary, Alberta, Canada

JOANN PHOEBE WESSMAN, RN, BS,
MS, PhD
Dean, Oral Roberts University
Anna Vaughn School of Nursing
Tulsa, Oklahoma

CONTENTS

1

INTRODUCTION

JULIE R. CLIFFORD

The attack is very short but like a storm. It usually ends within an hour. I have undergone all bodily infirmities and dangers, but none appear to be more griev-ous. Why not? Because to have any other malady is to be sick; to have this is to be dying.[1]

—Lucius Anneaus Seneca (4 B.C.–A.D. 65)

According to the American Heart Association (AHA), atherosclerotic heart disease is the leading cause of death in the United States and all of the Western world.[2] This complex disease affects not only the coronary arte-rial system but also the renal, cerebrovascular, and peripheral arteries as well as the iliac vessels and thoracic and abdominal aorta.[3] In North America, more than 1 million people die each year from an acute myo-cardial infarction (AMI). The average age of onset in men is approximately 50 years and in women, 60 years.[4,5] Although the exact cause of coronary artery disease remains a mystery, there are several theories currently being researched.[3,6] Early identification of those who are at risk is of great signif-icance to clinicians. Over the past 20 years, much effort has been directed at increasing public awareness of risk factors and at early identification of a coronary event. It has been clearly established that early detection and rapid treatment of acute myocardial infarction and other coronary events are the most effective ways to decrease mortality and morbidity. The com-bination of health promotion, risk factor reduction, and active participa-tion in the treatment plan has demonstrated that mortality from heart disease can be lessened if health care providers and consumers work co-operatively toward this common goal.

In today's health care environment—where resources are limited, costs are high, and rapid change is commonplace—many types of providers are involved in the continuum of care from prevention to in-tervention. There is a desire to increase primary care specialists, both

The author wishes to acknowledge the invaluable assistance of Elizabeth Nolan, MS, RN, CS in the development of this chapter.

1

physicians and nurses, to fill the need for first-line care, preventive care, and health education. In many settings nurses are, and will continue to be, the primary patient educators and therefore are expected to be knowledgeable, articulate, and accountable to consumers. Because patient care is multifaceted, nurses must exert leadership in a variety of settings and function as practitioner, researcher, and educator.

The purpose of this book is to provide clinicians with vital information about the numerous invasive and noninvasive tests that are used to diagnose cardiac disease. In addition to a description of the tests, specific patient care before and after each procedure is discussed. Each chapter has at least one patient education sheet that can be used directly for patient preparation. Application of most procedures as they are used in managed- or coordinated-care critical pathways is also included.

This chapter will provide a brief review of the heart's structure and function as well as an overview of the current management of cardiac disease. A review of the major clinical trials relative to the treatment of myocardial infarction and congestive heart failure will also be covered.

ANATOMY AND PHYSIOLOGY

The heart is a muscular organ, approximately 12 cm long and 9 cm wide, weighing between 300 and 400 grams. It is encased in fat that protects it and insulates the coronary arteries. The heart is situated obliquely in the chest between the lungs, with the upper portion or base at the level of the second rib and the apex angled down and left at the level of the fifth rib. The pericardial sac surrounds the heart and contains two layers filled with 10 to 30 ml of fluid that acts as a lubricant for the heart while it contracts and expands. The heart muscle is made up of three layers, which are illustrated in Figure 1.1.

1. *Endocardium*   The inner layer is in direct contact with blood circulating through the heart. Its smooth surface discourages clot formation on the inner surface of the heart.
2. *Myocardium*   The middle layer is composed of muscle fibers that perform the pumping action of the heart.
3. *Epicardium*   The outermost layer. The coronary arteries and veins are embedded in the epicardium.

Coronary Circulation

The coronary circulation originates from the aorta and can be quite variable within individuals. The myocardial blood supply is provided by the right coronary artery (RCA) and the left coronary artery (LCA), along with their respective branches. These arteries originate in

FIGURE 1.1

The three layers of the heart: endocardium, myocardium, and epicardium. The pericardium is a saclike structure that surrounds the heart.

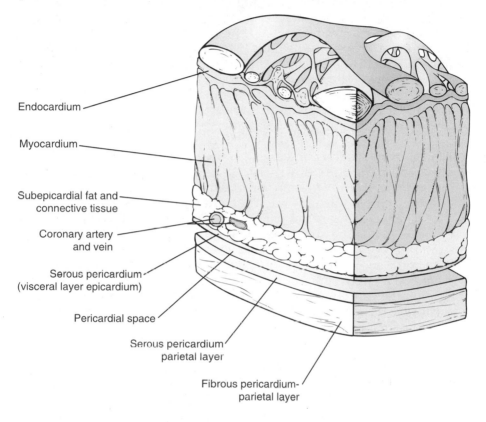

Endocardium

Myocardium

Subepicardial fat and connective tissue

Coronary artery and vein

Serous pericardium (visceral layer epicardium)

Pericardial space

Serous pericardium parietal layer

Fibrous pericardium-parietal layer

the aortic root, with the ostia located behind the aortic valve leaflets. Myocardial blood flow occurs mainly during the diastolic portion of the cardiac cycle. This is due to the squeezing and shortening effect on myocardial vasculature that occurs during systole. As the heart begins diastole the muscle relaxes; the leaflets assume their closed position as the aortic root pressure or systolic pressure rises. The result is that blood is forced down into the coronary arteries and myocardial perfusion takes place.

The LCA usually has three or four major segments or branches. The portion of the LCA from the ostium to the first point of major branching is designated the left main coronary artery (LMCA) or left main. The LMCA then commonly bifurcates into the left anterior descending (LAD) and the circumflex (Cx) arteries. In a significant number of subjects the artery will trifurcate and form the LAD, the Cx, and the intermediate arteries. This intermediate artery usually follows along the same path as either the first diagonal branch or the first obtuse marginal branch.[7,8]

Either the RCA or the LCA may give rise to a special coronary branch called the posterior descending artery (PDA), which supplies the major portion of the blood delivered to the inferior portion of the left ventricle. It is the presence of this branch on either the RCA or LCA that determines coronary dominance. In approximately 70% of individuals the PDA originates from the RCA; these individuals are termed "right dominant" with regard to anatomic myocardial circulation. In 10% of the population the PDA arises from the Cx and thus fulfills the criterion for "left dominance." The remaining individuals are referred to as "codominant" in that both the RCA and Cx provide a blood supply to the inferior wall. One further distinction is that the artery supplying blood to the AV node originates from the dominant artery[8,9] (Figure 1.2).

The cardiac veins lie superficial to the cardiac arteries. The coronary sinus is the largest component of the venous system and is located in the posterior portion of the right atrium. All of the major coronary veins empty into the coronary sinus except the anterior great cardiac vein, which empties directly into the right atrium.

There are four valves within the heart. The mitral and tricuspid (AV) valves divide the atria from the ventricles and are open during the diastolic filling phase of the cardiac cycle. The semilunar valves, also known as the aortic and pulmonic valves, exit the ventricles and are open when blood is ejected into the great vessels during systole. The mitral and tricuspid valves are attached to the myocardium via the papillary muscles and chordae tendineae. This rather complex structure is subject to damage from ischemia and infarct.

Mechanical Contraction

The purpose of the heart is to pump blood, and cardiac muscle is specialized for this purpose. Myocardial muscle is composed of

1. *Sarcolemma* A single membrane surrounding the myocardial cell and consisting of a thin, bimolecular phospholipid layer.
2. *Sarcoplasmic Reticulum* A membranous continuation of the sarcolemma. The sarcoplasmic reticulum is the repository for calcium ions used in the process of muscle contraction.
3. *Sarcoplasma* Intracellular proteinaceous fluid.
4. *Contractile unit* A muscle fiber divided into filaments composed of the contractile proteins actin and myosin interacting with troponin and tropomyosin. The filaments are further divided into thick filaments (composed of myosin) and thin filaments (composed of actin, troponin, and tropomyosin).[10]

Adapted from Principal Investigators of CASS and Their Associates. National Heart, Lung, and Blood Institute Coronary Artery Surgery Study. *Circulation.* 1981; 63 [Suppl 1]:1–81. Used by permission of the American Heart Association, Inc.

FIGURE 1.2

The coronary artery anatomy.

1. Proximal right
2. Midright
3. Distal right
4. Right posterior descending
5. Right posterolateral segment
6. First right posterior lateral
7. Second right posterior lateral
8. Third right posterior lateral
9. Inferior septal
10. Acute marginal
11. Left main
12. Proximal left anterior descending
13. Midleft anterior descending
14. Distal left anterior descending
15. First diagonal
16. Second diagonal
17. First septal
18. Proximal circumflex
19. Distal circumflex
20. First obtuse marginal
21. Second obtuse marginal
22. Third obtuse marginal
23. Left atrioventricular
24. First left posterior lateral
25. Second left posterior lateral
26. Third left posterior lateral
27. Left posterior descending

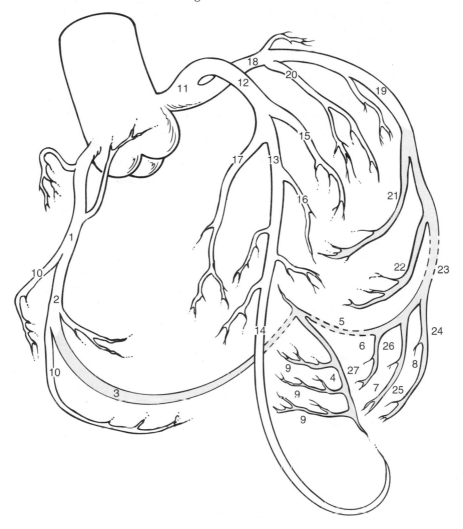

Circulating venous blood enters the right atrium via the inferior and superior vena cava. Coronary venous blood also enters the right atrium through the coronary sinus. Blood flows across the tricuspid valve into the right ventricle, across the pulmonic valve and into the pulmonary arteries, where it is transported to the lungs. In the lung alveoli, carbon dioxide is exchanged for oxygen. The average oxygen saturation for blood on the right side of the heart is 75%; after leaving the lungs the average saturation is 95%.[10]

Oxygenated blood returns to the left atrium via the pulmonary veins and passes through the mitral valve to the left ventricle. The healthy left ventricle ejects about 60% of its resting volume across the aortic valve into the aorta and on to the systemic circulation. The forward flow of blood is ensured by valves designed to prevent backward flow regardless of chamber pressures.[10]

Conduction System

The specialized system of cells known as the conduction system provides for a regular cardiac rhythm, and is designed to maximize the efficiency of each contraction. Each cycle is initiated by the generation of an action potential that begins at the sinoatrial (SA) node. The SA node is a subepicardial structure located in the posterior wall of the right atrium by the opening of the superior vena cava. Spindle-shaped and composed of closely packed cells in a fibrous tissue matrix, the SA node consists of cells that initiate electrical impulses. The normal rate of impulse formation in the SA node is 60 to 100 beats per minute in the adult.[10,11] Impulses travel through the atrium via specialized tracts called internodal pathways to the atrioventricular (AV) node. The AV node is a small subendocardial structure located in back of the right atrium, close to the septal leaflet near the tricuspid valve. In ninety percent of human hearts the AV node gets a dual blood supply from the AV nodal artery, a branch of the RCA, and from the septal branches of the LAD. The AV node and surrounding junctional tissue in the normal heart have an intrinsic rate of 40 to 60 beats per minute and can pace the heart if the SA node fails.[11]

The His bundle emerges from the AV node and divides into the right and left bundle branches. These branches provide a pathway for impulses to travel throughout the myocardium to their point of termination in the Purkinje fibers. Conduction defects anywhere within the His bundle or bundle branches can cause loss of atrial/ventricular synchrony and symptomatic bradycardia (Figure 1.3).

Properties of Cardiac Cells

There are four main physiological characteristics of the cardiac cells that allow for the integration of electrical and mechanical activity.

FIGURE 1.3

The electrical conduction system in the heart.

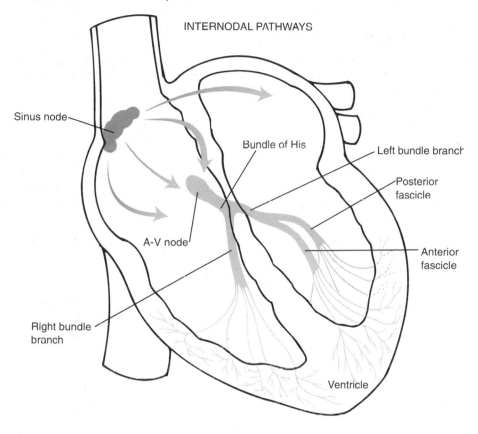

These are: (1) *excitability*, the responsiveness of the cell to an impulse; (2) *automaticity*, the ability to initiate an impulse; (3) *conductivity*, the ability to transmit impulses; and (4) *contractility*, the ability to respond to impulses with a pumping action.

OVERVIEW OF CARDIAC DISEASE

While a comprehensive review of cardiac disease is beyond the scope of this text, a brief discussion of the major types of cardiac disease is included here as a reference. Current research findings on treatment options and directions in future research will also be included. A brief review of the current literature related to quality of life for chronically ill cardiac patients is presented as well. Subsequent chapters will elaborate on specific diagnostic procedures, patient preparation and aftercare, and education plans. A variety of critical pathways encompassing a wide range of cardiac diseases and diagnostic tests are also included.

Atherosclerosis

Atherosclerosis of the coronary arteries is the leading cause of death in the United States.[2] Atherosclerosis is a multifactoral process that leads to a progressive degeneration of the integrity of the arterial wall and the eventual obstruction of the lumen.

The artery is composed of three layers: the intima, the media, and the adventitia (Figure 1.4). The *intima*, or innermost layer, is thin and comprised of connective tissue and smooth muscle cells. The *media* is the muscular wall of the artery and is comprised of smooth muscle cells that are surrounded by internal and external elastic fibers. The outermost layer, the *adventitia*, consists of a dense structure with numerous groups of collagen fibrils, elastic fibers, and fibroblasts. The adventitia is highly vascular, and contains its own blood supply and nerves. It is separated from the media by a sheet of elastic tissue called the external elastic lamina. During the aging process, the smooth muscle cells, collagen fibrils, and elastic fibers slowly proliferate and migrate to the intima, which leads to a thickening of the intima and forms the basic structure of the atherosclerotic lesion.[12] Clinical symptoms of ischemia usually occur as the lumen narrows in a spot that has developed an atherosclerotic lesion.

FIGURE 1.4

The structure of an artery and vein.

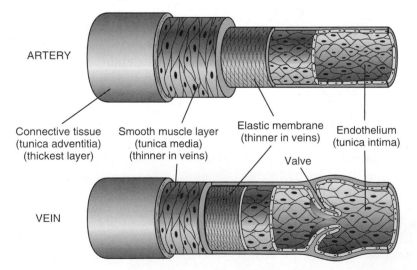

ARTERY

Connective tissue
(tunica adventitia)
(thickest layer)

Smooth muscle layer
(tunica media)
(thinner in veins)

Elastic membrane
(thinner in veins)

Endothelium
(tunica intima)

Valve

VEIN

Atherosclerosis is most often associated with medium-size arteries, such as the coronaries and the carotids. It may occur in a single coronary artery or may affect multiple vessels. The lesions may be anywhere in the coronary tree. Three types of lesions have been described in the process of atherosclerosis: fatty streaks, fibrous plaques, and complicated plaques.

The *fatty streak* consists of small numbers of intimal smooth muscle cells surrounded by lipid deposits, most of which are in the form of cholesterol and cholesterol esters. These fatty streaks can be found in childhood and are seen in people of all ages (but cause minimal or no vascular obstruction). By the time fatty streaks or smooth yellow lesions are visible there is histologic evidence of lipid deposits in the smooth muscle cells and in the macrophages of the intima. However, the deposits generally do not result in significant interruption of arterial blood flow. Whether these fatty streaks are precursors of plaque remains controversial. Plaque develops in areas where no fatty streaks have been apparent and fatty streaks do not always develop into plaque.[13]

Fibrous plaques are more advanced lesions. They are gross, white, raised lesions that protrude into the lumen of the vessel and eventually compromise arterial blood flow. Fibrous plaques consist of an accumulation of intimal smooth muscle cells, macrophages, and T-lymphocytes. There are both intracellular and extracellular deposits of lipids. Connective tissue or collagen, elastic fibers, and proteoglycans accumulate. These are the basic components of the plaque, which may have a fibrous cap that encloses the mass of connective tissue and lipids.

Complicated plaque and *advanced plaque* are terms used to describe plaque where calcification, thrombosis, hemorrhage, and/or rupture have occurred. This type of lesion is often associated with occlusive disease.[12] Complicated plaques are difficult to reduce with angioplasty, and may require more aggressive maneuvers such as atherectomy (Figure. 1.5).

RISK FACTORS FOR DEVELOPING CORONARY ARTERY DISEASE

The relationship between risk factors and coronary artery disease has been well documented by extensive epidemiological studies. The atherosclerotic process occurs gradually over time. It is very important for patients to understand that atherosclerotic heart disease is a chronic, incurable condition. Treating it effectively requires a commitment on the part of the patient to incorporate lifelong adaptive health behaviors.[12 15]

Of all the studies that have been done on the risk factors for developing coronary artery disease, the Framingham Study is undoubtedly the most well known and influential. It began in 1948 with 5209 women and men ranging in age from 30 through 52 years. Participants had com-

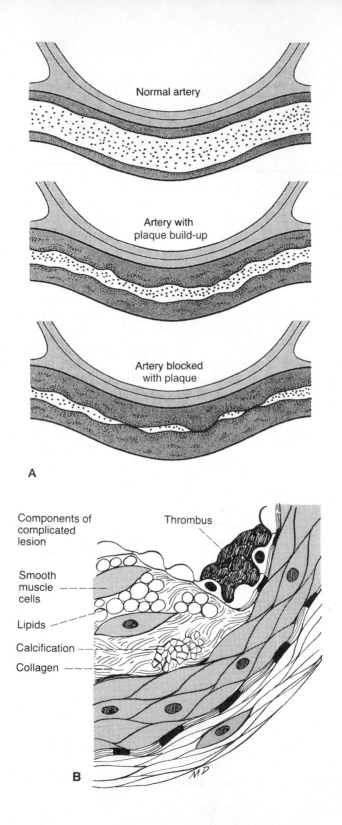

Normal artery

Artery with
plaque build-up

Artery blocked
with plaque

A

Components of
complicated
lesion

Thrombus

Smooth
muscle
cells

Lipids

Calcification

Collagen

B

plete history and physical examinations, ECGs, and blood tests, and were followed every two years. As of 1990, over 60% of the original participants were dead. As expected, the leading cause of death was cardiovascular disease.[13,16]

Over 40 years of cumulative data has provided clear evidence identifying various coronary risk factors. A risk factor can be thought of as "any habit or trait that can be used to predict an individual's probability of developing that disease."[15] The Framingham risk factors include hyperlipidemia, hypertension, cigarette smoking, diabetes mellitus, left ventricular hypertrophy, obesity, age, family history, and male gender. Despite the clear-cut relationship between these risk factors and the development of coronary disease, exact etiology of the genesis of atherosclerosis is still uncertain. The study further divides risk factors into modifiable and nonmodifiable factors.[13] Modifiable factors such as hypertension, hyperlipidemia, and smoking are treatable, and either reducing these factors or eliminating them results in a decreased risk for heart disease. Nonmodifiable factors such as gender, age, or family history are obviously not treatable but are important considerations in making the diagnosis of CAD. Consequently, educational efforts should focus on helping patients modify such risk factors. Further, public health concerns should focus on the prevention of heart disease through treatment or avoidance of the modifiable risk factors.

Hyperlipidemia

The first of the three modifiable risk factors is *dyslipidemia*, which is described as an abnormal metabolism of plasma lipids caused by genetics, diet, or a secondary disease process. The major classes of plasma lipids include cholesterol, cholesterol esters, triglycerides, and phospholipids. Although some plasma lipids are vital to normal cellular function, in many cases patients cannot adequately rid their bodies of excess lipids. Since lipids are insoluble in water, they are transported in the blood by molecules called lipoproteins.[17] Table 1.1 gives a brief description of the major types of lipoproteins.

FIGURE 1.5

Development of the atherosclerotic plaque. A. Blood flow through the lumen is impaired by the buildup of plaque. B. A complex fibrotic lesion is apparent within the lumen of the artery.

A. Adapted from Ignatavicius D, Workman L, Mishler M. *Medical-Surgical Nursing: A nursing process approach*, 2nd ed. Philadelphia: WB Saunders; 1995. Used with permission. B. Adapted from Luckmann J, Sorensen KC. *Medical-Surgical Nursing*, 3rd ed. Philadelphia: WB Saunders; 1987. Used with permission.

TABLE 1.1

Major Types of Lipoproteins

CHYLOMICRON
The largest of the lipoproteins. Composed primarily of triglycerides and found in the intestines, chylomicrons travel to the lymph system, where they are added to the venous system. They are acted upon by an enzyme called lipoprotein lipase (LPL) and are then further broken down into fatty acids for storage. Their end product consists mostly of cholesterol, which is taken up by the liver and then synthesized into very low density lipoproteins (VLDL). The more fat the molecule contains, the lower its density.

VERY-LOW-DENSITY LIPOPROTEIN (VLDL)
A smaller lipoprotein. VLDL is produced in the liver and contains primarily triglycerides.

LOW-DENSITY LIPOPROTEIN (LDL)
Made primarily of cholesterol. When LDLs are oxidized, they attract macrophages that turn the LDL cells into foam cells. Foam cells activate growth factors and secrete cytolytic substances, resulting in platelet activation and thrombus formation.

HIGH-DENSITY LIPOPROTEIN (HDL)
The smallest of the lipoproteins. HDLs are made primarily of protein and are produced by the liver and GI tract. They transport cholesterol away from the intimal wall to the liver for catabolism. Higher levels of HDL are associated with lower atherosclerosis risk.[14,15]

As a general rule, the LDL/HDL ratio is measured to estimate coronary risk. The focus of treatment for high-risk individuals is to reduce LDL. This is attempted through dietary low-fat prescriptions and through the use of hypolipidemic agents. Desirable ranges for lipoprotein levels are presented in Table 1.2.[18,19]

Smoking

A second major modifiable risk factor associated with coronary artery disease is cigarette smoking. Tobacco leaves were given as tokens of friendship by Native Americans to Columbus and his crew; they were rolled and smoked by Native Americans during religious ceremonies and

TABLE 1.2

Desirable Lipid Values

Total cholesterol/HDL ratio	< 3
LDL/HDL ratio	< 4.5
Triglycerides	< 200 mg/dl
LDL cholesterol	< 160 mg/dl in patients with no other risk factors
	< 100 in patients with CAD
HDL cholesterol	
men	> 35
women	> 40

used for medicinal purposes. It wasn't long before tobacco crops were growing and the cigarette industry was born.[20]

Only in the last fifteen or so years has smoking been associated with ischemic heart disease. The exact pathophysiologic mechanism behind the adverse effects of smoking is not clear. However, there are at least three major effects of cigarettes on the heart. First, it is believed that the harmful cardiovascular effects of smoking are in part due to increased endothelial permeability.[21] This results in injury to the intimal wall and to the accumulation of the components of the atheroma. When comparing smokers with nonsmokers, lower levels of HDL and higher levels of LDL and triglycerides were found.[21] Second, the Framingham study found that cigarette smoking had many effects on clotting factors and platelet functions. Fibrinogen levels were found to be significantly higher in smokers than nonsmokers. Interestingly, ex-smokers had fibrinogen levels that were the same as those who never smoked. Also, cigarette smoke generates carbon monoxide that replaces oxygen on the hemoglobin molecule, resulting in less circulating oxygen in the blood. Finally, the direct effect of nicotine is that of a stimulant: It results in the release of epinephrine and norepinephrine; and can lead to tachycardia, higher blood pressure, and increased oxygen consumption. In addition, cigarette smoking may aggravate arrhythmias.[22–25]

Hypertension

Hypertension completes the triad of the most common and significant risk factors.[25,26] A chronic blood pressure over 140/90 mmHg is associated with significant risk of coronary disease. Hypertension promotes the development of coronary disease by increasing left ventricular wall tension, which eventually causes hypertrophy, and by causing chronic vasoconstriction of the coronary arteries, which leads to intimal damage and atherosclerosis. Hypertensive patients also have an increased susceptibility to silent ischemia, sudden death, renal damage, and cerebral involvement. Hypertensive screening is important as people are often unaware that they have an elevated blood pressure, and progressive damage can occur for as long as 10 to 20 years. Untreated, half of patients with hypertension will die of coronary heart disease or congestive heart failure, while many others will suffer a stroke or renal failure.

ANGINA PECTORIS

"But there is a disorder of the breast marked with strong and peculiar symptoms, considerable for the kind of danger belonging to it, and not extremely rare, which deserves to be mentioned at length. The seat of it, and sense of strangling and anxiety with which it is attended, may make it not improperly be called angina pectoris."[27]

Dr. William Heberden was the first person to describe the sensation of classic angina, back in 1772, and his initial description still conveys the sensation most patients experience.[28] *Angina pectoris* is a clinical condition resulting from myocardial ischemia and is characterized by chest discomfort or discomfort from adjacent areas such as the right or left upper extremities, back, neck, or jaw. Stable or classic angina is described as chronic pain that occurs at reproducible levels of activity without changes in frequency or severity and is relieved by nitroglycerin.

Angina is usually described as a squeezing, burning, or strangling sensation, and often varies in intensity and character. It is usually brought on by activity or stress. The duration characteristically lasts 5 to 10 minutes, and for many patients may be relieved by resting. On an ECG, ST segments may appear depressed with inverted T waves.

Medical management of classic angina is directed at reducing myocardial oxygen demand and maximizing available oxygen supply. A wide range of drugs are used including nitrates, beta-blockers, calcium blockers, antiplatelet agents, and antihypertensive agents.

Prinzmetal's angina, also called variant angina, typically occurs between midnight and 9 AM, and is not precipitated by activity. There appears to be an association with smoking, and it occurs more often in men between the ages of 30 and 50.[29] Variant angina is associated with a moderate to severe reduction in diameter of a proximal coronary artery due to a spasm. It often causes ST elevation on an ECG. Patients with variant angina respond well to nitrates, calcium antagonists, and Prazosin, which is a selective alpha-blocker. It is important to distinguish variant angina from other forms of angina because beta-blockers may have a paradoxical effect on variant angina.

Unstable angina has been recognized as a separate entity for approximately 50 years. It is believed to be caused by microemboli in the coronary circulation. There are three subsets of unstable angina. The first, *progressive angina*, is characterized by a sudden change in severity, onset, or duration of pain. Pain does not occur at rest. *Angina at rest*, the second subset, is associated with increased mortality and increased risk of myocardial infarction. *Early postinfarct angina* occurs after myocardial infarction and is associated with recurrent infarcts and increased mortality.[30] In many cases, the pain persists longer than 15 minutes, is accompanied by ST elevations on the ECG, and is not usually relieved by nitroglycerin.[30]

Treatment of unstable angina is directed at relieving the pain, preventing an AMI, and revascularizing the heart whenever possible. Treatment with nitrates, beta-blockers, heparin, and antiplatelet agents including aspirin (ASA) is recommended. Ruling out a myocardial infarction and monitoring for arrhythmias are done rountinely when an angina patient presents to the hospital with chest discomfort of greater than 30 minutes duration unrelieved by nitroglycerin. Following relief of pain and stabilization of the patient, functional studies are performed to assess left ventricular responsiveness.

If functional studies are positive, coronary angiography is performed to identify coronary anatomy and define treatment options. Studies have shown that 10% to 20% of patients with unstable angina have left main disease, 40% have three-vessel disease, and the others will have one or two-vessel disease. Approximately 10% of patients who present with apparent unstable angina have coronary vasospasm.[27,30,31]

TREATMENT OF CORONARY ARTERY DISEASE

Revascularization procedures include angioplasty (PTCA) and coronary artery bypass grafting (CABG). While success rates are very high for each procedure, there are risk and cost issues to consider. PTCA versus CABG has been the subject of several clinical trials that are designed to evaluate the use of each in the treatment of CAD. See Table 1.3 for a list of the clinical trials that are currently under way. It is expected that these trials will eventually set the standard for revascularization in the setting of symptomatic coronary disease.[32]

Coronary Artery Bypass Grafting

Coronary artery bypass grafting is a surgically created detour designed to provide myocardial blood flow beyond an area of coronary blockage. A section of harvested saphenous vein is most often used to provide this detour, although one or both internal mammary arteries also can be grafted. Bypass surgery may involve grafts to several vessels (Figure 1.6).

TABLE 1.3

Ongoing Trials of PTCA Versus CABG in the Treatment of CAD

Acronym	Full Name
BARI	Bypass Angioplasty Revascularization Investigation
FAST	Emory Angioplasty vs Surgery Trial
RITA	Randomized Interventional Treatment of Angina
CABRI	Coronary Angioplasty Bypass Revascularization Investigation
GABI	German Angioplasty Bypass Intervention

The purpose of all of these studies is to evaluate the outcomes in patients with at least two-vessel disease who need revascularization. Patients are randomized into either PTCA or CABG groups. Postprocedure follow-up looks at death, myocardial infarction, recurring angina, exercise tolerance, and quality of life. Most of these studies have an enrollment period of several years and some have a follow-up period of up to 5 years postprocedure.

FIGURE 1.6

Typical insertion sites for vein grafts to coronary arteries.

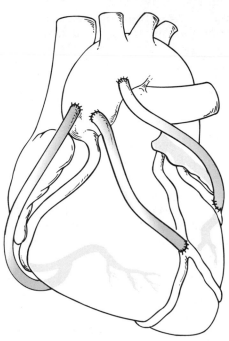

From Tilkian AG, Daily EK. *Cardiovascular Procedures: Diagnostic Techniques and Therapeutic Procedures*. St. Louis: Mosby-Yearbook Publishing; 1986:143.

Extensive data have been accumulated comparing the outcomes of bypass surgery with those of patients who are managed by medical therapy alone. One collaborative study, the Coronary Artery Surgery Study (CASS), reported average annual mortality rates of 1.5 and 2.1 percent in surgically and medically treated patients, respectively, with triple-vessel disease.[31,33,34] CABG improves survival in patients with hemodynamically significant left main coronary artery disease. Of patients with impaired left ventricular function (ejection fraction < 50%) and three-vessel disease at time of entry to CASS, those who went on to have surgery had a more favorable survival rate.

Percutaneous Transluminal Coronary Angioplasty

Percutaneous transluminal coronary angioplasty was first performed in 1977 by Dr. Andreas Gruentzig, who miniaturized a peripheral artery balloon catheter and used it to dilate a coronary artery in a male patient. Over the next 2 years, Dr. Gruentzig and his associates worked to improve both the technique and the equipment to allow for access and control within the coronaries. He then began to teach physicians worldwide about PTCA. By 1985, the use of PTCA in the treatment of CAD was widespread. Currently, over 500,000 procedures are performed in the United States each year.[35]

While the high initial success rates and low risks of PTCA cannot be argued, one significant drawback to the procedure has been the source of intense research and study. This is *restenosis*, a process that occurs in as many as 35% to 45% of patients undergoing angioplasty. Restenosis has proven to be a mighty foe. Despite a wide variety of techniques, pharmacologic agents, and intravascular devices, restenosis is still the biggest problem associated with PTCA and frequently is the reason for repeated procedures and proportionately higher costs. Coronary angioplasty and restenosis are discussed in greater detail in chapter 7.

MYOCARDIAL INFARCTION

Each year in America over 1 million acute myocardial infarctions occur, resulting in close to 500,000 deaths.[5] Too often, delays in treatment result in increased mortality and morbidity. Current research on the treatment of AMI focuses on salvaging the myocardium. This may be accomplished with the use of thrombolytic agents or angioplasty and is quite effective when treatment is initiated early. Several large-scale international trials have evaluated the efficacy of all the available thrombolytic agents as well as that of the available and investigational antithrombin and antiplatelet agents, and rescue angioplasty. A review of all of these studies is beyond the scope of this text; however, there is no doubt that early treatment of AMI protects the myocardium and preserves life.[36]

Myocardial ischemia results from a decreased blood flow to the myocardium due to atherosclerosis, vasospasm, platelet aggregates, or thrombus. Prolonged ischemia may result in tissue death. When this occurs, necrotic cells leak their contents into the surrounding tissue, affecting its ability to function.[5]

AMIs are usually classified by their location: inferior, anterior, lateral, septal, posterior, or right ventricular. The location of the MI depends on which artery is occluded. Additionally, the infarct may be classified using the ECG criteria, such as Q-wave and non Q-wave infarct.

The diagnosis of an AMI is usually based on the clinical presentation, serial ECGs, and serial cardiac enzymes. Upon physical examination, patients appear anguished, are restless, and frequently massage or clutch their chests. Clinically, findings can include hemodynamic instability, bradycardia or tachycardia, signs of congestive heart failure, new murmurs, extra heart sounds, or hypoxia. Pericardial rubs occur about 20% of the time and commonly appear on the second or third day. A persistent rub or one that appears 1 to 2 weeks after the infarct may be indicative of pericarditis (Dressler's syndrome).[10]

TREATMENT OPTIONS FOR ACUTE MYOCARDIAL INFARCTION

Current treatment for acute myocardial infarction is aimed at reducing tissue death by salvaging myocardium. Along with thrombolytic therapy, other interventions include rescue percutaneous transluminal coronary angioplasty (PTCA) and emergent coronary artery bypass graft (CABG) surgery.

Following the emergency procedures or stabilization of the patient, a focus on risk factor reduction and patient education should be done. Characterizing symptoms by type, location, duration and precipitating factors is helpful for the patient and the clinician as plans are made to detect and treat future symptoms rapidly. Identification of risk factors and development of a plan for treating other coexisting health problems are also important.

Thrombolytic Therapy

The most common cause of MI is thrombus.[6] When the vessel wall is injured or an atherosclerotic plaque ruptures, platelets adhere to the damaged area and begin the process of thrombus formation. Thrombin then acts on soluble fibrinogen and converts it to fibrin, which is an insoluble protein that forms a clot. The body attempts to dissolve this fibrin clot through a proenzyme called plasminogen that when activated becomes plasmin. Plasmin eventually dissolves the fibrin clot; however, by the time that occurs, the damage to the myocardium is done. Thrombolytic therapy is modeled after the normal thrombolytic process. Multiple clinical trials with thrombolytic therapy have demonstrated significant mortality reduction when compared to standard treatment.[6,36]

A number of clinical studies have demonstrated the success of early administration of thrombolytic agents. These drugs, when given within the first few hours of onset, help to recannulize the occluded vessel by lysing the clot, thus reestablishing adequate blood flow. The most dramatic results in reducing mortality are seen when thrombolytics are administered within the first 60 minutes after the onset of symptoms. From 4 through 12 hours, a small to moderate benefit is still seen.[36] This translates into decreased mortality and morbidity from AMI. By 12 hours after the onset of symptoms, the risks and costs of the therapy outweigh the benefits.[37,38]

The three major thrombolytic agents used are: tissue plasminogen activator (tPA), streptokinase (SK), and anisoylated plasminogen streptokinase activator complex (APSAC). Urokinase (UK) is used primarily during interventions in the catheterization laboratory, while prourokinase (scuPA) is still investigational. All of the thrombolytic agents can be further divided into fibrin-specific or nonfibrin-specific activators. tPA and scuPA are fibrin-specific, which theoretically results in less systemic fibrinolysis. APSAC, SK, and UK are nonfibrin-specific and may result in systemic anticoagulation.[6,36] Clinical trials have shown that all lytic agents reduce mortality. Whether or not one shows a superior benefit with regards to mortality is controversial. Overall, the patency rates are 60% to 70% using all agents as measured by coronary angiography.[36]

Streptokinase is a nonenzymatic bacterial protein that functions indirectly as a plasminogen activator. Streptokinase is administered intravenously, 1.5 million units over 60 minutes and has a half-life of 18 minutes. Allergic reactions, including antibody formation and a rare occurrence of anaphylaxis, are associated with SK.

Anisoylated plasminogen streptokinase activator complex is a thrombolytic agent developed to overcome some of the limitations of IV streptokinase. The APSAC molecule has greater specificity for fibrin than SK and can be given as a bolus. The pharmokinetic properties of APSAC result in a more sustained fibrinolytic activity than that of SK; the half-life of APSAC is 90 to 105 minutes.[6,36]

Urokinase (UK) is a naturally occurring plasminogen activator. Like streptokinase, urokinase does not have fibrin specificity. The major advantage of urokinase over SK is that UK is much less antigenic. The half-life of UK is 16 to 20 minutes.[6,36]

Tissue-type plasminogen activator (tPA), a second generation thrombolytic agent, is a plasminogen activator initially extracted from human tissue. Production of tPA using recombinant DNA techniques has made tPA widely available to researchers investigating its effectiveness in the treatment of strokes and emboli as well as coronary thrombi. Two types of tPA are commercially available, including one form that is made of altered human tPA.[39]

While tPA has a high affinity for fibrin and is relatively clot specific, there is some binding to circulating plasminogen, especially at higher doses. This can result in systemic bleeding problems and is common with all of the thrombolytic agents. Although tPA is a more effective clot-lysing agent than some others, it is also more likely to have a higher rate of reocclusion because of its short half-life [40] tPA is a highly successful thrombolytic agent in humans, with recannulization rates of 65% to 86%.[39] Additionally, because it is a human enzyme, rare antigenic responses have been noted. One potential drawback to the widespread use of tPA is the cost per dose.

ScuPA inactivates the endogenous circulating inhibitor of fibrin. Success rates at 90 minutes compare favorably to SK at about 70%, with a half-life comparable to tPA (about 5 minutes).[41]

Arrhythmias such as accelerated idioventricular rhythm, premature ventricular contractions (PVC), ventricular and supraventricular tachyarrhythmias, and heart block have been observed with successful reperfusion within the first few hours after administration of thrombolytics. These arrhythmias are believed to be caused by local tissue injury from oxygen free radicals that are formed at the site of injury and travel into the circulation after perfusion is restored. Arrhythmias tend to occur at the time lysis is achieved and are generally well managed with drugs, defibrillation, or pacing; in some cases, these reperfusion arrhythmias are self-limiting and no treatment is needed.[6,39]

The major risk associated with thrombolytic therapy is hemorrhagic complications. There have also been reported a much smaller incidence of immunologic complications, hypotension, and myocardial rupture.[42] Anaphylaxis is a very rare complication and occurs in about 0.5% of patients given streptokinase. Careful screening is vital prior to the administration of thrombolytics as they are contraindicated with any patient who has a recent history of bleeding. Bleeding complications from thrombolytics may be categorized into two types: superficial, where bleeding is seen at puncture sites or recent incisions, and internal, such as gastrointestinal, retroperitoneal, or cerebral bleeding. Superficial bleeding is treated conservatively while the thrombolytic drug is infused. Internal bleeding is a potentially life-threatening situation and is treated by immediately stopping the drug and providing aggressive resuscitation.

Adjunctive Therapy During Thrombolysis

Antithrombin Agents

Heparin is commonly used as an adjunct to thrombolytic therapy; given as an antithrombin agent. Studies have shown that the combination of antithrombin agents and fibrin-specific thrombolytics (tPA, scuPA) is critical in maintaining infarct vessel patency.[39] Generally, heparin is begun intravenously at a dose of 1000 U/hr concomitantly with or soon after the initiation of lytic therapy.

A new generation of antithrombin agents is currently under development. There are two promising agents currently in clinical trials. Hirudin, a derivative of leech saliva, was used in the TIMI-5 trials in conjunction with tPA and demonstrated statistically significant improvement in artery patency and mortality rates.[43] A more recent trial, GUSTO IIB, which used Hirudin in combination with tPA, SK, and APSAC, demonstrated a slightly beneficial effect with regard to mortality and recurrent ischemic events in patients with AMI and acute coronary syndromes.[44] The second agent, Hirulog, is a synthetic form of Hirudin and will be tested in several large scale clinical trials.

Antiplatelet Agents

Aspirin is now a standard antiplatelet agent used in the treatment of AMI. Multiple clinical trials have demonstrated reduced mortality associated with acute myocardial infarctions when aspirin is taken. A recently approved antiplatelet agent, ReoPro, which is a glycoprotein IIb, IIIa receptor blocker, has been shown to significantly reduce the incidence of recurrent ischemia and mortality in patients with coronary syndromes.[45]

PTCA in Myocardial Infarction

A number of clinical trials examined the risks, costs, benefits, and effects of performing PTCA on acute myocardial infarction patients for the purpose of obtaining a patent infarct vessel. The TAMI trials (Thrombolysis and Angioplasty in Myocardial Infarction) were the first to compare angioplasty and thrombolysis and generally concluded that patency was achieved at about the same rate in each procedure. However, higher cost and risks and the same rate of restenosis led researchers to conclude that PTCA should only be done in rescue situations where hemodynamic stability and pain relief could not otherwise be achieved.[46]

A more recent trial, PAMI, (Primary Angioplasty in Myocardial Infarction), used PTCA within the first 12 hours after the onset of symptoms. In comparison with thrombolytic therapy, this approach has resulted in fewer deaths and nonfatal cardiac events in the first 6 months after the angioplasty.[47] The PAMI, as well as the GUSTO IIB, study suggests that there is a role for primary angioplasty in the treatment of AMI. However, this role is limited because of the logistical difficulties in providing PTCA to patients immediately following an MI. Around-the-clock provision of interventional services is both costly and simply inaccessible for many patients outside large metropolitan areas.

Coronary Artery Bypass Grafting (CABG)

While it is not standard practice to perform CABG on an acutely infarcting patient, it is done in some settings as a treatment for unrelenting pain or cardiogenic shock in the acute infarction period. This is logistically difficult due to the time it takes to assemble an emergency operating team. Also, patients who have been treated with thrombolytic therapy are usually not considered for emergency CABG. In the studies that have been done on the success of CABG in the acute myocardial infarction patient, survival has been favorable at about 70%.

CONGESTIVE HEART FAILURE

Congestive heart failure (CHF) afflicts 2 to 3 million Americans. Nearly 300,000 people die from it each year and the incidence is rising. According to the American Heart Association, 400,000 new cases of CHF are diagnosed each year; it is the most common medical diagnosis in patients over 65 years.[2,48,49] (Congestive heart failure is listed most often as the reason for medical admissions to the hospital in patients over age 65.) Hypertension and coronary artery disease are the two most common causes of CHF in the adult population. Women are more likely than men to suffer from heart failure after myocardial infarction, especially if they have diabetes. The prognosis of heart failure is described by some as dismal: as high as a 50% mortality rate per year in those patients with very low ejection fractions (< 20%) and an overall mortality rate of 40% over 5 years.[49]

Congestive heart failure is associated with coronary artery disease and long-standing hypertension. It is characterized by ventricular dysfunction and decreased exercise tolerance. Many patients with CHF express a loss in quality of life, and generally experience a shortened life span.[49,50]

Heart failure occurs when the ventricle is no longer able to meet the oxygen demands of the tissues it supplies. Compensatory hemodynamics and neurohormonal mechanisms become exhausted.[48] Cardiac output is dependent on three things: systemic vascular resistance or afterload, venous return or preload, and contractility of the heart muscle. An increase in afterload or preload can result in too much work on the heart and result in hypertrophy and eventual heart failure. An overstretched muscle results in poor emptying; the resulting congestion, either pulmonary or systemic, results in a backup of fluid. Depending on whether the failure is right- or left-sided, symptoms may result in varying degrees of discomfort ranging from dyspnea to hypotension.[51]

In left-sided heart failure, ventricular end-diastolic volume will increase and the LV end-diastolic pressure will rise. The increased hydrostatic pressure in the pulmonary vasculature will result in fluid from the vascular space leaking into the alveoli, impairing gas exchange. Clinical signs include dyspnea, rales, orthopnea, a third heart sound, and restlessness.[51,52]

The most common cause of right-sided heart failure is left-sided heart failure. However, right-sided heart failure may occur independently as a result of right ventricular myocardial infarction, tricuspid or pulmonic valve disease, pulmonary emboli, or pulmonary hypertension. Clinical signs specific to right-sided heart failure are those of venous congestion, including jugular venous distention, hepatic congestion, dependent edema, and a low output state.[51,52]

Treatment is directed at improving hemodynamic parameters. Pharmacologic agents include diuretics, direct-acting vasodilators, positive inotropic agents, angiotensin-converting enzyme (ACE) inhibitors, and beta-adrenergic antagonists. Additionally, patients are monitored for life-threatening arrhythmias and treated with drugs or devices as necessary to prevent sudden death.[51,52]

Recently, large-scale studies have taken place to evaluate the effects of current treatments. Several studies are noteworthy and are listed in Table 1.4. In reviewing the results of these many trials, it becomes clear that treating CHF with ACE inhibitors in addition to vasodilators and diuretics is most likely to decrease mortality. In most of the trials the particular ACE inhibitor used was enalapril.

While drug therapy shows some promise in halting the devastating effects of CHF, it often is not enough to restore a patient's cardiac output to the degree needed for resuming an active lifestyle. In these cases, evaluation of the patient for transplant may be considered. Approximately 2500 patients per year in the United States receive new hearts. Most transplant recipients are men, ranging in age from newborn through 77 years. A current success rate of over 75% survival at 5 years post-transplant is due to the effectiveness of immunosuppressive drugs, the early and accurate detection of rejection, and highly successful organ procurement and preservation practices.[53]

Despite the impressive success of heart transplant in treating CHF, it is important to note the limiting factors. These include an enormous cost for the procedure itself as well as for lifelong medications and follow-up care. Another limiting factor is the number of donors, which each year is far exceeded by the number of potential recipients.[53] Much effort is needed to raise public awareness about the value of organ donation.

Cardiogenic Shock

The most serious form of congestive heart failure is cardiogenic shock. Cardiogenic shock usually occurs following a large myocardial in-

TABLE 1.4

Large-Scale Trials of ACE Inhibitor Therapy in CHF

Name of Study	Drug	Risk Reduction
SOLVD (Studies of Left Ventricular Dysfunction)	Enalapril	16%
CONSENUS (Cooperative North Scandinavian Enalapril Survival Study)	Enalapril	31%
SAVE (Survival and Ventricular Enlargement)	Captopril	19%
V-Heft-2 (Veterans Administration Vasodilator Heart Failure Trial)	Enalapril	38%

The purpose of these large-scale international trials was to evaluate the use of ACE inhibitors in treating congestive heart failure. The above studies are a sample of the current data, and the findings are consistent in all the studies. ACE inhibitors definitely result in a decrease in mortality along with an improvement in functional capacity and exercise tolerance. Patients generally report feeling better after starting ACE inhibitor therapy.

farction when there is severe loss of contractile fibers due to widespread cell death. It can also occur as a result of chronic ventricular tachycardia or pericardial tamponade, or from other types of degenerative muscle diseases of the heart.[51]

Cardiogenic shock occurs in about 10% to 15% of patients who suffer an AMI. Of these, only about 10% will survive. Despite aggressive, invasive measures and complex pharmacologic and ventilatory support, most patients simply cannot survive with the amount of damage that has occurred in their hearts. However, despite the dismal survival statistics, progress has been made in reducing the incidence of cardiogenic shock through prompt and aggressive revascularization, thrombolysis, and support of the acute myocardial infarction patient.

The process of cardiogenic shock evolves into three stages. In stage I, called compensated hypotension, the dysfunctional myocardial tissue results in decreased cardiac output. Hypotension triggers the arterial baroreceptors, which stimulate the catecholamine response in an attempt to restore tissue perfusion. Stage II, decompensated hypotension, is characterized by further necrosis, inadequate cardiac reserve, and even lower cardiac output. The compensatory mechanisms fail. By stage III, irreversible shock has reached the microcirculation and caused cellular membrane injury, which progresses to irreversible organ damage and death.[54,55]

Clinical presentation of the patient with cardiogenic shock includes a drop in systolic blood pressure to 30 mmHg below baseline or a sustained blood pressure less than 90 mmHg not attributable to any medications. Other symptoms are cold and clammy skin, cyanosis, altered sensorium, narrowing pulse pressure, cardiac index less than 2.2 L/min/m^2, urine output less than 20 ml/hr, and respiratory distress.[51,54,55]

Historically, treatment of cardiogenic shock has been difficult and largely unsuccessful in preventing death. Traditional methods of treatment include invasive hemodynamic monitoring, pharmacologic support with positive inotropes and vasopressors such as digitalis, dopamine, and dobutamine, and intra-aortic balloon counterpulsation. The focus is on protecting viable myocardium by raising the blood pressure, relieving pain, maximizing tissue oxygenation, increasing contractility, and reducing ventricular filling pressures. Mortality rates have been 80% to 90% and have shown virtually no improvement despite a variety of new drugs.[51]

Perhaps the most successful treatments for cardiogenic shock to date are emergency angioplasty and coronary bypass surgeries. A number of studies have shown that PTCA is successful about 70% of the time and that it improves mortality rates considerably. Of 313 patients who had emergent PTCA for cardiogenic shock, 55% survived.[56] This compares very favorably to the 10% to 15% survival rate in patients who do not get PTCA. In another series of 120 patients, survival was 72.5% following CABG.[56]

Cardiogenic Pulmonary Edema

Cardiogenic pulmonary edema, though less ominous than cardiogenic shock is a life-threatening condition that results from severe left-ventricular decompensation. It can result from an acute event such as a ruptured papillary muscle or myocardial infarction, or it can occur in a patient who has chronic congestive heart failure.

Hydrostatic pulmonary edema occurs in patients with heart failure. As volume and pressure increase on the left side of the heart, pressure rises in the pulmonary vasculature. Normally, the hydrostatic pressures in the pulmonary vasculature keep fluid within the blood vessel and prevent it from seeping into the interstitium of the lungs. When the hydrostatic pressure rises, the fluid leaves the vasculature and leaks into the lung. This leakage is irritating to the patient, who may cough and raise secretions that are frothy and pink tinged (due to red blood cells leaking into the lung from the high-pressure pulmonary vasculature). Patients will be dyspneic, orthopneic, and anxious. Altered mental status may be noted. Hypoxia triggers an increase in the heart and respiratory rates.

Treatment is aimed at stabilizing the patient hemodynamically and preventing further deterioration. The patient is placed in an upright position, and intravenous morphine is administered to promote vasodilation and rest. In addition, diuretics are given along with vasodilators to reduce systemic and pulmonary vascular pressures. Preload reducing agents, such as nitrates, and bronchodilators, such as theophylline, may also be given. Respiratory support may require the use of mechanical ventilation to increase alveolar ventilation and mean lung volume, allowing for more gas exchange. Both invasive measurement of vital signs and direct monitoring of pulmonary arterial and capillary wedge pressures during treatment are useful as a guide to therapy and also efficient.[51,55]

Cardiomyopathy

Cardiomyopathy is a term used to describe a group of diseases involving the heart muscle and characterized by myocardial dysfunction that may be idiopathic in nature or secondary to a specific systemic disease.[57] The three major types of cardiomyopathy are (1) dilated, (2) hypertrophic, and (3) restrictive.

Dilated Cardiomyopathy

Dilated cardiomyopathy (DCM) is the most frequently seen type of cardiomyopathy. Its earliest findings include left ventricular hypertrophy and contractile dysfunction. It often has an insidious onset, and affects more men than women. People of all ages can be affected; children have very poor outcomes.[58] Often no precipitating factor is identified. Toxins, metabolic aberrations, and infections have been associated with the development of DCM and are listed in Table 1.5; smoking has also been linked to DCM.[59]

In all cases the myocardium becomes damaged. Symptoms are related to the hypodynamic state. There is dilatation of the chambers and stretching of the myocardial fibers such that they lose contractile function to a significant degree. Patients then have symptoms of heart failure such as dyspnea and fatigue. DCM is usually degenerative, causing debilitating heart failure and eventual death. In most cases, death occurs within 5 years of the onset of symptoms.[57]

Hypertrophic Cardiomyopathy

Hypertrophic cardiomyopathy (HCM) is characterized by an asymmetrical and markedly hypertrophic left ventricle. In most cases, there is asymmetrical septal hypertrophy that may eventually obstruct blood flow out of the chamber, hence the term *hypertrophic obstructive cardiomyopathy*. Diastolic dysfunction occurs because the ventricle is unable to relax and fill normally. Cardiac output may be normal or increased initially but will eventually decline. Dyspnea of exertion, angina, presyncope, and ventricular arrhythmias are seen in these patients, as is sudden death.[60] Young patients without overt symptoms have a higher risk of sudden death.[61] In fact, HCM is the most common abnormality found in young athletes who die suddenly.[62]

Restrictive Cardiomyopathy

Restrictive cardiomyopathy is the least common type of cardiomyopathy. It is characterized by myocardial stiffness; the ventricular walls are rigid, impairing ventricular relaxation and filling. Systolic function is not usually affected.[57] It is important to make the differential diagnosis between pericarditis and restrictive cardiomyopathy since both conditions result in diastolic dysfunction and relatively normal systolic function. While it is possible to surgically treat pericarditis, there is no intervention for restrictive cardiomyopathy other than the use of pharma-

TABLE 1.5

Etiologic Factors in Dilated Cardiomyopathy

Toxins	Metabolic Aberrations	Infections
Alcohol	Hypertension	Viral
Cigarettes	Pregnancy	Bacterial
Cocaine	Thyrotoxicosis	Rickettsial
Bleomycin	Cardiac ischemia	Fungal
Adriamycin	Electrolyte imbalance	Parasitic

cologic agents to relieve symptoms. Restrictive cardiomyopathy is most likely to be seen in patients with amyloidosis or sarcoidosis where there has been an accumulation of abnormal substance (amyloid or sarcoid) within the myocardium. This type of cardiomyopathy is secondary to the systemic effects of the underlying disease.[57]

A good diagnostic workup is essential to the development of the most effective treatment plan for the patient with cardiomyopathy. Diagnostic tests will rule out other likely causes of the symptoms. For most patients, nearly every diagnostic test or procedure described in this text will be used to either make the diagnosis or follow the patient after treatment is begun.

There is no cure for cardiomyopathy. In many patients, cardiac transplantation is the only hope of long-term survival. In the 1989 International Heart Transplant Registry, cardiomyopathy was the reason for over 50% of the 10,000 transplants performed worldwide.[63] It is important to recognize the stresses that this condition places on patients and families. Waiting for a new heart may take weeks, months, or years. Physical deterioration, psychological stress, profound changes in interpersonal relationships, and serious financial worries are part of everyday life for those awaiting a donor heart. Providing support, education, and resources to help overcome some of these difficulties is part of the role of each member of the health care team.

Recent developments in implantable-assist devices may make the heart donor shortage less ominous in the near future. The battery-operated, fully-implantable, ventricular-assist device is currently being investigated in human subjects.

QUALITY OF LIFE STUDIES

As health care interventions become more technically sophisticated and complex, more patients are surviving and trying to regain a portion of their previous lifestyles. Unfortunately, these survivors are often plagued by the side effects of multiple drugs, the unpredictability of lifesaving devices, or the restrictions on activities. In an effort to better understand how chronically ill patients perceive their conditions and treatments, multiple studies have been conducted that examine the quality of life (QOL). Quality of life is fairly difficult to measure. It is multifaceted and subjective. Studies in both quantitative and qualitative measurements of QOL have been conducted on cardiac patients. Better understanding of the struggles, concerns, and perceptions of these patients can help health care providers choose effective treatment strategies and supportive interventions.

While there are a multitude of tools used to assess QOL, most researchers agree that the major components that should be studied include the perception of health, physical function, psychological function, and social relationships.[64] In five studies of cardiac patients with severe heart failure, measurement of quality of life indicators showed some significant areas of dissatisfaction.[65-68] The subjects included both pretransplant and post-transplant patients as well as those with advanced heart failure who were medically managed. Most patients reported decreased satisfaction with their QOL when they had symptoms that prevented them from completing activities of daily living. In addition, feelings of depression, anxiety, and hostility were also reported. In one study comparing post-transplant patients to pretransplant patients, the results in both groups were similar. Although the nontransplanted patients had poorer exercise tolerance, both groups were dissatisfied with their QOL and reported depression, anxiety, and hostility. In addition, the rate of employment was essentially the same and was thus not a distinguishing factor.[68]

QOL studies are also used to evaluate the effects of new drugs on the physical and psychological well-being of the patient. Health care providers are challenged to continue to work toward providing the most effective and safe treatments for cardiac patients. In a time of increasingly limited resources, it is vitally important that patients receive the type of interventions that will provide them with the most improvement in both mortality *and* quality of life.

REFERENCES

1. Julian DG, ed. *Angina pectoris* 2nd ed. New York: Churchill Livingstone; 1985.
2. American Heart Association. *Heart and Stroke Facts*. Dallas: American Heart Association; 1990.
3. Anderson HV, King SB. Modern approaches to the diagnosis of coronary artery disease. *Am Heart J*. 1992;123:1312–1323.
4. Hanisch PJ. Identification and treatment of acute myocardial infarction by electrocardiographic site classification. *Focus Crit Care*. 1991;18:480–488.
5. Mayberry-Toth B, Landron S. Complications associated with acute myocardial infarction. *Crit Care Nurs Q*. 1989;12(2);49–62.
6. Anderson HV, Willerson JT. Thrombolysis in acute myocardial infarction. *N Engl J Med*. 1993;329:703–709.
7. Walmsley R, Watson H. *Clinical Anatomy of the Heart*. New York: Churchill-Livingston; 1978.
8. McAlpine WA. *Heart and Coronary Arteries: An Anatomical Atlas for Clinical Diagnosis, Radiological Investigation, and Surgical Treatment*. Berlin: Springer-Verlag; 1975.
9. Canobbio MM. *Cardiovascular Disorders*. St Louis: CV Mosby; 1990.
10. Underhill SL, Woods SL, et al. *Cardiac Nursing*. 2nd ed. Philadelphia: JB Lippincott Co; 1989:27–85.
11. Ellenbogen KA, Peters RW. Indications for permanent and temporary cardiac pacing. In: Ellenbogen KA, ed. *Cardiac Pacing*. Boston: Blackwell Scientific Publications; 1992.
12. Ross R. The pathogenesis of atherosclerosis. In: Braunwald E, ed. *Heart Disease: A Textbook of Cardiovascular Medicine*. 4th ed. Philadelphia: WB Saunders; 1992; 1106–1124.

13. Cohn, PF, ed. *Diagnosis and Therapy of Coronary Artery Disease.* 2nd ed. Boston: Martinus Nijhoff; 1985.
14. Cohen JA. Reducing cholesterol: Strategies for increasing patient awareness. *Crit Care Nurs.* 1989;9(3):25–34.
15. Schell M. Cholesterol, lipoproteins, lipid profiles: A challenge in patient education. *Focus Crit Care.* 1990;17:203–211.
16. Levy D, Wilson PWF, Anderson KM, et al. Stratifying the patient at risk from coronary disease: New insights from the Framingham heart study. *Am Heart J.* 1990;119:712–717.
17. Farmer JA, Gotto AN. Risk factors for coronary artery disease. In: Braunwald E, ed. *Heart Disease: A Textbook of Cardiovascular Medicine.* 4th ed. Philadelphia: WB Saunders; 1992;1125–1160.
18. The Expert Panel. Report of the National Cholesterol Education Program Expert Panel on detection, evaluation, and treatment of high blood pressure in adults. *Arch Intern Med.* 1988;148:36–39.
19. LaRosa JC, Cleeman JI. Cholesterol lowering as a treatment for established coronary heart disease. *Circulation.* 1992;85:1229–1235.
20. Franklin RA. Smoking. *Nurs Clinics North Am.* 1992;27:631–641.
21. Roberts, WC. Atherosclerosis risk factors: Are there 10 or is there only 1? *Am J Cardiol.* 1989;64:552–554.
22. Nyboe J, Jensen G, Appleyard M, Schnohr P. Smoking and the risk of first acute myocardial infarction. *Am Heart J.* 1991;122:438–447.
23. Kannel WB, D'Agostino RB, Belanger AJ. Fibrinogen, cigarette smoking, and risk of cardiovascular disease: Insights from the Framingham Study. *Am Heart J.* 1987;113:1006–1010.
24. Kannel WB, Wolf PA, Castelli WP, et al. Fibrinogen and risk of cardiovascular disease. *J Am Med Assn.* 1987;258:1183–1186.
25. Caplan D. Smoking: Issues and interventions for occupational health nurses. *AAOHN Journal.* 1995;43:633–644.
26. Hockenberry B. Multiple drug therapy in the treatment of essential hypertension. *Nurs Clinics North Am.* 1991;26:417–436.
27. Heberden W. Account of a disorder of the breast. *Medical Transcriptions from the Royal College of Physicians.* 1772;2:59.
28. Kutcher MA: Unstable angina. Cardiovascular disease and chest pain (monograph), 2 (2). Kansas City, MO Biomedical Information Corp., 1986.
29. Antman E, Muller J, Goldberg S, et al. Nifedipine therapy for coronary artery spasm: Experience in 127 patients. *N Engl J Med.* 1980;302:12.
30. Braunwald E. Unstable angina: A classification. *Circulation.* 1989;80:410.
31. Wallace WA, Richeson JF. Unstable angina pectoris. *Clin Cardiol.* 1990;13: 679–686.
32. Gersh, BJ. Efficacy of percutaneous transluminal coronary angioplasty (PTCA) in coronary artery disease: Why we need randomized trials. In: Topol EJ, ed. *Textbook of Interventional Cardiology.* 2nd ed. Philadelphia: WB Saunders; 1994:265–269.
33. Myers WO, Davis K, Foster ED, et al. Surgical survival in the Coronary Artery Surgery Study (CASS) registry. *Ann Thor Surg.* 1985;40:245–260.
34. Whalen RE, Hurst JW. The surgical treatment of atherosclerotic coronary heart disease. In: Hurst JW, et al., eds. *The Heart.* 7th ed. New York: McGraw-Hill; 1990:1029–1039.
35. Hillegass WB, Ohman EM, Califf RM. Restenosis: The clinical issues. In: Topol EJ, ed. *Textbook of Interventional Cardiology.* 2nd ed. Philadelphia: WB Saunders; 1994:415–433.
36. The GUSTO Investigators: An international randomized trial comparing four thrombolytic strategies for acute myocardial infarction. *N Engl J Med* 1993;329:673–682.

37. Sleight P. Thrombolysis: State of the art. *Eur Heart J.* 1993;14 (Suppl G):41–47.
38. Lincoff AM, Topol EJ. The illusion of reperfusion: Does anyone achieve optimal reperfusion during acute myocardial infarction? *Circulation.* 1993; 87:1792–1805.
39. Topol EJ. Thrombolytic intervention. In: Topol EJ, ed. *Textbook of Interventional Cardiology.* Philadelphia, WB Saunders, 1994:68–111.
40. Stump DC, Califf RM, Topol EJ, et al. Pharmocodynamics of thrombolysis with recombinant tissue-type plasminogen activator. Correlation with characteristics of and clinical outcomes in patients with acute myocardial infarction. *Circulation.* 1989;80:1222–1230.
41. PRIMI Trial Study Group: Randomized double-blind trial of recombinant prourokinase against streptokinase in acute myocardial infarction. *Lancet.* 1989;1:863–868.
42. Califf RM, Fortin DF, Tenaglia AN, et al. Clinical risks of thrombolytic therapy. *Am J Cardiol.* 1992;69:12A–19A.
43. Cannon CP, McCabe CH, Henry TD, et al. for the TIMI-5 Investigators. Hirudin reduces reocclusion compared to heparin following thrombolysis in acute myocardial infarction: Results of the TIMI-5 Trial. *J Am Coll Cardiol* 1993;2(suppl A):A-136.
44. Topol EJ. Global use of strategies to open coronary arteries (GUSTO II). Hirudin versus heparin in acute coronary syndromes. Presentation at the 45th Annual Scientific Sessions of the Am College of Cardiology, Orlando, March 26, 1996.
45. Coller BS, Anderson K, Weisman HF. New antiplatelet agents: Platelet GP IIb/IIIa antagonists. *Thromb Haemost,* 1995;74:302–308.
46. Califf RM, Topol EJ, Stack RS, et al. for the TAMI Study Group. Evaluation of combination thrombolytic therapy and timing of cardiac catheterization in acute myocardial infarction. *Circulation.* 1991;83:1543–1556.
47. Grines CL, Browne KF, Marco J, et al. for the Primary Angioplasty in Myocardial Infarction Study Group. A comparison of immediate angioplasty with thrombolytic therapy for acute myocardial infarction. *N Engl J Med* 1993;328:673–679.
48. Packer M. Treatment of chronic heart failure. *Lancet.* 1992;2:92–95.
49. Funk M. Epidemiology of heart failure. In: Gould KA, ed. *Critical Care Nurs Clin North Am.* Philadelphia: WB Saunders; 1993:569–573.
50. Cuny J, Enger EL. Medical management of chronic heart failure: Direct-acting vasolidators and diuretic agents. In: Gould KA, ed. *Critical Care Nur Clin North Am.* Philadelphia: WB Saunders; 1993:575–587.
51. Ferguson DW, Abbound FM. The pathophysiology, recognition, and management of shock. In: Hurst JW, et al., eds., *The Heart.* 7th ed. New York: McGraw-Hill; 1990:442–461.
52. Braunwald E, Grossman W. Clinical aspects of heart failure. In: Braunwald E, ed. *Heart Disease: A Textbook of Cardiovascular Medicine.* 4th ed. Philadelphia: WB Saunders; 1992:444–465.
53. Dressler DK. Transplantation in end-stage heart failure. In: Gould KA, ed., *Critical Care Nursing Clinics of North America.* Philadelphia: WB Saunders; 1993:635–648.
54. Schlant RC, Sonnenblick EH. Pathophysiology of heart failure. In: Hurst JW, et al., eds. *The Heart.* 7th ed. New York: McGraw-Hill; 1990:387–418.
55. Levine BS, Laurent-Bopp D. Shock. In: Underhill SL, et al. *Cardiac Nursing,* 2nd ed. Philadelphia: JB Lippincott; 1989:868–879.
56. Topol EJ. Mechanical interventions for acute myocardial infarction. In: Topol EJ, ed. *Textbook of Interventional Cardiology.* Philadelphia: WB Saunders; 1994: 292–317.

57. Wynne J, Braunwald E. The cardiomyopathies and myocarditides. In: Braunwald E, ed. *Heart Disease: A textbook of cardiovascular medicine*. 4th ed. Philadelphia: WB Saunders; 1992.

58. Taliercio CP, Seward JB, Driscoll DJ, et al. Idiopathic dilated cardiomyopathy in the young: Clinical profile and natural history. *J Am Coll Cardiol*. 1985; 6:1126.

59. Hartz AJ, Anderson AJ, Brooks HL, et al. The association of smoking with cardiomyopathy. *N Engl J Med*. 1984;311:1201.

60. Gillum RF. Idiopathic cardiomyopathy in the United States, 1970–1982. *Am Heart*. 1986;111:752.

61. Maron BJ, Roberts WC, Edwards JE, et al. Sudden death in patients with hypertrophic cardiomyopathy: Characterization of 26 patients without functional limitations. *Am J Cardiol*. 1978;41:803.

62. Maron BJ, Epstein SE, Roberts WC. Causes of sudden death in competitive athletes. *J Am Coll Cardiol*. 1986;7:204.

63. Heck CF, Shumway SJ, Kaye MP, et al. The registry of the international society for heart transplantation: 6th official report. *J Heart Transplant*. 1989;8: 271–276.

64. Grady KL. Quality of life in patients with chronic heart failure. *Crit Care Nurs Clin North Am*. 1993;12:66–69.

65. Dracup K, Walden J, Stevenson L, et al. Quality of life in patients with advanced heart failure. *J Heart Lung Transplant*. 1992;11:273.

66. Muirhead J, Meyerowitz B, Leedham B, et al. Quality of life and coping in patients awaiting heart transplant. *J Heart Lung Transplant*. 1992;11: 265–271.

67. Grady KL, Jaloweic A, Grusk B, et al. Symptom distress in cardiac transplant candidates. *Heart Lung*. 1992;21:434.

68. Walden J, Stevenson L, Dracup K, et al. Heart transplantation may not improve quality of life for patients with stable heart failure. *Heart Lung*. 1989;18:497.

2

ELECTROCARDIOGRAPHY

MARGARET GILLIGAN
JOHN VAN RIPER

GLOSSARY

Aberrancy   Used to refer to conduction of an impulse outside the normal conducting pathway.

Axis   Refers to an imaginary line along which the wave of electrical depolarization travels. This concept is applied to the limb leads of the standard ECG.

Bipolar   On the ECG it refers to those leads that have positive and negative points of reference (e.g. standard leads I, II, III). In reference to pacemakers it is a pacing wire that has the positive and negative poles at the tip of the catheter.

Compensatory Pause   Used to describe the cessation of electrical activity that occurs after a premature depolarization. In premature ventricular contraction, the pause is usually equal to twice the basic rate of the dominant rhythm (i.e., two PP intervals) in which case it is termed *fully compensatory*.

Ectopic   Refers to an impulse arising from any focus other than the sinus node.

Fascicle   A division of the left bundle branch along which the electrical impulse travels. There are two main divisions of the left bundle branch: the left anterior and the left posterior fascicles. Some authorities differentiate a third, the septal branch (fascicle).

Infarction   Death of myocardial tissue as a result of oxygen deficit.

Intrinsicoid Deflection   Occurring in the initial portion of the QRS complex, it represents the change from maximal positivity to maximal negativity (or vice versa).

Ischemia   A transient and reversible insult to the myocardium as a result of insufficient oxygen supply to the heart tissue.

Isoelectric Line   The baseline of the ECG from which all wave measurements begin and end.

Mean Vector   Refers to the average direction of the heart's electrical forces.

Paroxysmal   An event that begins abruptly and usually ends in the same manner. Frequently used in reference to tachyarrhythmias.

PMI   Point of maximal impulse. The place on the chest where the apical pulse is felt.

Polymorphic   Refers to the multiple configurations associated with a multifocal ectopic rhythm.

Precordial Leads   Electrocardiographic tracings obtained from leads placed on the chest wall (e.g. V_1).

Supraventricular   Originating at or above the atrioventricular junction.

Unipolar   On the ECG it refers to those leads that have a designated positive electrode (e.g. aVR, aVL, aVF), with the negative point of reference determined by the remaining two leads.

Vector   A representation of the electrical activity of the heart indicating both direction and magnitude.

The electrocardiogram (ECG) is perhaps the most widely used diagnostic tool in today's health care environment. It is noninvasive and painless for the patient and relatively inexpensive. It requires minimal patient co-operation and operator skill and may be done quickly in a variety of settings. The ECG is used as a screening tool, as a guide to therapeutic intervention, and as a definitive diagnostic tool.

Coupled with additional equipment such as exercise machines, recording devices, and other diagnostic technologies, the ECG provides an ongoing assessment of cardiac rhythm, ischemic changes, or other aberrations during the testing period. While it is used primarily to diagnose and treat diseases of the heart, the ECG can be used to detect certain pulmonary and extracardiac events as well.

This chapter focuses on ECG interpretation, from basic rhythms to advanced disease states. Skilled interpretation of the ECG is an essential part of caring for acutely ill cardiac patients. Early diagnosis and rapid interventions, especially in the patient with ischemic heart disease, can be lifesaving.

ECG LEADS

The electrocardiogram, or ECG, can be a useful and accurate diagnostic tool if interpreted with care and knowledge. Relatively inexpensive and particularly advantageous because it is noninvasive, the ECG can render much information about the gross anatomy as well as the pathological processes of the heart. By using strategically placed electrodes, one can collect a great deal of information about chamber enlargement or strain, myocardial infarction or injury, conduction abnormalities, dysrhythmias, drug effects, and electrolyte imbalances. The patient lies in a supine position during the recording of the ECG, reducing the effect physical rotation of the heart has on electrical direction and promoting patient relaxation and comfort. The supine position also reduces the amount of artifact or "noise" caused by muscle fatigue or disease and sets a standard for future comparison. The machinery involved is portable and current models offer computerized storage of data.

Our understanding of electrical forces and the points on the body where they are best detected, is founded on the work of Willem Einthoven, a Dutch scientist who is recognized as the father of the electrocardiogram. This concept of measuring electrical potential between two parts or areas of the body is based on a triangular pattern and is referred to as Einthoven's triangle (Figure 2.1). Note that by drawing in the sides of the triangle to their center points and bisecting the six angles that are formed, the six diagonals produced correspond to the six leads of the standard frontal-plane ECG. This is referred to as the *hexaxial reference system*. These six leads are then divided between the bipolar leads (I, II, III) and the unipolar leads (aVR, aVL, aVF).

The bipolar leads measure electrical potential between two relatively distinct points (lead I = +left arm/−right arm; lead II = +left leg/−right arm; lead III = +left leg/−left arm). Depending upon the net di-

FIGURE 2.1

Einthoven's triangle and its relationship to the body. Note that the polarity of a lead (i.e., axis) is fixed at the three points of the triangle. The R electrode is attached to the right arm, the L to the left arm and the F point is usually taken to be the left leg. In lead I, the right arm is negative and the left arm is positive, while in lead III the left arm is negative and the left leg is positive.

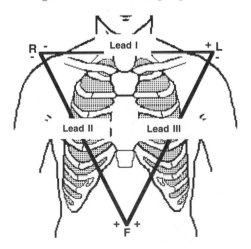

rection of the heart's electrical forces at any given time, an upward deflection is inscribed on the ECG if the majority of the vector is traveling toward the positive pole of the axis; and a downward deflection, when the majority of the vector is traveling away from the positive pole of the lead axis. If the majority of forces are traveling perpendicular to a certain lead axis (e.g. lead II), a biphasic deflection will occur (positive and negative forces are equal) in that lead.

The unipolar leads are "augmented vector" leads, hence the first two letters, *aV*. The third letter refers to the position of the positive pole [R = right (arm); L = left (arm); F = foot (left leg)]. The negative pole of a unipolar lead is actually an area or sector that lies somewhere between the remaining two axes. For example, if we take lead aVR (right arm positive), the negative reference point would be the area between the L and F points. These two points can be thought of as tied together and thus represent a more general area of negative reference than do bipolar leads.

Precordial or V leads are thought of as "probing electrodes" and measure potentials between specific (special) locations and a general body area. They are unipolar in nature and their usefulness is due to their selective area placement (Figure 2.2). The precordial leads track across the anterior and lateral aspects of the left ventricle. Normally, there is a progressive increase in the size of the R wave from V_1 into the late V leads (V_4 and V_5). This change in R wave morphology is referred to as R wave progression and reflects the increasing contribution of left ventricular forces in the ECG complex.

WAVE IDENTIFICATION

The naming of the major elements of the standard ECG (i.e. PQRST) occurred as a result of the influence French mathematician René Descartes had on Einthoven's thought processes. Descartes used a mathematical representation known as the *P point* in many of his formulas and series. Einthoven received his medical training at the University of Utrecht in Holland, which most certainly meant that he was well schooled in mathematics and the other sciences. It is believed that Einthoven chose the letter *P* as a result of his scientific background.[1] From this beginning a worldwide convention was established for the identification of events recorded on the standard ECG.

The P Wave

The first wave in the ECG is the *P wave*, representing the spread of depolarization through the atria via internodal pathways. It is normally upright in leads I, II, aVF, and V3 through V6; inverted in aVR, V1, and V2 (sometimes); and variable in leads III and aVL.[2] The P wave is usually rounded, and deviation from this is generally considered abnormal.

FIGURE 2.2

Common placement of the precordial (V) leads. Lead V_1 is placed in the fourth right intercostal space, and V_2 in the fourth left intercostal space. Lead V_3 is placed halfway between V_2 and V_4, with V_4 in the fifth left intercostal space at the midclavicular line. Lead V_5 is placed in the fifth intercostal space on the anterior axillary line, and V_6 in the fifth intercostal space on the midaxillary line. Proper and consistant placement of these leads is essential for a reliable reading.

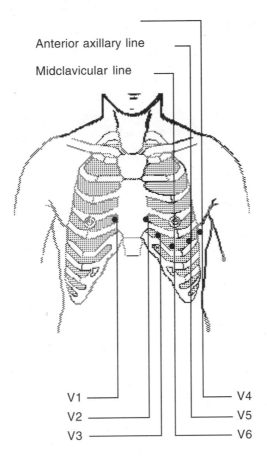

Increased amplitude or width is evidence for atrial hypertrophy, dilatation, enlargement, or nonspecifically diseased atrial muscle. Also, inversion of the P wave in a lead where it is normally upright can be seen in AV junctional rhythms or with atrial ectopic beats. Atrial repolarization occurs within the QRS complex and is usually not seen.

The wave of depolarization spreads to the AV node through the common bundle, down the bundle branches to the Purkinje fibers and, finally, to the ventricular myocardium. Ventricular depolarization occurs and is represented by the QRS complex. A labled diagram of these events is provided in Figure 2.3.

FIGURE 2.3

Components of the QRS complex. The P wave represents atrial depolarization, the QRS ventricular depolarization, and the T wave ventricular repolarization. The U wave represents an altered repolarization pattern and may be a normal variant. Normal interval durations vary with the QRS ranging up to 0.11 second; and the PR between 0.12 to 0.20 second. The ST and QT intervals vary with heart rate.

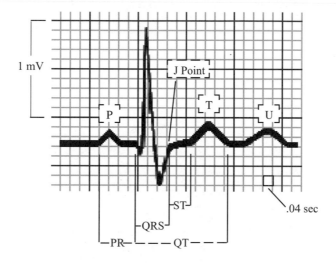

The QRS Complex

In a *QRS complex* the first *downward* deflection after the P wave is the Q wave. If there is no initial downward deflection, then a Q wave does not exist. The first *upright* deflection after the P wave is the *R wave, regardless of the presence or absence of the Q wave.* Any negative deflection following an R wave is referred to as an *S wave.* Special designations (i.e. qR, rSR', QS), along with a diagram of the basic QRS complex, are shown in Figures 2.3 and 2.4.

Some authorities consider the QRS complex the most important in the ECG. The width of the QRS interval gives information about intraventricular conduction disturbances such as bundle branch block and, more specifically, fascicular block. Ventricular hypertrophy can be determined by measuring QRS amplitude. The frontal-plane electrical axis can also be determined by comparing the QRS complexes.

The T Wave

The *T wave,* which comes after the S wave, represents ventricular repolarization. It follows the QRS complex and is normally upright and rounded in the frontal-plane leads (except for aVR, which is normally downward). Changes from this pattern can indicate myocardial ischemia,

FIGURE 2.4

The wave representing ventricular depolarization does not always have the commonly referred QRS configuration. Various possible QRS configurations are named using the rules for wave identification set forth in the text.

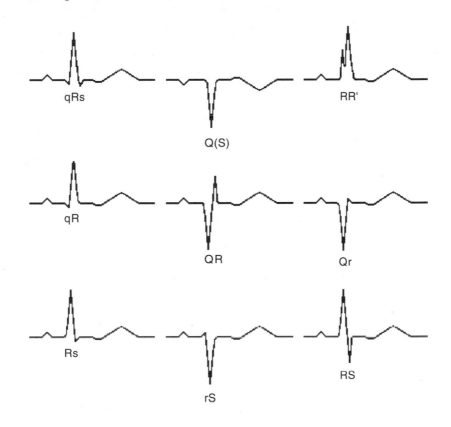

electrolyte disturbances, or pathological conditions. In obese persons the T wave can assume a flattened appearance that is reversible if the weight is lost.

The U Wave

A *U wave* can sometimes follow a T wave. This represents late ventricular repolarization, although it can indicate a pathological state[3] (Figure 3). It is normally of very low voltage but can be easily discerned when potassium levels are deficient. Its polarity is often reversed by myocardial ischemia and left ventricular overload secondary to hypertension or aortic or mitral regurgitation.[4] Negative U waves might also be an indication of significant left main coronary obstruction.[5]

INTERVALS

The *PR interval* marks the time from the beginning of atrial depolarization to the beginning of ventricular depolarization, including the activation of the Purkinje fibers. It is measured from the beginning of the P wave to the beginning of the QRS complex (Figure 2.3). The PR is normally isoelectric but can become displaced in acute pericarditis or atrial infarction.[2] The normal range for the PR interval is 0.12 to 0.20 seconds. Greater than 0.20 seconds is considered first-degree AV block; less than 0.12 seconds may indicate accelerated AV conduction or may be a normal variation.[2]

The *QRS interval* ranges from 0.04 to 0.11 seconds and is measured from the point where the first wave lifts off the isoelectric line to the point where the last wave touches back down to the isoelectric line (Figure 2.3).

The *QT interval* represents ventricular depolarization and repolarization. It is measured from the beginning of the QRS complex to the end of the T wave (Figure 2.3). It varies with heart rate, sex, and age. Usually the QT interval should be less than half of the preceding RR interval to be considered within normal limits. Prolonged QT interval can be associated with hypocalcemia, while a shortened QT is termed *early repolarization* and may be associated with hypercalcemia.

ST Segment

Immediately following the QRS complex is the *ST segment*. It starts at the point where the QRS complex returns to baseline. This is called the J-point or junction point (Figure 2.3). Usually the ST segment is isoelectric, but it may be slightly above or below the baseline. It slopes gradually into the T wave, forming a small curve. If the ST segment is completely horizontal, myocardial ischemia should be considered.

ELECTRICAL AXIS

The *QRS axis* refers to the average direction of depolarization of the ventricles. This is called the mean vector and represents the sum of electrical potentials during depolarization. It is the orientation of the heart's electrical activity to the frontal plane. The axis may be deviated to the left or to the right due to the actual position of the heart in the chest or because of disruptions in electrical activity. The hexaxial reference system is most commonly used for the determination of electrical axis (Figure 2.5). The frame is divided into 30° increments from 0° to 180° if moving in a clockwise direction, or from 0° to −180° if moving counterclockwise. Although

FIGURE 2.5

The hexaxial reference system.

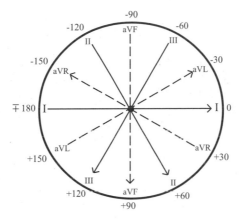

some variations in range exist, an axis of 0° to +90° is normal, whereas +90° to −90° is right axis deviation (RAD) and 0° to −90° is left axis deviation (LAD).

The easiest and least time-consuming approach to determining the QRS axis is to use all six limb leads and employ the vectorcardiographic approach. First consider which lead is most equiphasic (or isoelectric), then look at the lead that is perpendicular to it. If the perpendicular lead is positive then the axis is at the positive pole of that lead. If the perpendicular lead is negative then the axis is at the negative pole of that lead. Infrequently all six frontal-plane leads are equiphasic, making it impossible to determine electrical axis and resulting in what is called an *indeterminate axis*. An indeterminate axis is not necessarily abnormal, it is just not measurable.

Axis should be determined according to the patient's age and body build. Young and thin individuals may have a slight right axis shift, whereas obese or elderly individuals frequently have left axis deviation. Neither condition in these instances has much clinical significance.[3] Mechanical shifts may occur in pregnancy, abdominal tumor, or ascites and give the appearance of LAD. Hyperkalemia, left bundle branch block, or left anterior fascicular block are also associated with LAD. Right bundle branch block (RBBB), left posterior fascicular block, and dextrocardia are some causes of RAD. RAD is almost always present in right ventricular hypertrophy. It is important for the clinician to know how to calculate axis in order to more completely assess the cardiac patient. A sudden onset of RAD can indicate pulmonary embolism and/or infarction. The 12-lead ECG should be used along with other diagnostic testing to help complete the clinical picture (Figure 2.6).

FIGURE 2.6

(A) Left axis deviation. Using Lead II as the most biphasic lead, aVL would then be perpendicular to Lead II. On the hexaxial circle the positive pole of aVL is −30°. Thus, left axis deviation is present. (B) Right axis deviation. Using Lead I as the most biphasic lead, the perpendicular lead is aVF. The positive deflection of aVF gives an axis of +120°. Thus, right axis deviation is present.

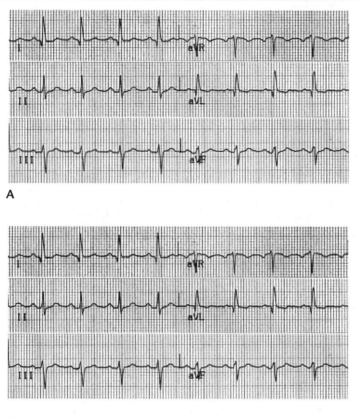

A

B

CHAMBER ENLARGEMENT

Atrial Hypertrophy

Left atrial hypertrophy is a thickening of the left atrial wall. Because it was once most commonly caused by mitral valve disease, especially mitral stenosis, the P waves are called *P mitrale*. Although mitral valve disease is not nearly as prevalent as it was, left atrial hypertrophy is now often seen in patients with systemic hypertension. The changes in the P wave configuration are caused by the increased muscle mass in the chamber. This is evidenced by wide (≥ 0.12 seconds) and notched P waves in leads I, II, and aVL and/or a wide, deep negative component to the P wave in one of the chest leads (V_1 and V_2) (Figure 2.7).

Right atrial hypertrophy is a thickening of the right atrial wall. It is commonly caused by chronic pulmonary disease; thus the P waves are called *P pulmonale*. The P waves are usually tall (> 2.5 mm) and have a "witches hat" peak in leads I, II, aVF and sometimes V_1 and V_2. If right atrial hypertrophy (RAH) is caused by various congenital heart diseases, the term *P congenitale* is used (Figure 2.8).

Thickening of both the right and left atrial walls is called biatrial enlargement. Since different portions of the P wave are affected by each atrium's depolarization, recognition of this pathology is not difficult. Bilateral atrial hypertrophy should be considered when the signs of both right and left atrial enlargement coexist. In general, the following criteria must be met for a diagnosis of biatrial hypertrophy to be made:[6]

1. The presence of tall, peaked P waves (> 1.5 mm) in the right precordial lead (V_1) and a wide, notched P wave in the limb leads or far left precordial leads (V_5 and V_6)
2. An increase in both the amplitude (2.5 mm or greater) and duration (0.12 seconds or longer) of the P wave in the limb leads
3. The presence of a large, biphasic P wave in V_1 or V_2 with the initial positive component greater than 1.5 mm and the terminal negative component reaching 1 mm in amplitude and 0.04 seconds in duration

FIGURE 2.7

Left atrial hypertrophy. Note that the P wave in Lead V_1 is distinctly biphasic, while the P in Lead II is wide and notched.

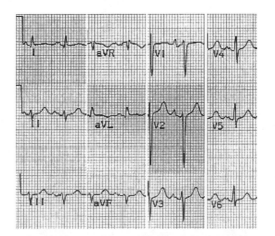

FIGURE 2.8

Right atrial hypertrophy. Note the tall, peaked P waves in leads II and III.

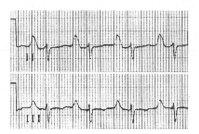

VENTRICULAR HYPERTROPHY

Normally the left ventricular wall is three times as thick as the right ventricular wall. Also, the electrical potential of the left ventricle is about ten times greater than that of the right ventricle. This produces an electrocardiogram with pronounced differences between the right and left ventricles, as evidenced by progressive increments of R wave amplitude from leads V_1 through V_6. If left ventricular hypertrophy exists, this relationship is exaggerated even more. The increase in myocardial thickness produces an increased positive voltage in the leads over the affected area and an increased negative voltage in the leads opposite the hypertrophied area. Criteria for determining left ventricular hypertrophy varies somewhat but the following is generally accepted.[3,6]

    1. R wave in V_5 or $V_6 \geq 26$ mm
    2. R wave in V_5 or V_6 plus S wave in $V_1 \geq 35$ mm
    3. R wave in lead I ≥ 15 mm
    4. R wave in I plus S wave in III ≥ 25 mm
    5. R wave in aVL ≥ 13 mm or R wave in II, III, or aVF ≥ 20 mm
    6. Delayed intrinsicoid deflection of 0.045 sec in V_5 and V_6
    7. Secondary T wave changes (strain pattern) in leads V_5 through V_6 with ST segment depression; T wave inversion in leads I, II, and V_4 through V_6
    8. Mean QRS axis of 0 to $-30°$ (left axis deviation)

    The most reliable diagnostic criteria appears to be secondary T wave changes with a tall R wave in either V_5 or V_6 and a deep S wave in V_1. Diagnosis of left ventricular hypertrophy should be made with caution in individuals without strain patterns because high voltage in the chest leads is common in thin and healthy individuals.[3] The most common cause of left ventricular hypertrophy is hypertension. Other causes include aortic stenosis and/or insufficiency, hypertrophic cardiomyopathy, or coarctation of the aorta (Figure 2.9).

FIGURE 2.9

Left ventricular hypertrophy. Note the ST depression in Leads I, aVL, V_5, and V_6. There is an associated deep S wave in Lead V_2. Left axis deviation is present.

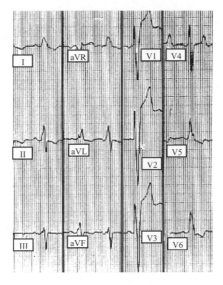

When right ventricular hypertrophy exists, the picture described above is reversed. The R waves become very pronounced in the right precordial leads while deep S waves appear in the left precordial leads. If the right ventricular wall does not surpass the left in size, the hypertrophy may go unnoticed. Right ventricular hypertrophy is commonly seen in congenital lesions such as tetralogy of Fallot, pulmonic stenosis, and transposition of the great vessels. Acquired valve diseases such as mitral stenosis or tricuspid insufficiency may cause RVH. However, the most common cause of RVH is chronic obstructive pulmonary disease—especially emphysema.

Right axis deviation (RAD) is one of the criteria of right ventricular hypertrophy, although RAD may also be the result of other disorders such as left posterior fascicular block. Other criteria for right ventricular hypertrophy are:[1,2]

1. Tall R wave in V_1. The voltage of the R wave in V_1 plus the voltage of the S wave in V_5 or V_6 is $\geq$ 10 mm.
2. RR' pattern in V_1.
3. Deep S waves in leads I, aVL, and V_4 through V_6. The S wave in I, II, and III is > R wave.
4. RAD of +110° or more.
5. Secondary T wave changes in leads V_1 through V_3. Depressed ST segment with upward convexity, inverted T waves in leads

FIGURE 2.10

Right ventricular hypertrophy. Note the right axis deviation and the tall R wave in lead aVR.

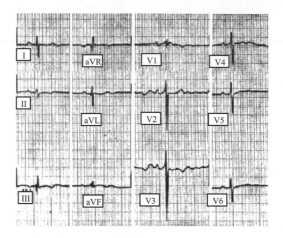

I, III, aVF, and V_1 through V_3 secondary to right ventricular strain.

6. Delayed intrinsicoid deflection in lead V_1 of 0.035 seconds.

It should be noted that other conditions can mimic right ventricular hypertrophy on the ECG. These include a vertical heart, right bundle branch block, posterior wall myocardial infarction, Wolff-Parkinson-White syndrome, and left posterior fascicular block (Figure 2.10).[6]

Just as with the atria, biventricular hypertrophy can exist. This is difficult to diagnose because the increased electrical forces cancel each other out. The best criteria is left ventricular hypertrophy (per voltage) in the chest leads and right axis deviation in the limb leads or vice versa. This condition is frequently caused by congenital heart disease and cardiomyopathies, as well as by advanced heart disease. Generally, chamber enlargement may indicate a chronic disease process. When examining the patient at the bedside, the clinician may use the knowledge of chamber enlargement to explain additional heart sounds as well as displaced point of maximal impulse (PMI).

MYOCARDIAL ISCHEMIA, INJURY, AND INFARCT

The three stages of myocardial perfusion abnormalities have been demonstrated by occlusion of the coronary arteries in experimental animals and appear to be analogous to coronary artery disease in humans. The stages are *myocardial ischemia*, a transient, reversible event producing such changes in ST segments and T waves (e.g. depression or inversion); *myocardial injury*, the intermediate stage that often manifests as ST segment elevations; and *myocardial infarction*, permanent irreversible damage to heart muscle that often produces changes in the QRS complex.

The ECG leads can determine the location of myocardial ischemia, injury, and infarct. For instance, inferior involvement can be diagnosed by examining leads II, III, and aVF, and anterior wall involvement by observing the precordial leads V_1 through V_6. These leads face the area of involvement so the changes seen are indicative changes. The changes that occur in leads that face the opposing surface of the area of the heart that is involved are reciprocal changes. These changes are usually exact reversals of the changes that occur in the leads directly over the injury.

Etiology of ischemia, injury, and infarct can be traced most commonly to coronary artery disease; other causes include trauma, anemia, or coronary vasospasm. The three characteristic changes—T wave inversion, ST segment elevation, and the appearance of Q waves—are seen on the ECG in approximately 80% to 85% of patients with proven myocardial infarction.

Ischemia can be defined as a lack of sufficient blood supply from coronary arteries to the surrounding myocardium. It is reversible damage

FIGURE 2.11

Myocardial ischemia. Note the deep, symmetrical, inverted T waves. These are referred to as ischemic T waves and are characteristic of myocardial ischemia.

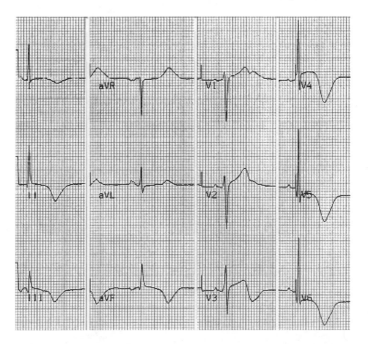

FIGURE 2.12

ST segment elevation. Note the ST elevations in leads V_2 and V_3, indicative of myocardial injury involving the anterior wall of the heart.

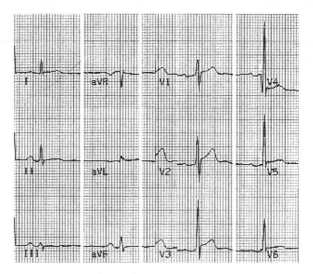

and appears on the ECG as inverted T waves or ST segment depression. On an ECG all leads should be routinely checked for T wave inversion and ST depression, but keep in mind that the T wave is always normally inverted in aVR and can be normally inverted in leads III and V_1 (Figure 2.11).

Myocardial injury, the stage beyond ischemia, is also reversible and can produce either ST segment depression (as with subendocardial injury) or ST elevation (seen with subepicardial injury). If both layers are injured then ST elevation will be seen (Figure 2.12).

Myocardial infarction refers to the necrosis of myocardial tissue due to prolonged lack of blood supply as a result of coronary thrombosis. Most infarcts occur either in the ventricular septum or left ventricular free wall. Right ventricular infarctions are difficult to diagnose because the mean QRS vector toward the right ventricle is very small compared to the left ventricle and thus does not significantly alter the QRS configuration. Recording of right precordial leads (e.g. V_{2R}, V_{3R}, V_{4R}) helps to confirm the diagnosis.

MI LOCATION

It is first necessary to define the areas of the left ventricular chamber that will be discussed. They are the anterior, septal, apical, inferior, lateral, and posterior walls. The term *inferior* is applied to the surface of the heart that rests above the diaphragm. Combinations of these areas may be referred to as anteroseptal, anterolateral, inferolateral, and so on.

Q Wave Infarctions

The changes that are produced as a result of infarct usually occur in a series of stages that allow the evolution of the infarct to be observed. First, the leads over the area of injury will show ST elevation lasting not more than 72 hours. During the first 24 hours significant Q waves also develop in the same leads over the area of infarction. (Abnormal Q waves are identified as those with a depth ≥ 0.04 sec or with a width ≥ 25% of the R wave. All others are considered insignificant.) Sometimes, it is possible to document an MI's hyperacute phase, which is recognized as high ST elevation without the presence of Q waves. This is usually seen only for the first 4 through 6 hours after the onset of chest pain. During the fully evolved acute phase, the ST segment is still elevated; T wave inver-

FIGURE 2.13

Acute anterior wall myocardial infarction. Note the elevated ST segments and Q waves in precordial leads V_2 through V_5, indicating an acute, evolving anterior MI.

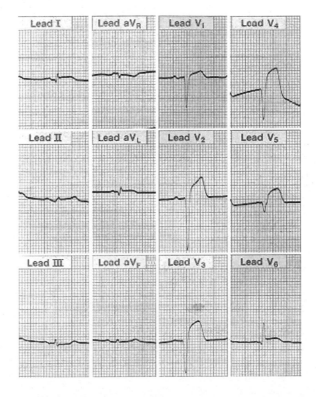

sion occurs in the same leads over the infarcted area and may last as long as 7 to 10 days (Figure 2.13 and 2.14). After 72 hours, the ST segment will become depressed in the lead over the area of the infarct. Finally, in the chronic phase, the ST segment returns to baseline while the T wave returns to normal, and the Q wave remains (Table 2.1). These are the changes that are seen in the leads directly over the infarcted areas. Reciprocal changes include ST depression in the leads opposite the infarction. It is usually possible to differentiate evolving MIs from old ones. For in-

FIGURE 2.14

(A) Evolving inferior wall myocardial infarction. Note the Q waves in II, III, and aVF along with the elevated ST segments. (B) Evolving anteroseptal myocardial infarction. Note the Q waves in precordial leads V_1 through V_4 along with elevated ST segments and inverted T waves in leads V_2 through V_4.

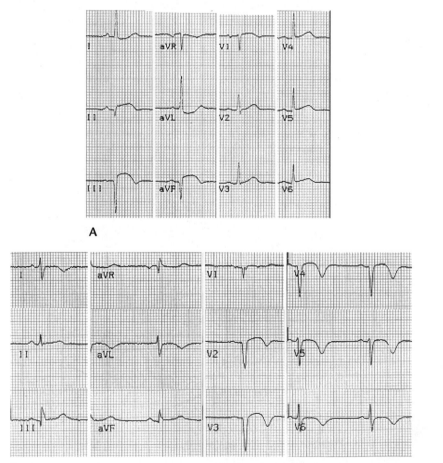

A

B

TABLE 2.1

Progressive Phases of Acute MI

Phase	ECG Changes
Hyperacute (lasts 4–6 hours)	Elevation of the ST segment Tall, wide T waves
Fully evolved acute phase	Pathological Q waves Elevated ST segment Tall, wide T waves
Chronic	Pathological Q waves ST segments return to normal

stance, if the ST segment is elevated the infarct can be called "acute." If a Q wave is seen with the ST segment at baseline but T waves are inverted, the infarct can be termed "age indeterminate" (i.e. somewhere in the evolution process). When a Q wave is visualized in a lead where it should not normally be, the ST segment is returned to baseline, and the T wave is upright, the infarct can be considered "old."

Serial ECGs are important to document the evolution of the MI. For instance, inverted T waves seen with abnormal Q waves (i.e. Q waves not normally found in a particular lead) may persist for months or even years, making it impossible to determine the relative age of an infarct. Thus, a comparison to a previous ECG is extremely helpful when one is looking for or assessing the evolution of an MI.

Non–Q Wave Infarctions

Non–Q wave infarctions occur in about 25% of all acute myocardial infarctions. It is believed that they are partial-thickness infarcts. The ECG changes that occur are ST elevations, depressions, and deep T wave inversions that will eventually resolve. No Q wave is seen. Many patients with non–Q wave myocardial infarctions suffer repeated episodes of postinfarction chest pain and are more likely to have recurrent infarcts[6] (Figure 2.15).

ECG CHANGES SEEN IN ACUTE MYOCARDIAL INFARCTION

Anterior	Q or QS in V_2 through V_4
Anteroseptal	Q or QS in V_1 through V_3
Anterolateral	Q or QS in I, aVL, and V_4 through V_6
Lateral	Q or QS in I, aVL, V_5, and V_6
Inferior	Q or QS in II, III, and aVF

| Posterior | Tall R waves in V_1 through V_3 |
| Right ventricle | Q or QS in V_{1R} through V_{6R} |

Note that a true posterior infarction may produce reduction of the S wave in V_1 through V_3 rather than actual tall R waves. Also remember that these changes must be seen in at least two of the leads over the suspected area of infarct. Changes in only one lead are not diagnostic of acute infarct (Figure 2.16).

Myocardial infarction changes may occur in more than one area of left ventricular free wall. For instance, an inferolateral MI will have ST elevation with T wave inversion and Q waves in leads II, III, aVF, and V_4 through V_6. An anteroinferior MI will have ST elevation and T wave inversion with the appearance of Q waves in leads V_2 through V_6 and II, III, and aVF. An anteroseptal MI will produce Q waves in leads V_1 and V_2 with loss of the initial R wave.

Right ventricular infarctions can often go undiagnosed. This is because the standard 12-lead ECG is oriented to the left ventricle. However, the right ventricle can be effectively evaluated for MI by simply reversing the placement of the standard precordial leads so that they traverse the right side of the chest. From this position, the same evolutionary changes can be identified that would be evident in a left ventricular infarct (ST elevations, T wave inversions, and Q waves).

Finally, a ventricular aneurysm may provide ECG changes that suggest its existence. Pathological Q waves, elevated ST segments, and inverted T waves that persist for 3 months or longer may be indicative of a ventricular aneurysm. Aneurysms are usually associated with the ante-

FIGURE 2.15

Non–Q wave myocardial infarction. This patient presented with chest pain unrelieved by nitroglycerin. Note the inverted T waves in leads I, aVL, and V_3 through V_6. No Q waves are present, but cardiac enzymes confirmed the presence of a myocardial infarction.

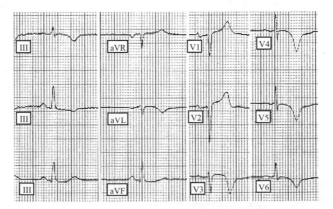

FIGURE 2.16

Posterior wall myocardial infarction. Note the tall R wave in leads V_1 through V_3. These are mirror-image changes that would correspond to the Q wave if the leads were directly over the infarcted area. The rear (posterior) portion of the heart is an area not directly recorded on the standard 12-lead ECG.

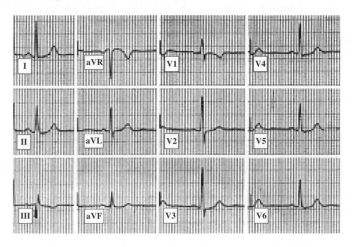

rior wall of the heart, specifically the anteroseptal region. Ventricular aneurysms may be the site of ventricular arrhythmias (particularly ventricular tachycardia).[7,8,9]

MISCELLANEOUS ECG CHANGES

The state of one's physical health or body size can have a major impact on the ECG taken at a particular time. For instance, a grossly obese person or one who is pregnant may have a marked left axis deviation. Pregnancy may also produce precordial T wave inversions. Long-distance runners have been shown to have a RBBB pattern as well as a marked sinus bradycardia. Many disease states have characteristic effects on the ECG. Hypothermia, for example, produces a marked bradycardia as well as prolongation of all intervals and elevation of the ST segment, especially in the precordial leads. Central nervous system disorders such as subarachnoid hemorrhage, meningitis, and cerebral thromboembolism may manifest on the ECG as ST elevation, prolongation of the QT interval, T wave abnormalities, and various supraventricular tachyarrhythmias. Hyperthyroidism is associated with various supraventricular tachycardias, including atrial fibrillation with rapid ventricular response. Hypothyroidism can produce pericardial effusion with low-voltage QRS complex and P wave. The low P wave may be missed and the rhythm mistaken for an AV junctional rhythm. Pulmonary embolus, pericardial tamponade, and other chest disorders may result in tachycardias, low-voltage ST and T wave changes, and arrhythmias. The point is to bear in mind all possible factors that could or should produce changes on the ECG tracings. The interpreter should consider that a previous ECG may be useful if not necessary for comparison or that further tracings may be needed to complete the diagnostic picture, as with MIs. Another important factor that could cause erroneous interpretation is misplaced or improperly placed leads. If lead placement is in doubt another ECG should be done. Marking the chest for the first ECG and using the same spots for future ECGs help eliminate this problem.

Dextrocardia

One very unusual ECG pattern is the one associated with dextrocardia. Most dextrocardias are mirror-image positions where the heart is anatomically reversed in the chest (oriented to the right and associated with anatomical reversal of other viscera as well). The 12-lead ECG will reflect minimal muscle mass on the left side. For example, the precordial leads will show a diminishing R wave progression, with V_1 having the largest R wave and V_6 having the smallest one. At first glance. the patient with dextrocardia would appear to have his precordial leads on in reverse order. To properly assess this patient the V leads should be placed across the right precordium, and the right and left arm leads should be reversed.

DRUG AND ELECTROLYTE EFFECTS

Digitalis

Digitalis can be responsible for many changes on the ECG. The ST segments can become depressed, characteristically sagging in nature but with an upward concavity often associated with inversion of the T wave, especially in the left precordial leads or in those leads with tall R waves. The T wave can be biphasic but is usually nonsymmetric. The QT interval is frequently shortened and U waves may appear with an increased amplitude. These changes are not associated with digitalis toxicity, rather they indicate a "digitalis effect" (Figure 2.17).

Digitalis toxicity is the cause of many arrhythmias on the ECG and should be suspected if these arrhythmias are seen along with the digitalis effect, but digitalis toxicity should never be diagnosed solely on the basis of the ECG. Patients with digitalis toxicity will demonstrate cardiac arrhythmias 80% to 90% of the time, with ventricular bigeminy the typical arrhythmia seen. An AV junctional tachycardia and type I second degree AV block (Wenckebach) may also be seen. However, digitalis intoxication can produce every known cardiac arrhythmia and even various combinations of arrhythmias.[3]

FIGURE 2.17

The digitalis effect. Note the junctional rhythm and the scooped, rounded shape of the ST segment, both characteristic of digitalis use.

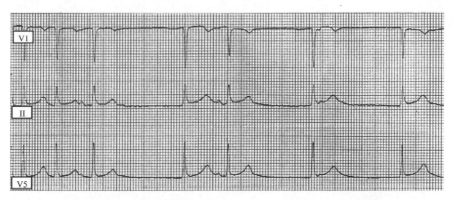

The AV junctional tachycardia that results from digitalis toxicity is related to enhancement of the automaticity of the junctional pacemakers. These patients often have an underlying atrial fibrillation.

Quinidine

Quinidine also causes classic changes on the ECG. Most commonly the QT interval becomes prolonged (in contrast to the effect of digitalis). Quinidine may also prolong the QRS complex and lead to the ominous "R-on-T phenomenon" [a premature ventricular contraction (PVC) that occurs on the T wave of the normal beat during the refractory period and often results in ventricular tachycardia] or to torsades de pointes. T waves may become depressed, widened, notched, and eventually inverted. Quinidine produces nonspecific changes in the ST segment. Blocks of any type may occur, especially SA block or even atrial standstill.

Potassium

Potassium is an electrolyte that is vital to normal cardiac function; abnormal levels commonly produce arrhythmias. The earliest and most common finding in hyperkalemia (5.5–7.5 mEq/L) is tall, tent-shaped, peaked T waves. These T waves are best visualized in leads II and III and in the precordial leads (Figure 2.18). Sometimes anterior or posterior fascicular block may occur at these serum concentrations. When hyperkalemia progresses (7.5–10.0 mEq/L) the P wave tends to flatten out and widen; the PR interval becomes prolonged and the ST segment becomes depressed. Eventually the P wave disappears and the height of the T wave decreases. At concentrations greater than 10 mEq/L, the QRS com-

FIGURE 2.18

Elevated serum potassium. Tall, peaked T waves may be seen as the serum potassium rises. Lengthening of the PR interval and widening of the QRS complex may also occur.

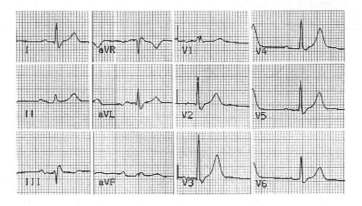

plex widens and the development of ventricular tachycardia and ventricular fibrillation becomes inevitable.

Hypokalemia produces changes on the ECG as well. Serum concentrations below 3.0 mEq/L manifest as an increase in the size of the U wave. A depressed ST segment and lowering of the T wave may combine with the increased prominence of the U wave to give rise to the illusion of a prolonged QT interval. Actually, it is the width of the T wave that has changed—not the length of the ST component of the QT interval. Diagnostically, a prominent U wave is defined as a U wave equal to or taller than the T wave in the same lead, especially in leads V_2 through V_4 (Figure 2.19). A prominent P wave (leads II, III, aVF) may be evident as the serum potassium continues to fall. The P wave is described as being similar in appearance to the P wave found in P pulmonale. Eventually, as hypokalemia progresses, the PR interval lengthens, though only slightly, and the QRS becomes widened. The ST segment is markedly depressed and T wave inversion is evident. Cardiac arrhythmias occur as a dangerous complication of hypokalemia, the most common being complex ventricular ectopy, supraventricular tachycardias, ventricular tachycardia, and ventricular fibrillation.[10]

Calcium

Hypocalcemia commonly produces a prolonged QT interval due to the lengthening of the ST segment. The T wave may remain relatively normal, or it may flatten or become inverted. Cardiac arrhythmias are rare, although prolonged QT intervals are associated with the R-on-T phenomenon and with torsades de pointes (Figure 2.20).[6]

Hypercalcemia commonly produces a shortening of the QT interval. This is usually associated with a shortened or nearly absent ST seg-

FIGURE 2.19

Low serum potassium. The prominent U wave, seen best in leads V_2 through V_4 in the example above, is common when serum potassium falls below 3.0 mEq/L.

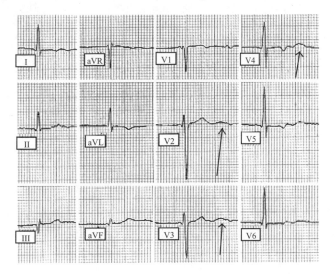

ment. Less frequently the PR interval and QRS complex become prolonged, but these changes are usually minor. Arrhythmias are rare, but PVCs, ventricular tachycardia and fibrillation, sinus arrest, and sudden death have been documented, mostly due to rapid IV administration of calcium (Figure 2.21).[11] Hypercalcemia may also result in increased contractility, increased oxygen consumption, and ischemia in some individuals with coronary artery disease.

DISEASE STATES

Mitral Stenosis

Mitral stenosis or P mitrale produce a specific pattern of change on the ECG. Leads I and II show a wide, notched P wave while lead III produces flat, biphasic, or inverted P waves. When the P mitrale pattern is seen with right axis deviation, mitral stenosis should be considered.

Aortic Stenosis

In mild cases of aortic stenosis the ECG may be normal, but with severe disease the ECG will show left ventricular hypertrophy with a pattern of systolic overloading. Systolic overloading (also called pressure overload) presents a tall monophasic R wave in V_1 or a diphasic RS, Rs, or

FIGURE 2.20

Hypocalcemia. Note the prolonged QT interval of 0.48 second.

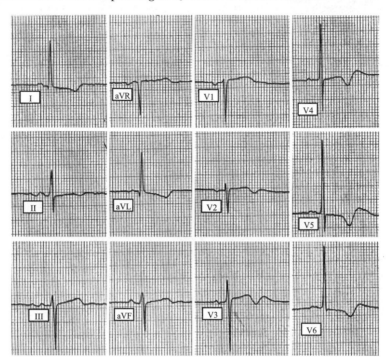

qR complex. The T wave will usually be inverted.[12] In severe cases of aortic stenosis, left bundle branch block may be present.

Combined mitral and aortic involvement demonstrates hypertrophy of both ventricles. Right ventricular hypertrophy may be produced with pulmonic stenosis, a relatively common congenital defect in children and adults. When the right ventricular pressure is greater than or equal to the left ventricular pressure, an rR or qR is present in V_1 with secondary T wave changes in V_1 through V_3. If the right ventricular pressure is less than left ventricular pressure, Rs or rS in V_1 will be seen. P congenitale, which consists of tall, peaked P waves in leads I and II with tall, positive P waves in the right chest leads (V_1 and V_2), is seen frequently. Tricuspid stenosis can be suspected with right atrial enlargement associated with a prolonged PR interval. An rSR' pattern with low voltage may be seen in V_1.

Cor Pulmonale

Acute cor pulmonale, which can be the result of a massive pulmonary embolism, may imitate an inferior infarction. Usually a Q wave will develop in lead III along with an elevated ST segment and T wave inversion. Lead I develops reciprocal changes: the appearance of an S wave,

FIGURE 2.21

Hypercalcemia. Note the increased voltage of the QRS complex and the short QT interval.

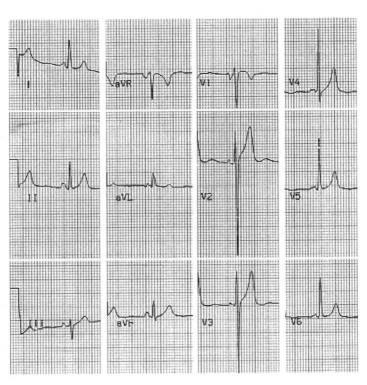

ST depression, and an upright T wave. The major difference between cor pulmonale and inferior infarct is that lead II does not develop a Q wave or ST elevation; rather it looks similar to lead I. A transient RBBB may also appear. The changes mentioned above will resolve more quickly than an infarct would: a few hours or days compared to a few weeks or months.[2]

Cor pulmonale is more commonly seen as a chronic condition and is manifested on the ECG by a rightward shift greater than 30° of the QRS complex; inverted, biphasic, or flattened T waves in leads V_1 through V_3; ST depression in leads II, III, and aVF; and a right bundle branch block. Often the P pulmonale pattern is seen. Right ventricular hypertrophy may also be seen.[2]

Pericarditis

Pericarditis generally involves ST segment elevation with an upward concavity in several leads. This is due to the profuse nature of the disease. As pericarditis progresses, inverted T waves are seen as the ST segment flattens out. In the early stages of pericarditis, the ECG changes can be mistaken for those of acute myocardial infarction. However, there are typically no reciprocal changes and no Q waves. Low voltage is caused by the thickening of the pericardium, especially in chronic or constrictive pericarditis (Figure 2.22).

Pericardial Effusion

Pericardial effusion is classically associated with low QRS complex voltage and ST segment elevation. If the effusion coexists with tamponade, total electrical alternans is almost always present.[6,13] Total electrical alternans appears as a regular alteration in the configuration (height) of the ECG complex. Every complex originates from the same pacemaker and the RR intervals usually remain regular.

Cardiomyopathy

Cardiomyopathy can produce arrhythmias and ECG changes. Frequently, left ventricular hypertrophy is seen with hypertrophic or dilated

FIGURE 2.22

Pericarditis. This 52-year-old patient presented with chest pain 2 weeks following an acute anterior wall MI. Persistant ST elevations in the anterior and lateral leads, negative cardiac enzymes, and pain relief using nonsteroidal anti-inflammatory drugs complete the profile for acute pericarditis.

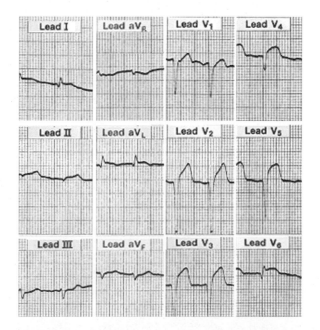

cardiomyopathy. Also, any combination of bundle branch block may be seen, such as right or left bundle branch block, anterior or posterior fascicular block, bifascicular or trifascicular block. Sudden death is the most frequent cause of death in cardiomyopathy. It has been found that patients with a history of nonsustained ventricular tachycardia are eight times more likely to die suddenly than patients without ventricular arrhythmias,[6] however antiarrhythmic therapy does not significantly reduce that risk. Use of implanted cardioverter defibrillators has demonstrated improved survival in these patients. Supraventricular tachyarrhythmias occur frequently, usually in the form of atrial fibrillation. SA disease and high grade AV block are rare complications.[14,15] End-stage cardiomyopathy can produce enlargement of any chamber. Hypertrophic cardiomyopathy can produce left axis deviation along with LVH. Also, Q waves may be present in 20% to 25% of patients with hypertrophic CMP that do not appear to be related to an infarct.[16] These changes are commonly seen in the anterolateral leads (I, aVL, V_4 through V_6) and are believed to be due to septal hypertrophy.[6]

Pulmonary Embolism

Pulmonary embolism and infarct demonstrate inverted T waves in leads V_1 through V_3 (right ventricular strain pattern) and right axis deviation. The "S1, Q3, T3" pattern (S wave in lead I with Q waves and inverted T waves in lead III) with concomitant Q waves in leads I and aVF is common. At times a transient RBBB may appear along with the S1, Q3, T3 and right axis deviation. Sinus tachycardia is almost always present, although paroxysmal multifocal atrial tachycardia may be observed (Figure 2.23).[3]

FIGURE 2.23

Pulmonary embolus (PE). The sudden appearance of a large S wave in lead I and a q wave in lead III, accompanied by clinical symptoms, may be indicative of an acute PE.

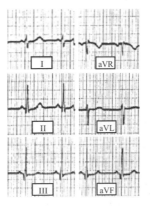

THE SINUS NODE: NORMAL AND ABNORMAL FUNCTION

The *sinus node*, located in the roof of the right atrium near the junction with the superior vena cava, is the physiological pacemaker of the heart. It has an intrinsic rate of 60 to 100 bpm. Infants and young children may have a normal rate considerably higher than this, and healthy, well-conditioned adults may have a slower than "normal" heart rate. When a rhythm originates from the sinus node within the specified rate range, and is conducted through the normal pathways, it is called *normal sinus rhythm*. If the sinus node fires at a rate less than 60 bpm but is conducted normally, the rhythm is called *sinus bradycardia*. At rates faster than 100 bpm and normally conducted, the term *sinus tachycardia* is applied (Figure 2.24).

Sinus Arrhythmia

Sinus arrhythmia originates in the sinus node and is conducted normally but irregularly. The PP and RR intervals vary by more than 0.16 second.[3,6] The PR interval usually remains normal at 0.12 to 0.20 seconds.

Sinus arrhythmia is most frequently associated with the respiratory cycle. As inspiration occurs the sinus rate gradually increases. With expiration the rate slows. This respiratory sinus arrhythmia is commonly seen in healthy children and young adults, and can be eliminated by breath holding. Normally, no treatment is necessary, although atropine can be used if the rate decreases markedly and is associated with symptoms. In older adults sinus arrhythmia is often an early manifestation of sinus node disease (Figure 2.25).

FIGURE 2.24

The various presentations of a sinus-driven rhythm. **A** = sinus rhythm at a rate of 100 bpm; **B** = sinus bradycardia at a rate of 35 bpm; **C** = sinus tachycardia at a rate of 110 bpm.

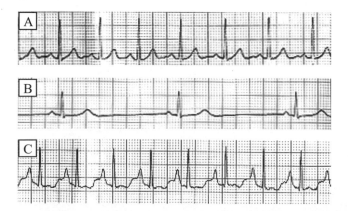

FIGURE 2.25

Sinus arrhythmia. Note the irregularly irregular RR intervals.

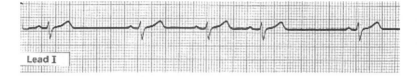

Sinus Arrest

Sinus arrest is a result of the failure of the sinus node to form an impulse. There is no P wave, nor is there a QRST complex for the duration of the pause. If the arrest is prolonged, escape beats from the AV junction or ventricles may appear as a measure to increase cardiac output (Figure 2.26).

Sinus arrest should be differentiated from SA block by determining if the long pause is a multiple of the basic PP interval. In sinus arrest the PP interval is greatly variable and there is no demonstrable relationship between the pause and the basic PP cycle. Conversely, SA block manifests a PP interval that either is a multiple of the basic PP interval or demonstrates a regular irregularity. Sinus arrest may be the result of increased vagal tone or carotid hypersensitivity. Drugs to be considered as etiologic factors include digitalis, quinidine, and calcium channel blockers.

Sinoatrial Block

Sinoatrial (SA) block occurs when there is failure of an impulse to be transmitted from the sinus node to the atrium. It is classified into first, second, or third degree SA block.

First degree SA block occurs when a delay is present in the time between when a sinus impulse is formed within the node and when that impulse actually arrives at the atrial tissue. This cannot be seen on the surface ECG since only the *activation* of atrial tissue is recorded (i.e. the P wave).

FIGURE 2.26

Sinus arrest. The sinus node has failed to initiate an impulse and the result is several seconds of asystole terminated by a junctional escape beat.

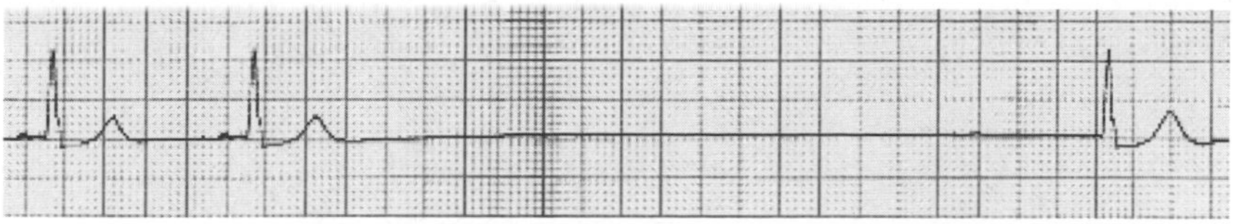

Type I second degree sinus node block (Wenckebach) occurs when a progressively longer delay occurs between impulse formation in the node and atrial tissue activation, until an impulse fails to reach the tissue altogether. This appears on the ECG as progressively shorter PP intervals, group beating, and pauses between beats that are less than twice the shortest PP interval (Figure 2.27).

Type II SA block is recognized by long, regular cycles between P waves. These cycles are usually exact multiples of the basic PP interval. Type II second degree SA block results when a sinus impulse fails to arrive at the atrial tissue; therefore, no P wave is seen. Generally the QRS complex and T wave are absent as well (Figure 2.28).

Third degree sinus block or sinus arrest is characterized by long pauses. These pauses are not a multiple of the sinus rate. They may last up to 60 seconds and are occasionally interrupted by a junctional escape beat. After the pause, the sinus node resumes, however, in some patients, the pause is long enough to result in syncope.

SA block is most commonly the result of digitalis toxicity. Other causes include quinidine toxicity, hyperkalemia, salicylate poisoning, coronary artery disease, acute infections, hypersensitive carotid sinus, or increased vagal tone.[3]

Sick Sinus Syndrome

Sick sinus syndrome (SSS) is a condition in which a variety of sinus node dysfunctions may be seen, including bradycardias, paroxysmal tachycardias, sinus arrest, or blocks as well as delayed sinus recovery time. Occasionally conduction defects exist in both the SA and AV nodes. Bradycardia-tachycardia syndrome (BTS) occurs when bursts of an atrial tachycardia are interrupted by bradycardic periods. These episodes appear as periods of very slow or absent rhythms (Figure 2.29).

Sick sinus syndrome is often caused by ischemic heart disease, cardiomyopathy, amyloidosis, collagen disease, or surgical injury, or it may be the result of processes associated with advancing age. In most

FIGURE 2.27

Sinus Wenckebach. There is a progressively shorter PP interval ending in a pause that is less than twice the shortest PP interval.

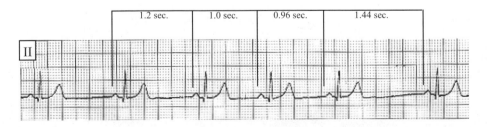

FIGURE 2.28

Type II sinoatrial block. One complete PQRST cycle is missing (arrow).

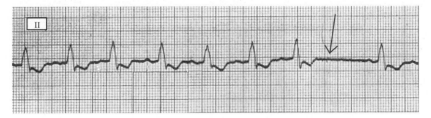

cases, the cause is not evident and the disease is then classified as idiopathic.

Clinically, the patient may present with syncope or near syncope, palpitations, angina, or dizziness and may show progressive congestive heart failure. Syncopal attacks associated with SSS are called Stokes-Adams attacks. Treatment is aimed at maintaining a steady heart rate either with medications or with an artificial permanent pacemaker.

ATRIAL ARRHYTHMIAS

Premature Atrial Contractions

Premature atrial contractions (PACs) or atrial extrasystoles have three distinguishing features. The first is a premature P wave that is sometimes inverted. This is followed by a normal QRST complex, if the beat is not conducted aberrantly. Last, the pause following the PAC is usually not fully compensatory (Figure 2.30).

FIGURE 2.29

Bradycardia-Tachycardia Syndrome (BTS): In the continuous lead II strip above, notice the hallmark characteristics of this syndrome: (1) rapid atrial tachyarrhythmias (in this case coarse atrial fibrillation); and (2) periods of slow atrial or ventricular rates. These paroxysms may be the result of both SA and AV node disease. The tachybrady episodes are, by definition, sudden in onset and sporadic in occurrence.

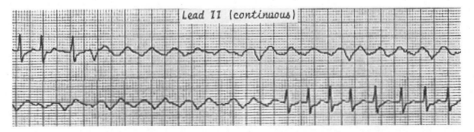

FIGURE 2.30

Premature atrial contraction. This is a lead II showing a normally conducted premature atrial contraction (PAC). Note the deformation of the preceding T wave by the premature P wave.

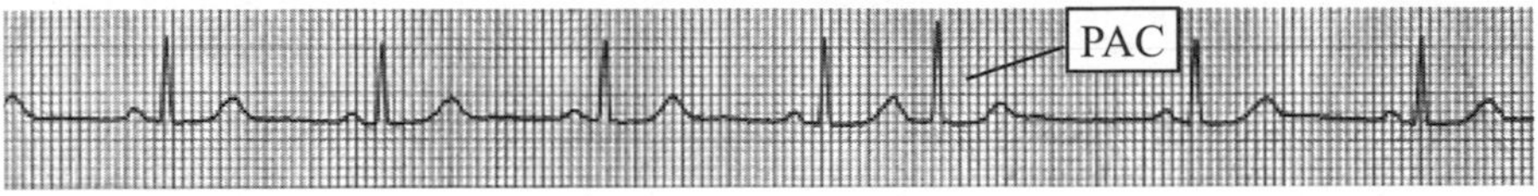

Atrial premature contractions can originate anywhere within the atria but are usually outside the sinus node. This will cause the P wave to have a different configuration. Atrial bigeminy occurs when every sinus beat is followed by a PAC. Atrial trigeminy occurs when every third beat is a PAC (Figure 2.31).

Atrial Flutter

Atrial flutter is a rapid, regular discharge from a single atrial focus, causing a hallmark flutter wave that replaces the P wave. This flutter wave has a sawtooth or "picket fence" configuration and is discharged at a rate of 250 to 350 bpm (Figure 2.32). Since the ventricles are unable to conduct at a rate this fast due to the refractory period of the AV node, the ventricular response is much slower (120 to 180 bpm). The ventricles usually respond to the even-numbered waves, producing AV ratios of 2:1, 4:1, or 6:1 in a regular fashion if the AV conduction is regular, or in irregular fashion if the AV conduction is irregular.

Atrial Fibrillation

Atrial fibrillation is believed to be caused by the rapid and repetitive firings of ectopic atrial foci. This happens at a rate of 350 to 650 bpm. Because of the rapid rate and repetitiveness of the discharge, the

FIGURE 2.31

Atrial trigeminy. Every third beat is a premature atrial contraction.

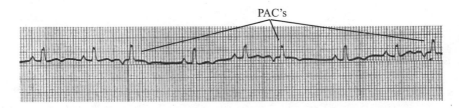

FIGURE 2.32

Atrial flutter. Two examples of atrial flutter with a variable ventricular response. Note the sawtooth appearance of the waves representing atrial activity. The designation *F* (flutter) wave is used when referring to these instead of the usual P wave.

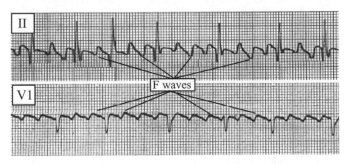

atria appear to be quivering rather than contracting. The ventricles tend to respond in an irregular manner because the AV node is in various states of refractoriness due to electrical bombardment by multiple atrial foci.

Fibrillatory waves have either a coarse or fine configuration (coarse fibrillatory waves are greater than 1.0 mm in height). Untreated atrial fibrillation almost always has a rapid ventricular rate of 120 to 180 bpm. Coarse atrial fibrillation tends to have a slower atrial rate.[3] The ventricular rate usually slows with digitalization, especially when the atrial fibrillation is associated with congestive heart failure (Figure 2.33).

FIGURE 2.33

Slow atrial fibrillation. (**A**) demonstrates what is commonly referred to as coarse atrial fibrillation or atrial fib/flutter. Note the undulating baseline activity. (**B**) shows fine atrial fibrillation. Note the lack of observable baseline activity and the irregularly-irregular ventricular rate.

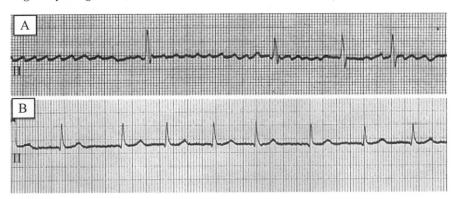

Atrial Tachycardia

Atrial tachycardia is very rare and originates from an ectopic site somewhere in the atria other than in the sinus node. Conduction of the ectopic atrial impulses is usually normal through the ventricles. Usually each P wave is followed by a QRS complex if the tachycardia is uncomplicated. Atrial tachycardia can occur as paroxysms or may be chronic. If it occurs as a paroxysm there may be a pause after the tachycardia is terminated so that the sinus node may regain its function. Atrial tachycardia is then defined as a run of six or more PACs at a rate of 140 to 220 bpm. Paroxysmal atrial tachycardia (PAT) is a sudden burst of unifocal PACs. If the burst occurs at a rate less than 180 bpm it is likely that all the atrial impulses will be conducted through the AV node. If the rate is greater than 180 bpm, the AV node may be refractory to some of the atrial impulses and all the P waves may not be conducted. This is known as atrial tachycardia with block (Figure 2.34). Atrial tachycardia may be produced from multiple foci and is then termed *multifocal atrial tachycardia* (MAT). Diagnosis is made when there are two or more ectopic P waves with different configurations at an atrial rate of 100 to 250 bpm. Multifocal atrial tachycardia is usually associated with chronic lung disease (Figure 2.35).

Paroxysmal supraventricular tachycardia (PSVT) is an umbrella term for any sudden burst of tachycardia that originates from above the level of the ventricles and stops as abruptly as it starts (Figure 2.36). Two distinct mechanisms of PSVT are defined by Marriott as *reentrant* and *ectopic*.[2]

FIGURE 2.34

(A) Atrial tachycardia at a rate of 150 beats per minute (B) atrial tachycardia with atrioventricular block. Note the nonconducted P waves at a rate of 176 beats per minute.

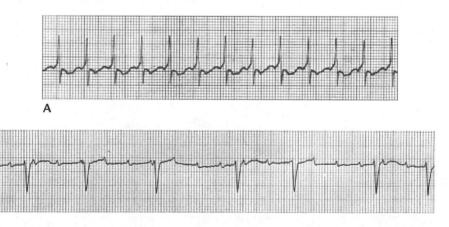

A

B

FIGURE 2.35

Multifocal atrial tachycardia. The rhythm is characterized by a rapid atrial rate with multiple P waves of varying morphology arising from different locations in the atria.

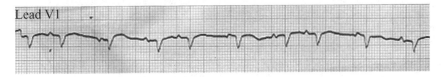

Reentrant PSVT is very common and can involve either the sinus or AV nodes. It often involves an AV nodal bypass tract. The tachycardia may begin with a single premature beat and may result in a circuitous pathway through atrial muscle, the AV node, and/or the ventricles. The ectopic mechanism for PSVT includes atrial tachycardia and atrial fibrillation as well as the very rare AV junctional tachycardia. It is necessary to distinguish the mechanism causing the tachycardia in order to use such treatments as the surgical Maze procedure or intracardiac radiofrequency catheter ablation. These evaluations are made during electrophysiologic testing, which is discussed in chapter 8 of this text.

One other form of atrial arrhythmia is wandering atrial pacemaker (WAP). This results from impulse formation from a variety of foci within the atria and can occur as often as every beat. The PP interval is usually irregular and the P wave configuration is variable (Figure 2.37).

FIGURE 2.36

Supraventricular tachycardia. The 12-lead ECG above shows a paroxysmal supraventricular tachyarrhythmia at a rate of about 190 bpm. Discrete atrial activity cannot be seen so a precise determination of the mechanism is unclear. In such circumstances it is frequently easier to describe what the arrhythmia is not (i.e. ventricular in origin) and so the term *supraventricular* is applied.

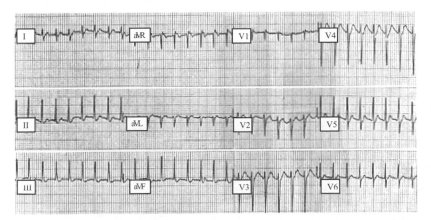

FIGURE 2.37

Wandering atrial pacemaker. Note the varying P wave morphology. The third beat in the tracing above is a premature ventricular contraction (PVC).

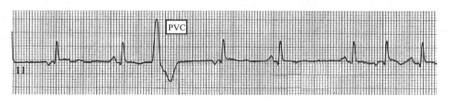

THE AV JUNCTION

A *junctional rhythm*, which originates from the AV node or common bundle, may occur as a primary rhythm or in response to SA or AV block (see previous section) in the form of junctional extrasystoles or escape beats. The intrinsic rate of the AV node is 40 to 60 bpm, although a junctional rhythm can be found at higher rates and is called *accelerated junctional rhythm* (Figure 2.38). Junctional rhythms are usually not seen because the normal sinus node rate is 60 bpm or greater. Therefore, junctional escape beats or junctional rhythm are more commonly seen when the sinus rate is depressed. AV junctional rhythm may be preceded or followed by retrograde P waves, depending on the location of the ectopic focus in the AV node and the condition of the antegrade and retrograde conduction pathways (Figure 2.39).

Premature junctional contractions (PJCs) are early beats that originate in the junctional tissue. This ectopic impulse will conduct both antegrade (toward the ventricles) as well as retrograde (toward the atria).

FIGURE 2.38

(A) Junctional bradycardia at a rate of 35 bpm (B) accelerated junctional rhythm at a rate of 68 bpm

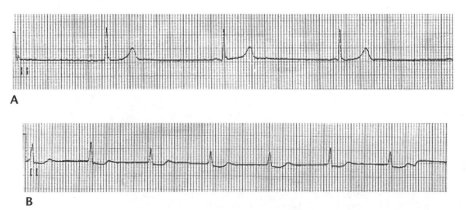

A

B

FIGURE 2.39

Accelerated junctional rhythm with retrograde conduction producing P waves after the main QRS complex.

P waves

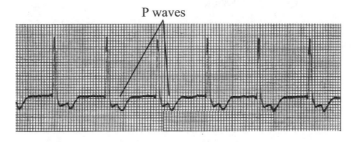

Junctional beats may have a P wave immediately in front of the QRS complex or immediately after it (retrograde P). Often a P wave can not be identified and the assumption is that one has not been initiated or that it is "buried" in the QRS complex.

An AV junctional rhythm can occur in healthy as well as diseased hearts. When a junctional escape beat occurs as a result of sinus node suppression, sinus arrest, or SA block that terminates quickly, the rhythm is considered insignificant. When the rhythm occurs as a result of complete heart block or SA block of long duration, the patient is usually symptomatic and requires treatment (Figure 2.40).[3]

AV/HIS CONDUCTION FAILURES

The impulse that originates in the sinoatrial node is conducted through the atria to the atrioventricular (AV) node. When conduction pathway

FIGURE 2.40

Sinus arrest with junctional escape. The long pause is not a multiple of the underlying sinus rate, thus indicating a sinus arrest. The junctional escape rhythm reestablishes a basic heart rhythm.

failure occurs here, it is usually termed *AV block* and is described in grades or degrees.

First Degree AV Block

The mildest form of AV block is first degree AV block. It is diagnosed when the PR interval is greater than 0.20 seconds. (Remember that normal is 0.12 to 0.20 sec.) This means that conduction *through* the AV node is prolonged. It is due to prolongation of the relative refractory period in the AV node. This condition usually requires no treatment (Figure 2.41).

Second Degree AV Block

Second degree AV block is diagnosed when one or more atrial impulses fail to reach the ventricles. There are several varieties of second degree AV block.

Wenckebach or type I block occurs at the AV junction after a period of progressively lengthening PR intervals until, finally, a P wave is not conducted. The pause following the dropped beat allows the AV node to repolarize so that the next atrial impulse is conducted normally. Type I AV block is not considered life threatening and is not treated. It is usually associated with acute reversible conditions like rheumatic fever, digitalis effect, or propranolol effect. It can also be associated with AMI (Figure 2.42).

Type II AV block is much more serious. This condition is characterized by the alternation of normally conducted P waves with nonconducted P waves. This is called 2:1 block and is the most common form of this disturbance. The PR intervals in the conducted beats are unchanged. The block is usually below the level of the bundle of His, although it can occur at this level. A block originating at the HIS bundle would produce a normal QRS complex, as opposed to the pattern seen with a block at the level of the bundle branches (Figure 2.43).

FIGURE 2.41

Sinus rhythm with first degree atrioventricular node block. Note the PR interval of 0.32 sec.

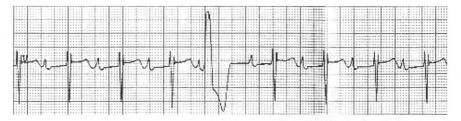

FIGURE 2.42

Type I second degree AV block. Note the progressively lengthening PR intervals until a QRS is "dropped." The PP intervals remain constant at 0.80 second (75 bpm).

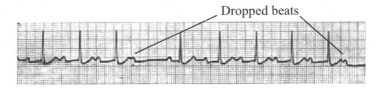

It may be difficult to discern Wenckebach from Type II block when the block is 2:1. If the width of the QRS is normal, Wenckebach is most often suspected. When the QRS is widened it is due to block below the bundle and is most often related to type II. However, type II 2:1 block may appear with a normal QRS complex.[6] Also, when the patient's atrial rate is increased with either exercise or atropine, the AV block with Wenckebach will tend to decrease, while type II AV block will increase.

Advanced or high grade second degree AV block occurs when two or more consecutive atrial impulses fail to be conducted (e.g. 3:1, 4:1). As in type II block, the PR interval remains constant in the conducted beats. The atrial rate remains normal or close to normal. In both type II and high grade second degree block the ventricular rate is slower than the atrial rate (Figure 2.44).

Third Degree AV Node Block

Third degree or complete heart block is diagnosed when no atrial impulses are conducted through the AV node. This is most often caused by trifascicular block in the bundle branches rather than a block at the AV node, although blockage can occur at that level. On the ECG the P wave and QRS complex occur independent of each other. That is, normal atrioventricular conduction is blocked and the P waves are unrelated to the QRS complexes. There is ventricular depolarization due to one of two things: the AV node may take over the pacemaker function, resulting in a junctional escape rhythm; or some ectopic site in the ventricles be-

FIGURE 2.43

Type II second degree AV block. Note that every other P wave is not conducted to the ventricles. The PR intervals of the conducted beats remain constant at 0.32 sec.

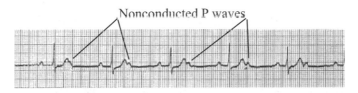

FIGURE 2.44

High grade second degree AV block. Note the consistant and prolonged PR interval in the beats that are conducted. This is an example of a 3:1 atrial/ventricular conduction ratio.

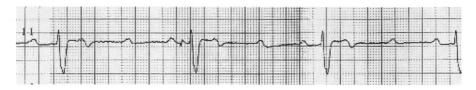

comes the pacemaker, causing an idioventricular rhythm (Figure 2.45). The inherent rate in the AV node is 40 to 60 bpm while the ventricular rate is 20 to 40 bpm. A normal atrial rate is usually seen coexisting with a much slower ventricular rate. The QRS complex generally will be normal if it originates in the AV junction but will be wide and bizarre if the impulse originates in the ventricles.

Clinically, second and third degree heart blocks result in a compromised cardiac output. Especially in complete heart block, perfusion to the vital organs may be greatly reduced. Treatment for third degree heart block is aimed at increasing the heart rate to maintain a normal cardiac output. Discontinuation of myocardial depressants and/or digitalis preparations is indicated with type II to prevent progression to high grade block or complete block. Treatment with an artificial pacemaker is generally indicated in type II block and is almost always indicated in high grade or complete heart block.

BUNDLE BRANCH BLOCK

Right Bundle Branch Block

Normal activation of the ventricles begins at the common bundle and then travels down the left bundle branch, which then activates

FIGURE 2.45

Third degree AV block. The P waves are visible at a rate of 50 bpm. The QRS complexes are visible at a rate of 30 bpm and are initiated from a site in the AV junctional tissue. There is no conduction relationship between the atria (P waves) and the ventricles (QRS complexes).

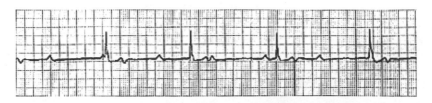

the septum, causing left to right depolarization. If the impulse finds the right bundle branch blocked, right ventricular depolarization must occur following depolarization of the left ventricular Purkinje fibers. Right bundle branch block (RBBB) produces a characteristic morphologic pattern in the precordial leads: an rSR′ or M pattern in the right (V_1 through V_3) precordial leads and a deep, wide S wave in the left precordial leads (V_4 through V_6) (Figure 2.46). This is due to the slowed depolarization of the right ventricle. Usually in RBBB the first portion of the QRS complex retains its natural appearance due to normal early septal activation. It is the second portion of the QRS complex that is affected. As the septum is activated from left to right, a large S wave is produced in lead I. Usually, forces from right ventricular depolarization balance the septal activation from left to right, but if the right bundle branch is blocked, thereby delaying right ventricular depolarization, the impulse moving through the septum is allowed to oppose the left ventricular activation.

Once left ventricular depolarization is finished there is nothing to oppose the right ventricle when it finally depolarizes. This is seen as a large and wide R wave in lead V_1. For this reason RBBB is usually a triphasic complex on the 12-lead ECG, with a QRS of 0.12 seconds or greater. Secondary ST-T wave changes occur as a result of repolarization of the right bundle branch. The T wave will have an opposite deflection from the later portion of the QRS complex. These are not indicators of myocardial disease but are merely changes produced by the block and are thus called secondary changes.

Left Bundle Branch Block

Left bundle branch block (LBBB) is a blockage in the main portion of the left bundle branch. Again, an impulse travels from the SA node

FIGURE 2.46

Right bundle branch block. Note the QRS width of 0.12 sec, the triphasic qRS pattern in lead V_1, and the wide S wave in leads I, aVL, V_5, and V_6.

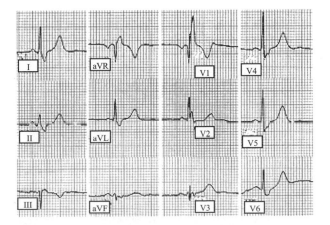

to the common bundle and begins to move down the left side to begin depolarization. When the impulse finds the left bundle branch blocked it changes direction and activates the septum from right to left. Then the Purkinje network of the right ventricle is activated. This obviously is a dramatic change from the normal intraventricular conduction. The activation of the septum from right to left produces an initial R wave in V_6 because the mean vector is traveling toward it. As the impulse travels through the free wall of the left ventricle via the intraventricular septum a large S wave is recorded in V_1 and an R' wave in V_6, giving the appearance of a notched QRS complex (Figure 2.47).

The characteristic findings in bundle branch block are: a QRS complex greater than 0.12 seconds in both right and left BBB; a predominantly positive QRS configuration with the rSR' configuration in V_1 and wide S

FIGURE 2.47

Left bundle branch block. Note the wide monophasic complex in leads I and V_6 along with the inverted T waves in leads I, aVL, V_5, and V_6.

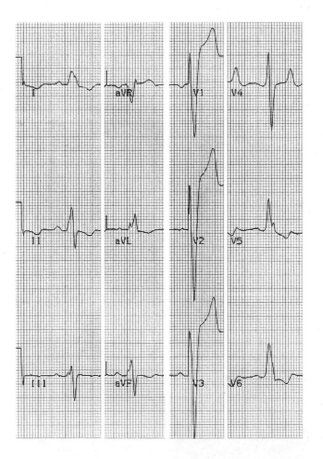

wave in lead I for RBBB; and a predominantly negative QRS configuration in V_1 with a wide, notched QRS complex in I, V_5, and V_6 in LBBB. Both forms of bundle branch block will have secondary ST depression and T wave inversion representative of repolarization changes.

Bundle branch block is sometimes intermittent, although this usually means that permanent BBB is ensuing.[2] However, intermittent BBB is often related to the ventricular rate. Right or left BBB can develop if the rate increases so that an impulse from the common bundle finds either side refractory to that impulse. The rate at which normal conduction changes is called the *critical rate*. When block occurs at the critical rate it is known as *rate-dependent BBB*. Rarely, BBB exists when the ventricular rate slows rather than speeds up. This is a "paradoxical critical rate" and the condition is termed *bradycardia-dependent BBB*. If BBB occurs intermittently without a change in ventricular rate it is called *rate-independent right or left BBB* (Figure 2.48).

Fascicular Blocks

In most people, the left bundle branch consists of two divisions: the anterior or superior portion, which runs toward the anterior papillary muscle, and the posterior or inferior portion, which moves in the direction of the posterior papillary muscle. Some people also have a septal fascicle in addition to the anterior and posterior ones. When any of these divisions is blocked the term *fascicular block* is used.

Left Anterior Fascicular Block

Normally, both divisions or fascicles depolarize almost simultaneously, but if the anterior fascicle is blocked the impulse travels down the posterior fascicle, activating the Purkinje network between the fascicles. The anterior portion of the left ventricle is depolarized via this network. This change in activation of the anterior portion of the left ventri-

FIGURE 2.48

Rate-dependent bundle branch block. At a sinus rate of 75 bpm the characteristic bundle branch block pattern becomes evident. As the sinus rate slows to 60 bpm, normal ventricular conduction returns.

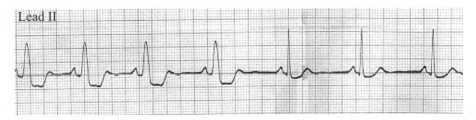

cle records some characteristic findings on the ECG: a small q wave in lead I with a smaller r wave in lead III occur because of the initial rightward and downward pull. As the impulse then travels toward the anterior portion of the left ventricle it moves away from lead III, resulting in a deep S wave there, and directly toward lead I, where it records a large R wave (Figure 2.49). There must also be marked left axis deviation in order to diagnose left anterior fascicular block. There is usually no prolongation of the QRS interval unless a preexisting right bundle branch block is present.

Left Posterior Fascicular Block

When the posterior fascicle is blocked the left ventricle is activated by the intact anterior fascicle. The impulse goes through the Purkinje fibers between the two fascicles and then activates the posterior portion of the left ventricle. Initially the QRS vector is leftward and upward because of depolarization through the anterior fascicle. It then moves downward as the posterior portion of the left ventricle becomes activated. Therefore, lead III will record a small q wave initially while Lead I records a small r wave. As the mean QRS vector changes to activate the posterior portion of the left ventricle the impulse travels toward lead III, recording a large R wave, while lead I records a large S wave because the wave of depolarization is moving opposite it. Because the impulse is conducted inferiorly and rightward a right axis deviation of about +120° is produced. Once again there is no prolongation of the QRS complex (Figure 2.50).

FIGURE 2.49

Left anterior fascicular block. Note the small q and tall R waves in lead I, the small r and deep S waves in lead III, and the presence of left axis deviation.

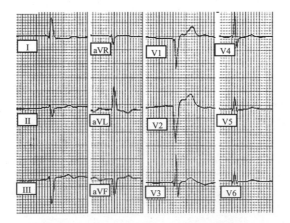

FIGURE 2.50

Left posterior fascicular block. Note the small r and large S waves in lead I, the small q and tall R waves in lead III, and the presence of right axis deviation.

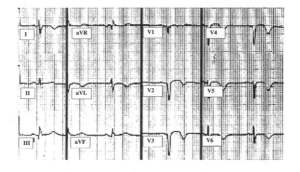

The term *bifascicular block* is used when two fascicles are blocked simultaneously. This can include RBBB with left anterior or posterior fascicular block, RBBB or LBBB with first degree AV block, or alternating RBBB and LBBB. The QRS complex in these cases will be prolonged because of the accompanying RBBB (Figure 2.51).

Trifascicular block is defined as a RBBB plus alternating left anterior and left posterior fascicular blocks. Trifascicular block is usually associated with a type II AV block. Bifascicular block with some degree of AV node block may also be a manifestation of trifascicular block (Figure 2.52). Trifascicular block usually requires treatment with a permanent pacemaker.

FIGURE 2.51

Bifascicular block

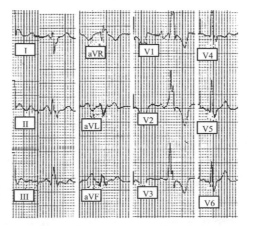

FIGURE 2.52

Trifascicular block. A complete left bundle branch block and first degree atrioventricular node block are present.

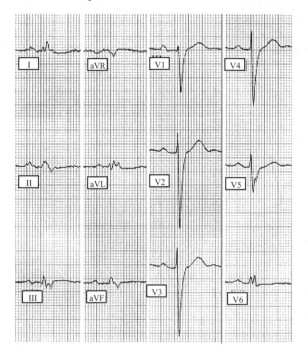

ABNORMAL CONDUCTION PATHWAYS

Preexcitation

Abnormal conduction pathways, such as those involved in preexcitation or aberration, are a common source of arrhythmias. Preexcitation syndromes imply that a portion of the ventricular myocardium is activated via a "bypass tract" before it normally would have been. One common type of preexcitation is Wolff-Parkinson-White (WPW) syndrome. WPW is characterized by a short PR interval (< 0.12 sec) and a delta wave (the slurred initial component of the QRS complex) that makes the QRS complex look wider than normal (Figure 2.53). Patients with WPW are often prone to supraventricular tachycardias such as atrial fibrillation and atrial flutter. For further discussion see chapter 8.

Aberration

Aberration is another form of abnormal intraventricular conduction. This is simply the temporary, abnormal ventricular conduction of a supraventricular impulse, which is usually due to a change in heart rate.

FIGURE 2.53

Preexcitation. Note the delta wave producing a widened QRS complex and a shortening of the PR interval.

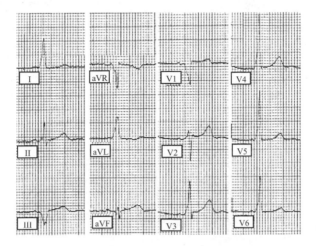

For the most part aberration is in and of itself benign, but serious consequences may result if aberration is misdiagnosed and treated as if it were malignant. More specifically, runs of aberrantly conducted beats can be mistaken for ventricular tachycardia and treated as such. Aberration is seen with supraventricular rhythms such as sinus tachycardia, atrial fibrillation or flutter, accelerated AV nodal rhythm, and paroxysmal atrial tachycardia. It is dependent upon three important events: unequal refractory periods of the bundle branches, critical premature impulse formation, and the length of the preceding RR interval. Usually the left bundle branch recovers first; thus the aberration takes the morphological form of RBBB in 80% of the cases.[2]

If and when a supraventricular premature impulse is produced one of three things will occur. First, the premature impulse may be blocked because it found both bundle branches refractory to an impulse (blocked PAC). Second, the impulse may be conducted normally because both bundle branches have repolarized and were able to accept the wave of depolarization (normal PAC). Last, if the impulse is conducted early enough so that at least one bundle branch has recovered but not late enough to find them both recovered, the impulse will be conducted aberrantly (aberrantly conducted PAC).[17]

Characteristically, an aberrantly conducted beat will have a QRS complex less than 0.14 sec. Ventricular ectopy is usually greater than 0.14 sec. The aberrantly conducted beat will often be preceded by a P wave indicating the supraventricular origin of the impulse. The QRS complex usually has the classic triphasic morphology of RBBB in V_1 (rsR') and a qRS in V_6. Also, aberrantly conducted beats often have the same initial vector as that of the other normally conducted beats around it (Figure 2.54, Table 2.2).[2,18]

FIGURE 2.54

Premature atrial contractions (PACs). In (**A**) above (lead V_1), the third and eighth complexes are aberrantly conducted PACs. Note that the aberrant beat assumes the morphology of a right bundle branch block, which is common. The P wave can be seen as a notch in the T waves of the preceeding beats. In (**B**) (lead II), a P wave can be seen in the T wave of the fourth conducted complex. Note that there is no associated QRS complex with this P wave and it is therefore referred to as a "blocked" PAC.

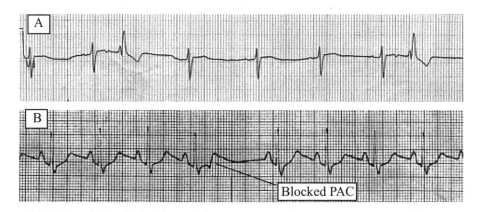

VENTRICULAR RHYTHMS

Idioventricular Rhythms

Ventricular escape beats can originate from anywhere in the ventricle. They may be seen when there is sinus bradycardia, sinus arrest, SA block, or AV block. These escape beats can be grouped together. When six or more ventricular escape beats occur consecutively the term *idioventricular rhythm* is used to describe them. The intrinsic rate of the ventricles is

TABLE 2.2

Differentiation of Ventricular Ectopy and Aberrant Conduction

Ventricular Ectopy	Aberration
QRS morphology: wide and bizarre looking, usually monophasic	QRS morphology: usually an rSR′ in lead V_1 and a qRS configuration in lead V_6
QRS width: greater than 0.14 sec in duration	QRS width: less that 0.14 sec in duration
Associated rhythm: sinus or other supraventricular rhythm	Associated with a long-short cycle (Ashman's phenomenon) or supraventricular prematurity
Initial deflection: usually different from the patient's basic beat, often pointing in the opposite direction in the lead being viewed	Initial deflection: usually in the same direction as the patient's basic complex in the lead viewed

between 20 and 40 bpm but it may be as slow as 15 bpm or as fast as 50 bpm. The QRS complex in this rhythm is abnormally wide, usually exceeding 0.16 sec. Most often there is complete AV dissociation and the ventricular rhythm is regular (Figure 2.55).

Premature Ventricular Contraction

Early beats that originate from an ectopic focus in the ventricular myocardium are called *premature ventricular contractions* or PVCs. These may arise from one focus (unifocal) or from several foci (multifocal). Since they do not follow normal pathways of conduction, these QRS complexes are wide (> 0.12 sec) and bizarre looking, and usually of the opposite deflection from the normal sinus beat. They are never associated with a P wave and are almost always followed by a fully compensatory pause. Although PVCs may be found in healthy individuals, organic heart disease should be suspected when PVCs are complex in origin. If every other beat in a sinus rhythm is a PVC the rhythm is termed *ventricular bigeminy*; every third beat is *ventricular trigeminy*; every fourth beat is *ventricular quadrigeminy* (Figure 2.56). PVCs can occur singly or in pairs (ventricular couplet), threes (ventricular triplet), or groups of four or five (salvos) (Figure 2.57).

Groups of consecutive beats should be regarded cautiously as they can lead to *ventricular tachycardia*, which is defined as six or more consecutive PVCs. In the patient with ischemic heart disease or electrolyte imbalance, a PVC on the T wave of the preceding beat may provoke ventricular tachycardia (the R-on-T phenomenon).

Ventricular Tachycardia

The QRS complex in ventricular tachycardia is usually wide and bizarre like the PVCs and extrasystoles. The ventricles will beat rapidly

FIGURE 2.55

Idioventricular rhythm. Note the very slow rate (approx. 30 bpm) and wide QRS. No P waves are visible. An idioventricular rhythm is the most primitive escape rhythm.

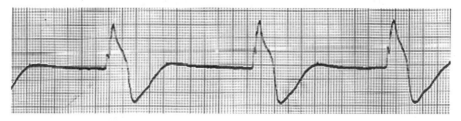

FIGURE 2.56

(**A**) is an example of ventricular bigeminy, in which every other beat is of ventricular origin. (**B**) shows ventricular trigeminy, in which every third beat is of ventricular origin. (**C**) shows PVCs arising from different locations in the ventricle. These are called multifocal PVCs.

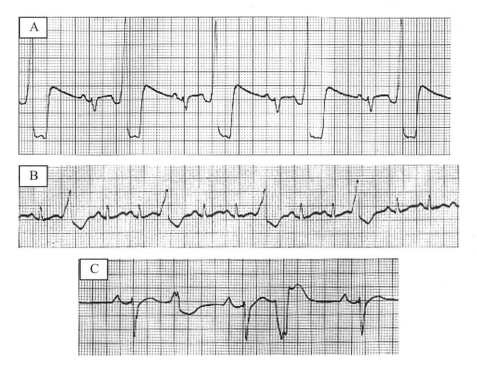

and independently of the P waves. The rate of ventricular tachycardia is usually between 180 and 250 bpm but may be slowed by drug therapy, and the rhythm is usually regular although some irregularity may be present (Figure 2.58). Ventricular tachycardia may arise from one ectopic focus or from multiple foci. The coexisting, underlying atrial rhythm is usually sinus rhythm. On occasion the sinus impulse will be able to meet the impulse from the ventricle via antegrade conduction and produce a ventricular fusion beat. Ventricular tachycardia is life threatening and can degenerate into ventricular fibrillation. It is commonly seen in acute myocardial infarction and in other chronic diseases of the heart.

Torsades de Pointes and Polymorphic Ventricular Tachycardia

Torsades de pointes (TdP), literally "twisting of the points," is a type of ventricular tachycardia where the QRS complexes change their

FIGURE 2.57

In (**A**) there is a pair of ventricular beats commonly referred to as a couplet. (**B**) shows a short burst of ventricular tachycardia interspersed in a baseline sinus rhythm.

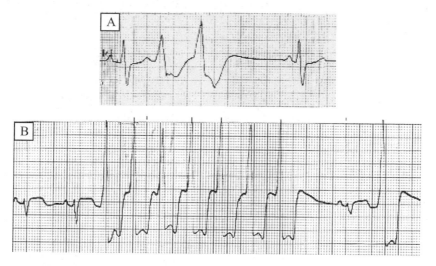

amplitude and appear to twist around the isoelectric line. It is sometimes poetically referred to as the "cardiac ballet." The rate is usually 200 to 250 bpm. Torsades de pointes is usually associated with a long QT interval and is frequently seen during quinidine or other antiarrhythmic drug therapy (Figure 2.59). Polymorphic ventricular tachycardia (PVT) is the diagnosis reserved for those patients who do not have a long QT interval but have the characteristic pattern of multiformed ventricular tachycardia. It may be treated like conventional ventricular tachycardia using ACLS guidelines. Torsades de pointes may be self-limiting, lasting only 5 to 25 seconds, or it may require DC countershock. Patients with TdP should discontinue the offending antiarrhythmic agent causing the prolonged QT interval. Often magnesium sulfate can be used to help terminate the rhythm in addition to DC countershock.[6]

Ventricular Fibrillation

Frequently ventricular tachycardia can degenerate into ventricular flutter and/or fibrillation. These two arrhythmias are life threatening because virtually no blood is ejected into the systemic circulation. Ventricular flutter is characterized by very rapid firing of a ventricular focus (rate of 150 to 300 bpm) at a fairly regular rhythm. At this point no atrial activity can be recognized (Figure 2.60). The QRS complexes appear to run into each other, making ST-T waves impossible to identify. Ventricu-

FIGURE 2.58

Examples of ventricular tachycardia (VT). (**A**) is an example of a very rapid form of VT often referred to as ventricular flutter. In most cases, the patient will not maintain consciousness or pulse. (**B**) is a type of VT commonly known as slow VT. It may be accompanied by adequate perfusion and an acceptable blood pressure. Note the wide complexes and the regular rate.

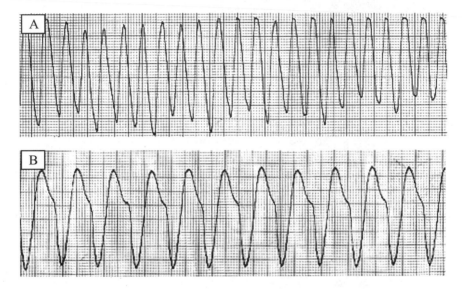

lar fibrillation is characterized by a chaotic, irregularly irregular ventricular rhythm. Fibrillatory waves replace the QRST complex, with the rate occurring at a very large range: 250 to 500 bpm. During ventricular fibrillation, no useful cardiac output is generated. Both ventricular flutter and ventricular fibrillation are treated with DC shock, although these arrhythmias may be terminal despite aggressive medical intervention. The best results are obtained when the patient receives DC countershock

FIGURE 2.59

Torsades de pointes.

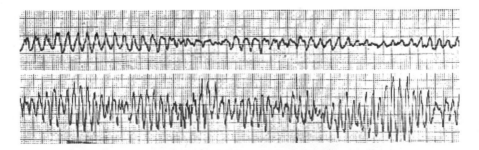

FIGURE 2.60

Ventricular fibrillation.

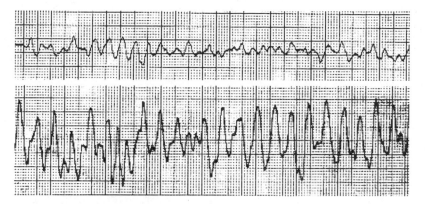

within 2 minutes of the onset of the arrhythmia. This helps to ensure survival of the heart muscle as well as the brain.

SIGNAL-AVERAGED ELECTROCARDIOGRAPHY

The signal-averaged ECG is a specially filtered, computerized ECG that is designed to pick up very small oscillations or electrical potentials. These potentials generally occur late in the QRS complex and are under 40 mV in amplitude with a duration of greater than 40 msec. They have been shown to be highly correlated with the risk of ventricular tachycardia in certain populations of patients, particularly those with ischemic heart disease, myocardial infarction, chronic heart failure, or cardiomyopathy. A high percentage of patients with syncope and late potentials were positive for ventricular tachycardia in one recent study. Some researchers use signal-averaged ECGs to screen high-risk patients for ventricular tachyarrhythmias. In patients with bundle branch blocks or ventricular pacemakers, signal averaging is of unknown value or significance.

TILT TABLE TESTING IN PATIENTS WITH SYNCOPE

Syncope may affect people of all ages. It is not necessarily associated with structural heart disease or with arrhythmias but may mimic these presentations. When syncope occurs in the noncardiac patient, it may be the result of decreased venous blood return to the heart that begins a cascade of compensatory reactions, beginning with the release of endogenous catecholamines. Decreased venous return can be caused by a number of events, including excessive fluid loss (profuse sweating or bleeding), hypotension, drugs, or emotional stress. The terms *vasodepressor syncope* and *neurocardiogenic syncope* are used to describe this event.

The actual events that produce the syncopal episode are as follows. First, there is decreased venous return to the right heart from the fluid loss. This limits the available supply of blood to the left heart, which reduces cardiac output. The reduced cardiac output stimulates catecholamine release, which increases contractility. Concurrently, parasympathetic stimulation occurs, which serves to limit sympathetic stimulation, increase myocardial electrical stability, and protect against ventricular fibrillation. However, vagal stimulation also promotes peripheral arteriole vasodilatation and bradycardia. This peripheral vasodilatation leads to increased venous pooling and hypotension, which produce the loss of consciousness. Generally patients recover within a few moments if they are placed in a supine position.

Patients who suffer from neurocardiogenic syncope can be diagnosed using the tilt table test. A tilt table can be rotated from a flat position to a 70° tilt in a few seconds. The abnormal result to tilting is a drop in heart rate and blood pressure, which are a result of peripheral vasodilatation. Normal individuals have an increase in heart rate and little to no change in blood pressure when they are tilted. Patients with suspected vasodepressor syncope are typically given isoproterenol during tilting to simulate sympathetic stimulation.

Once a positive tilt table test is observed, the patient may be treated with beta-blockers, certain antidepressants, or disopyramide to block catecholamine response and thereby prevent the chain of events that produces the transient loss of consciousness. By using this very effective and relatively inexpensive method of testing, the patient is treated quickly and without the need for any invasive procedure. An additional benefit is that the tilt table test is readily done on an outpatient basis.[19,20]

EXERCISE ELECTROCARDIOGRAPHY

The exercise electrocardiogram is valuable in the evaluation of chest pain. An early diagnosis of coronary artery disease can be made with this noninvasive technique at a relatively small cost to the patient. The exercise ECG can also evaluate the exercise tolerance of a known cardiac patient and the efficacy of medical or surgical treatment. Originally introduced as the Master "2-step" exercise test in 1929, only measurements of pulse and heart rate were used to evaluate cardiac function. In 1941, however, Master and Jaffe noted the importance of preexercise and postexercise electrocardiograms in detecting coronary insufficiency. In 1940 Riseman proposed continuous ECG monitoring during the test. Yu and associates emphasized the necessity of continuous monitoring in 1952 and also described a motor-driven treadmill used to exercise patients. It was not until approximately 1955 that the motor-driven treadmill gained wide acceptance for both clinical and research use.

A variety of protocols may be used to evaluate the patient with known cardiac disease (Table 2.3). Exercise is geared toward developing a target heart rate, which is a percentage of the patient's expected maximum heart rate based on his or her age. An arm crank ergometer was developed for patients who are unable to walk on the treadmill. In the past, patients who were totally unable to exercise were paced through a right atrial or esophageal pacing lead. However, since atrial pacing has resulted in more false positives and false negatives than the standard treadmill, current diagnostic tests for such a patient would include a stress echocardiogram or thallium study.[3] The following has been suggested as a standard to be used in selecting an exercise protocol:[3]

1. The initial workload should be well within a given individual's anticipated physical working capacity.
2. The workloads should be increased gradually rather than abruptly and should be maintained for a sufficient length of time to achieve a near-physiologic steady state, which is approximately 3 minutes for each workload level.
3. The exercise protocol should not cause any excessive mental or physical stress beyond tolerable workloads.

TABLE 2.3

Exercise Testing Protocols

Stage	Speed (MPH)	Grade(%)	Minutes	Mean METS	Total Time
BRUCE REHABILITATION PROTOCOL					
1	1.7	10	3	3.0	3
2	2.5	12	3	6.0	6
3	3.4	14	3	7.6	9
4	4.2	16	3	10.7	12
5	5.0	18	3	16.3	15
6	5.5	20	3	19.5	18
7	6.0	22	3	22.7	21
NAUGHTON (MODIFIED BRUCE) REHABILITATION PROTOCOL					
1	1	0	2	1.6	2
2	2	0	2	2.0	4
3	2	3.5	2	3.0	6
4	2	7.0	2	4.0	8
5	2	10.5	2	5.0	10
6	2	14	2	6.0	12

Most treadmill tests involve a series of periodic increases in both speed and grade. The Bruce protocol is the most widely used in patients who have not yet had a cardiac event, while the Naughton or modified Bruce protocol is used in patients with known cardiac disease.
(Reproduced with permission from Bardsley WT, Mankin HT. Exercise Testing. In: Brandenburg RO, Fuster V, Giuliani ER, McGoon DC. eds. *Cardiology Fundamentals and Practice.* Chicago: Yearbook Medical Publishers; 1987.)

4. Continuous ECG monitoring (at least a two-channel recorder) with periodic (at least 1-minute intervals) recording of the rhythm strips throughout the entire exercise period and for at least 6 to 8 minutes during the postexercise period is essential. In addition, periodic (1 to 3-minute intervals) measurement of blood pressure before, during, and after exercise (for 6 to 8 minutes postexercise) should be done in conjunction with continuous evaluation of signs and symptoms.

The purpose of the exercise ECG is to stress the myocardium, thus increasing the oxygen demand, and then evaluate the ability of the coronary arteries to respond to the increased demand. This is done by monitoring the ECG, the patient's pulse and blood pressure, and any symptoms such as fatigue, SOB, chest pain, palpitations, and diaphoresis as well as the general appearance of the patient.

Patients exercise until they reach a target heart rate that is somewhere near or at 85% of the predicted age-adjusted maximal heart rate. A positive test is diagnosed when there is ST segment depression of 1 to 2mm, 0.08 seconds beyond the J-point.[2]

When to Terminate the Exercise ECG

The patient should be exercised at maximal levels in order to obtain a higher percentage of positive results. The test can be stopped when the patient reaches 85% of the predicted maximal heart rate (age adjusted); however, it may be terminated because the patient is experiencing significant symptoms such as severe chest pain, dyspnea, marked fatigue, or dizziness. If the patient develops ST segment elevation equal to or greater than 1 mm or depression equal or greater than 2 mm, complex ventricular arrhythmias, ventricular fibrillation, or hypertension (systolic pressure > 220 mmHg, diastolic pressure > 110 mmHg) or if there is a failure of the blood pressure to rise as the workload is increased, (> 20 mmHg) the test should be stopped. Other indications for premature termination of the test are leg cramps, persistent supraventricular tachyarrhythmias, and, of course, the appearance of ECG changes associated with acute myocardial injury.

Other highly suspicious ECG changes include horizontal or downsloping ST segment (depression ≤ 1mm), upsloping ST segment (depression ≥ 2mm beyond 0.08 seconds from the J-point), appearance of a third or fourth heart sound or murmur, hypotension, frequent ventricular premature contractions, ventricular tachycardia induced by only mild exercise, or exercise-induced angina.

There are multiple causes of false positive results in the exercise ECG. There are conflicting reports about the effects of digitalis in producing false positives.[21,22,23] Sketch noted that the ST changes induced by digitalis during the exercise ECG were indistinguishable from genuine ischemia. A patient receiving thiazide-type diuretics may lose potassium stores without alterations in the resting ECG, but characteristic hypokalemic changes, such as increased height of U waves with a depressed ST segment, may become apparent after exercise.[24] Wolff-Parkinson-White syndrome, mitral valve prolapse, hyperventilation, cardiomyopathy, idiopathic hypertrophic subaortic stenosis (IHSS), myocarditis, rheumatic heart disease, and hypertensive heart disease may all cause false positive results on the exercise ECG test.[25,26,27]

Patient Preparation

Patient preparation for the exercise ECG includes the following instructions:

1. Both men and women should wear loose-fitting trousers or shorts with a front-buttoning shirt and comfortable, low-heeled shoes. Women should also wear a bra, but *not* pantyhose. Hospitalized patients should wear pajamas and either well-fitting slippers or comfortable shoes.
2. All prescribed medications should be taken unless otherwise advised by the physician.
3. An overnight fast is recommended, although a very light meal may be consumed no sooner than 2 hours before the test. This is to prevent the diversion of blood to the digestive tract, which could result in inaccurate results or discomfort. No alcohol, butter, cream, coffee, or tea should be ingested. Patients should refrain from smoking for at least 1 hour prior to the test.
4. Exercise is usually done on a treadmill, with gradual increasing of the grade and speed. A bicycle or stair-step exerciser is sometimes used.
5. The patient should be instructed to inform the physician monitoring the test of any untoward symptoms such as chest pain, palpitations, vertigo, ataxia, and visual or gait disturbances.

Following the stress test, an assessment of the patient's tolerance of exercise should be done. Ask how long the patient was able to exercise, or if any untoward symptoms such as palpitations, chest pain, shortness of breath, or dizziness occurred during the test. A period of rest after the stress test is usually appreciated by the patient.

CONTINUOUS AMBULATORY MONITORING

Continuous ambulatory monitoring may be helpful when a patient reports symptoms that may be caused by an arrhythmia and have not been documented on a regular 12-lead ECG. Using a typical bipolar recording system (modified to lead V_4 or V_5), various bradyarrhythmias and tachyarrhythmias as well as conduction disturbances and ST-T changes may be observed. The leads are connected to a portable electrocardiographic monitor. The signal is recorded on magnetic tape for 10, 12, or 24 hours for later reading by a technician. This permits the patient to go about his or her daily activities and allows the physician to gain information about what abnormalities can be induced by these activities. One important aspect of ambulatory monitoring is the patient diary. In it, the patient records each activity, the time of the activity, and any symptoms or absence of symptoms associated with it. This lets the physician correlate symptoms with arrhythmias as well as arrhythmias with certain activities. Continuous ambulatory monitoring, or the Holter monitor technique, may be done on an inpatient or outpatient basis. The cost of a Holter recording is relatively small—about twice the cost of an ECG. The Holter monitor can be used to evaluate artificial pacemaker function or the efficacy of antianginal or antiarrhythmic drugs; it is also useful in correlating symptoms such as syncope, lightheadedness, palpitations, chest pain, or dyspnea with arrhythmias. Myocardial ischemia can be evaluated by observing the ST segment for depression or elevation that correlates with episodes of angina. Paroxysmal bursts of tachyarrhythmias, especially those associated with the WPW syndrome, are also easily documented via the Holter technique.

Patient Preparation for the Holter Monitor

The patient should be instructed about how the monitor is applied and what information is to be gained from its inclusion into the diagnostic workup. The patient should be told what activities are acceptable and which activities should be avoided, such as bathing, swimming, or any activity that has the potential for interfering with lead adhesion or function. Instructions should be given on how to complete the accompanying diary. The patient should be told not to touch the electrodes during the monitoring period and to keep both the recorder and the electrodes dry. Preventing the recorder from falling or being struck helps ensure the reliability of the device. It is also important to tell the patient how to remove the Holter monitor after the recording period is over.

Event Recorders

Event recorders are devices used to document specific events that are associated with patient symptoms. Patients are instructed to activate the device whenever they feel an episode of dizziness, palpitations, or other symptom that may be caused by an arrhythmia. After the event has been recorded, or after several events are recorded, the device is returned to the physician, who plays it back to reveal the rhythm that was occurring at the time of the symptoms. When possible, patients are asked to keep a written record of symptoms and surrounding activities to help discern if certain activities were related to the arrhythmia.

PACEMAKERS

Artificial pacemakers, first introduced in 1959, have undergone tremendous changes as modern technology has increased generator life while decreasing the size and allowing for external programmability. Because of the complex nature of pacemakers and their capabilities, the InterSociety Commission for Heart Disease Resources (ICHD) introduced a 5-letter code for identification of the sensed and paced chambers, the pacing mode and certain programmability, and special functions the pacemaker may have. Both the North American Society for Pacing and Electrophysiology (NASPE) and the British Pacing and Electrophysiology Group (BPEG) have proposed a generic code based on the ICHD format.[28] Often, only the first three or four letters of the code are used.

On the ECG, the pacemaker impulse is recognized by the so-called pacemaker spike or artifact, a sharp, narrow vertical line with a duration normally less than 2 msec. The morphology of the waveform after the pacemaker spike is usually distorted, causing an ectopic-looking complex. Depending upon where the pacemaker lead is placed, the P waves and QRS complexes will generally reflect the location. For instance, because the pacemaker lead is located in the right ventricle, the QRS complexes take on the appearance of complete left bundle branch block. An atrial lead near the sinus node can produce P waves that are similar to normal sinus beats. All pacemakers consist of a pulse generator and leads that are usually placed in the heart transvenously.

In bipolar leads the negative electrode is located at the tip of the catheter and the positive electrode is approximately 1 cm proximal to this. The electrical current travels from the negative electrode to the positive electrode to complete the circuit. In unipolar leads the active electrode or cathode is located at the tip of the catheter while the indifferent electrode, the anode, consists of the exposed metal portion of the pulse generator. The electrical current flows from the cathode to the anode via tissue and body fluids. A larger spike will usually be seen with the unipolar lead because of the greater distance the electrical current must travel.

Pacemaker Types

The Ventricular Demand (VVI) pacemaker is a commonly used pacemaker. As indicated by the code letters, both sensing and pacing occur in the ventricle. The pacemaker will deliver an impulse to the ventricle after a set escape interval if no depolarization in the ventricle is sensed. In keeping with the inhibition mode, the pacemaker function is suppressed if the patient has spontaneous ventricular depolarization. The pacemaker does not compete with the patient's own heart rate; it fires only when needed.

On the ECG, a VVI pacemaker will produce complexes that will be widened in the typical LBBB pattern. The spike-to-spike interval is constant, usually at a set rate of 72 bpm. If the patient's own rate is greater than the programmed rate of the pacemaker, the complexes will be those of the patient's baseline rhythm and the presence of a pacemaker will not be visible on the ECG. Sometimes both spontaneous depolarization and pacemaker-stimulated depolarization may be seen. The interval from a spontaneous beat that is followed by a paced beat is called the escape interval and is usually slightly longer than the spike-to-spike interval.

The *AV sequential (DVI) pacemaker* paces both the atrium and the ventricle, senses the ventricle only, and acts in the inhibited mode. It can pace the atrium alone; the atrium and ventricle sequentially; or, in the presence of preserved atrial activity and AV block, the ventricle alone. If there are normally conducted beats or PVCs that occur before the preset escape interval, the pacemaker is inhibited. If no ventricular depolarization is sensed then the atria will be paced. After the atrial spike, if the patient's AV conduction time and subsequent QRS complex appears before the programmed AV interval, the ventricular channel of the pacemaker will be suppressed. If, however, there is delayed conduction and no ventricular depolarization is sensed, the ventricle will be paced to provide atrioventricular sequential stimulation. This is an uncommitted-type AV sequential pacemaker. In the committed type of DVI pacemaker, ventricular pacing will occur whether or not there is spontaneous ventricular depolarization.[6] Competition occurs when the patient's spontaneous atrial rate is faster than the programmed pacemaker rate (Figure 2.61).

AV sequential pacemakers were designed to preserve sequential depolarization of the atria and ventricles to maintain an adequate cardiac output (i.e. preservation of atrial kick). This type of pacemaker also has an upper-rate control mechanism to prevent tracking of supraventricular tachyarrhythmias. There are several types of upper-rate control mechanisms, including a Wenckebach-type blocking, a 2:1 blocking pattern, and rate smoothing.[29,30]

The *atrial synchronous ventricular inhibited (VDD) pacemaker* provides atrioventricular synchrony by sensing atrial activity. If ventricular depolarization fails to occur within a preset interval, ventricular pacing occurs. This pacemaker is able to sense PVCs or accelerated idioventricular rhythms, thereby avoiding competition. An added feature of these units is that they have independent minimum and maximum rates. A

FIGURE 2.61

Dual chamber pacing.

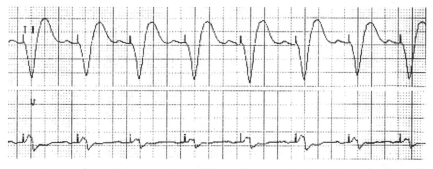

lower rate may be set to preserve AV synchrony during sinus rhythm, but a higher rate may be used to achieve a satisfactory exercise heart rate, especially with young patients (Figure 2.62). This can be noninvasively programmed.[28]

The *AV (DDD) pacemaker* is capable of pacing and sensing both the atrium and ventricle and can operate in either the inhibited or triggered mode. In this way it can operate as a VDD-type or DVI-type pacemaker. Many parameters can be programmed into the pacemaker, including minimum and maximum rates, AV delay, atrial and ventricular output and sensitivity, atrial and ventricular refractory periods, and AV intervals.[31]

One problem with this pacemaker—and with any pacemaker with atrial sensing capabilities—is the occurrence of the so-called pacemaker-mediated or endless loop tachycardias. These are caused by the presence of retrograde P waves, which are the result of reverse atrial depolarization from a paced ventricular beat. The P wave is sensed by the

FIGURE 2.62

Atrial-triggered ventricular pacing. Note the sinus P wave at a rate of 75 bpm followed by a paced QRS complex.

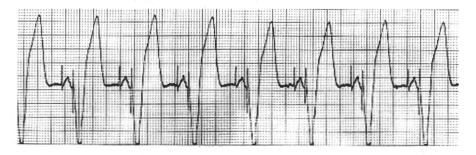

atrial pacemaker lead, triggering ventricular depolarization that again results in retrograde atrial depolarization. This can repeat itself, resulting in a reentrant or loop tachycardia. The incidence of this may be minimized but not obliterated by careful evaluation of the patient's ventriculoatrial conduction prior to implantation and by lengthening the atrial refractory period.

Rate responsive pacing (VVIR, DDDR) is one of the newer developments in pacing technology and represents an attempt to make pacing technology truly responsive to physical need. The most common rate responsive pacemaker senses muscle vibrations in the body via a piezoelectric crystal within the shell of the pacemaker. As the intensity of these vibrations increases, the pacing rate is also increased. Thus, mild muscle activity is associated with mild elevations in heart rate while vigorous excercise will produce higher rates. Minimum and maximum rates are programmed upon implantation and can be changed using an external programmer. Since the pacemaker is able to alter its output in response to varying activity levels ranging from low to medium to high, it can be programmed so that it meets the patient's needs. A low threshold would respond to muscle vibrations of small magnitude such as those associated with walking, while a medium threshold screens out signals of small amplitude in favor of more strenuous activity. A high threshold would not respond until strenuous activity was done. Generally a baseline rate of 60 bpm and an upper rate limit of 150 bpm are used, but the best results are achieved when a patient's individual needs, activity levels, and underlying disease process are used to determine appropriate settings.[31]

In addition to pacemakers that sense muscle movement, a variety of other sensors exist. Core body temperature, thoracic chest excursion, and respitory rate sensors can be used to guide heart rate in rate responsive pacemakers.

Programmability

Programmability refers to the ability to noninvasively alter certain pacemaker parameters. An external programmer is placed on the patient's chest over the area of the pulse generator. The programmer transmits a coded impulse to the generator, which decodes it and then reacts in a predicted manner.[28] All modern pacemakers are programmable and are easily altered to accommodate the patient's need.

ECG Signs of Pacemaker Malfunction

Malfunctions with the demand-type pacemakers may involve sensing ability, pacing ability, or both. This discussion will deal with ventricular demand pacemakers.

Sensing is the ability of a pacemaker to determine the presence or absence of spontaneous electrical discharge within the sensed chamber (i.e. the ventricle). If the pacemaker is undersensing it loses its ability to detect ventricular depolarization. This may result in the pacemaker performing like a fixed rate asynchronous pacemaker.

Undersensing can be intermittent. Fusion beats and pseudofusion beats are sometimes mistakenly attributed to pacemaker undersensing. Fusion beats occur when the ventricle is simultaneously depolarized from both the pacemaker and some spontaneous focus. Pseudofusion beats are when a pacemaker spike is inscribed within a QRS complex on the ECG. The pacemaker spike does not cause depolarization because it falls in the absolute refractory period of the ventricle, after the onset of spontaneous depolarization but before sufficient intracardiac voltage has been generated.[6]

Oversensing, though uncommon, can occur when there are tall P or T waves that are mistaken for R waves, thereby causing the pacemaker to be reset. Also, skeletal muscle potentials are commonly mistaken for myopotentials.

Pacing failure is usually readily evident on the ECG during periods when pacing is occurring or should be occurring. Severe changes in spike amplitude should be considered abnormal and may be the result of current loss through the pacemaker lead, with wire fracture being a common cause. With decreased spike amplitude, failure of the pulse generator is more likely. Although changes in the depolarization pattern may indicate an underlying myocardial process, Q waves in leads I and/or aVL may indicate slight displacement of the pacemaker lead.[26] A dominant R wave in lead V_1 is nearly always abnormal and strongly suggests perforation of the right ventricle by the pacing catheter.

Failure to capture is diagnosed when a pacer spike occurs during the appropriate period (not during a refractory period) but produces no depolarization. This is most frequently caused by displacement of the

FIGURE 2.63

Pacemaker failure.

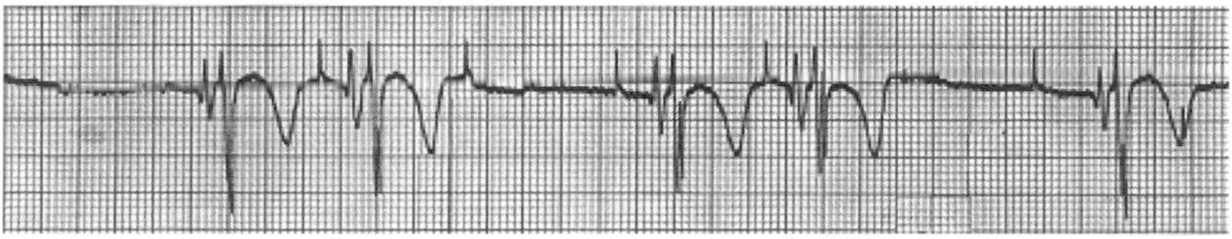

pacing catheter although drug and electrolyte imbalances should be ruled out (Figure 2.63).

Pacemaker failure can be caused by battery failure or component failure of the pulse generator. This is commonly seen as a lowering of the pacing rate. If the patient's own rhythm is higher than the pacemaker rate a magnet may be applied to the chest wall over the pacemaker. This causes the pacemaker to operate in the fixed rate, allowing for an accurate cal-

---

PATIENT EDUCATION BOX 2.1

Permanent Pacemaker Implantation

The purpose of a permanent pacemaker is to help restore and maintain a normal heart rate. It will take about 2 hours to implant the device.

BEFORE THE PROCEDURE

Do not eat or drink anything after midnight the evening before the operation unless instructed to do so by your doctor or nurse.
Take your medication as prescribed unless you are instructed to do otherwise.

DURING THE PROCEDURE

The pacemaker will be inserted under the skin in your upper right or left shoulder area.
The doctor will numb the area first (local anesthetic).
A small incision will be made and a small "pocket" will be created to hold the generator (pacemaker battery).
The pacemaker wire is threaded into your heart and attached to the generator. It is tested to be sure it works and then the incision is closed. A bandage is put over the area.
You will be awake throughout the entire procedure.

AFTER THE PROCEDURE

Your heart rhythm will be monitored for a day or two. A chest x-ray will be done.
After a day or so, the dressing can be removed.
You will be given instructions about how much you can use the arm on the side where the pacemaker has been placed. Generally, lifting your arm above your head is prohibited for one to two weeks.
Prior to discharge, the follow-up plan should be discussed with you. Remember to carry your pacemaker ID card with you at all times.
Any questions you have about returning to your prepacemaker activities should be discussed with your doctor or nurse.

culation of the pacemaker rate. Current pacemakers have telemetry messages that indicate battery failure to the programmer.

Indications for Pacing

Pacemakers were originally used to treat Stokes-Adams attacks and complete heart block. Now, however, with a variety of programming options, the indications for permanent artificial pacing have been expanded to include antitachycardia pacing, symptomatic bradycardia pacing, and in some cases arrhythmia control when medications are unsuccessful or contraindicated. Pacemakers are used to treat sick sinus syndrome, chronic atrial fibrillation or atrial flutter with AV block and slow ventricular rate, and impaired AV conduction or bundle branch block.[32,33]

Patient Preparation for a Pacemaker

For some patients, a permanent pacemaker is both threatening and life saving. Many patients are alarmed by their dependence on a device, but relieved by the improvement in their overall well-being. It is very important for the patient to understand why a pacemaker was selected as the most effective treatment.

Information about how the pacemaker works may alleviate fear or anxiety. (See Patient Education Box 2.1.) Having a demonstration pacemaker on hand to let the patient look at and touch may be helpful. Information such as the battery life expectancy of a pacemaker and a general idea of routine follow-up also helps to lessen fears about the impending implantation. The length of the procedure, the use of local anesthesia, the location of the generator, and the sensations that might be experienced are usually of interest to patients. There will be limited use of the extremity involved for a short time and some mild discomfort at the implantation site (Figure 2.64).

Prior to discharge, patients should be reminded that they should always carry their pacemaker ID card. They should know if any occupational conditions will affect pacemaker function. For example, large running diesel engines, certain vibrating construction equipment, and large magnetic fields may affect the pacemaker. On the other hand, household appliances, including microwave ovens, are safe for pacemaker patients to use. Any questions regarding the safety of machinery specific to pacer function should be directed to the implanting physician or to the vendor. Patients who travel by air should know that their pacemaker will be detected when they walk through the airport metal detector and that security personnel may require their pacemaker ID card to be displayed. The metal detectors will not be harmful to the pacemaker.

FIGURE 2.64

Critical pathway: permanent pacemaker implantation.

Collaborative Problems	Nursing Diagnoses	Expected LOS
• Syncope	• Anxiety	
• Dsyrhythmia	• Alteration in comfort	Admission Date
	• Impaired skin integrity	
	• Potential for infection	
	• Potential for altered self-concept	Discharge Date

Night/Morning Before	Day of Procedure	Day of Discharge
MEDICAL		
Assessment	**Assessment**	**Assessment**
• Include allergies, health hx	• Assess change from baseline	• Assure labs and ECG WNL
• Labs, physical exam, ECG	• Read CXR	
Medical Orders	**Medical Orders**	**Medical Orders**
• Diet: Regular, NPO after MN	• Resume diet	• D/C IV
• IV access	→	
• Labs, ECG	• ECG & CXR after procedure	• Write prescriptions and F/U appts
• Order routine meds	• Antibiotic after procedure × 5 doses	• D/C monitor, D/C to home
• Telemetry monitoring	→	
	• Sling to affected arm × 24 hrs	
	• Mild pain reliever	
BOTH		
Patient and Family Education	**Patient and Family Education**	**Patient and Family Education**
• About PPM insertion	• Activity limitations (arm use)	• Reinforce activity limitations, importance of
• Reinforce with pamphlets and videotapes	→	attending F/U appts, and importance of
• Obtain consent		notifying MD if symptoms reoccur

Discharge Planning
- Consider referrals for social services, dietary home care

NURSING

Assessment
- Health hx
- VS, telemetry, heart sounds, lung sounds, labs, anxiety
- Assess for SOB, lightheadedness
- Assess shoulder site

Nursing Orders
- IV access
- Administer medications
- Telemetry monitoring
- Up as tolerated

Discharge Planning
→
- Provide pacer ID card (temp) and booklet

Assessment
→

- Monitor drainage, change dressing prn

Nursing Orders
→
- Obtain stat ECG for change in rhythm
- Bed rest × 3 hrs; do not raise affected arm—up as tolerated
- Pressure dressing to shoulder site
- Apply sling × 24 hrs

Discharge Planning
- Make final arrangements for F/U care
- Assure pt. has pacer ID card and booklet; anticipate receipt of permanent ID card in mail

Assessment
- Assure WNL

- Assure absent
- Remove pressure dressing; assure steri-strips intact; teach patient or family care of site

Nursing Orders
- D/C IV
- Provide medication schedule
- Assure WNL, then D/C
- Do not raise affected arm above shoulder level for 2 weeks after D/C to home
- D/C (see above)
- D/C
- Provide and/or review D/C instruction

References

1. Grauer K, Curry R Jr. *Clinical Electrocardiography: A Primary Care Approach*. 2nd ed. Oradell, NJ: Medical Economics; 1992.
2. Marriott HJL. *Practical Electrocardiography*. 8th ed. Baltimore: Williams & Wilkins; 1988.
3. Chung EK. *Electrocardiography: Practical Applications with Vectorial Principles*. 3rd ed. Philadelphia: Harper and Row; 1985.
4. Kishida H, Cole JS, Surawicz B. Negative U wave: A highly specific but poorly understood sign of heart disease. *Am J Cardiol*. 1982;49:2030–2036.
5. Gerson MC, McHenry PL. Resting U wave inversion as a marker of stenosis of the left anterior descending artery. *Am J Med*. 1980;69:545–550.
6. Chou TC. *Electrocardiography in Clinical Practice*. 3rd ed. New York: Grune & Stratton; 1991.
7. Cheng TO. Incidence of ventricular aneurysm in coronary artery disease. An angiographic appraisal. *Am J Med*. 1971;50:340–355.
8. Cokkinos DV, Hallman GL, Cooley DA, et al. Left ventricular aneurysm: Analysis of electrocardiographic features and postresection changes *Am Heart J*. 1971;82:149–157.
9. Goldberg MJ. Left ventricular aneurysm. *Br J Hosp Med*. 1982;27:143–154.
10. Knochel JP. Diuretic induced hypokalemia. *Am J Med*. 1984;77(5A):18–27.
11. Bellet S. *Clinical Disorders of the Heartbeat*. 3rd ed. Philadelphia: Lea and Febiger; 1971.
12. Aronow WS, Kronzon I. Prevalence and severity of valvular aortic stenosis determined by Doppler echocardiography and its association with echocardiographic and electrocardiographic left ventricular hypertrophy and physical signs of aortic stenosis in elderly patients. *Am J Cardiol*. 1991; 67:776–777.
13. Usher BW, Popp RL. Electrical alternans: Mechanisms in pericardial effusion. *Am Heart J*. 1972;83:459–463.
14. Canedo MI, Frank MJ, Abdulla AM. Rhythm disturbances in hypertrophic cardiomyopathy: Prevalence, relation to symptoms and management. *Am J Cardiol*. 1980;45:848–855.
15. McKenna WJ, Chetty S, Oakley LM, et. al. Arrhythmia in hypertrophic CMP: Exercise and 48 hour ambulatory electrocardiographic assessment with and without beta adrenergic blocking therapy. *Am J Cardiol*. 1980;45:1–5.
16. McMartin DE, Flowers NC. Clinical electrocardiographic correlations in diseases of the myocardium. *Cardiovasc Clin*. 1977;8:191–199.
17. Schamroth L. *The Electrocardiology of Coronary Artery Disease*. 2nd ed. London: Blackwell Scientific Publications; 1984.
18. Conover MH, Marriott HJL. *Advanced Concepts in Arrhythmias*. 2nd ed. St. Louis: CV Mosby; 1989.
19. Fitzpatrick A, Sutton R. Tilting towards a diagnosis in recurrent unexplained syncope. *Lancet*. 1989;1:658–660.
20. Lagi A, Vannucchi P, Annatoli G. The tilting cardiovascular response in orthostatic syncope. *Ital J Neurol Sci*. 1992;13:203–207.
21. Tonkon MJ, Lee G, DeMaria AN, et al. Effects of digitalis on the exercise electrocardiogram in normal adult subjects. *Chest*. 1977;72:714–718.
22. McHenry PL, Richmond HW, Weisenberger BL, et al. Evaluation of abnormal exercise electrocardiography in apparently healthy subjects: Labile repolarization (ST-T) abnormalities as a cause of false positive responses. *Am J Cardiol*. 1981;47:1152–1160.
23. Gettes LS, Sapin P. Concerning falsely negative and falsely positive electrocardiogram responses to exercise [editorial]. *Br Heart J*. 1993;70:205–207.

24. LeWinter MM, Crawford MH, O'Rourke RA, et. al. The effect of oral propranolol, digoxin, and combination therapy on the resting and exercise electrocardiogram. *Am Heart J.* 1977;93:202–209.
25. Strasberg B, Ashley WW, Wyndham CR, et. al. Treadmill exercise testing in the Wolff-Parkinson-White syndrome. *Am J Cardiol.* 1980;45:742–748.
26. Gardin JM, Isner JM, Ronan JA, et. al. Pseudoischemic "false positive" ST segment changes induced by hyperventilation in patients with mitral valve prolapse. *Am J Cardiol.* 1980;45:952–958.
27. Kemp GL, Ellestad MH. The significance of hyperventilation and orthostatic T wave changes on the electrocardiogram. *Arch Intern Med.* 1968;121: 518–523.
28. Medina R, Michelson EL. Update on cardiac pacemakers: Description, complications, indications, and follow-up. *Cardiovasc Clin.* 1985;16:177–213.
29. Furman, S. *Dual-chamber Pacing and Pacemakers.* Chicago: Yearbook Medical Publishers; 1990.
30. Barold S, Mugica J. *New Perspectives in Cardiac Pacing.* Mount Kisco, NY: Futura Publishers; 1991.
31. Ellenbogen K. *Cardiac Pacing.* Boston: Blackwell Scientific Publications; 1992.
32. Braunwald E. *Heart Disease: A Textbook of Cardiovascular Medicine.* 4th ed. Philadelphia: WB Saunders; 1992.
33. Goldberger A. *Clinical Electrocardiography: A Simplified Approach.* 4th ed. St. Louis: CV Mosby; 1990.

3

LABORATORY TESTS

CATHERINE GAGE RICCIUTI
JUDITH RADKE

GLOSSARY

Anion   A negatively charged ion.
Cation   A positively charged ion.
Chvostek's Sign   Spasm of facial muscles following a tap on one side of the face over the area of the facial nerve; indicative of hypocalcemia.
Isoenzyme   One of several forms in which an enzyme may exist in various tissues. Although they are similar in catalytic qualities, isoenzymes may be separated from one another by special chemical tests.
Lipoprotein   Conjugated proteins consisting of simple proteins combined with lipid components (e.g. cholesterol, phospholipids, and triglycerides).
Serotonin   A powerful vasoconstrictor substance found in various cells of the body, including platelets.
Thromboxane   A substance involved in the coagulation process that causes platelet aggregation and vasoconstriction.
Trousseau's Sign   Muscular spasm resulting from pressure applied to nerves and vessels of the upper arm. It is indicative of hypocalcemia and latent tetany, and also occurs in osteomalacia.

Laboratory diagnostic tests can be of critical importance in the assessment of the cardiac patient. The determination of myocardial infarction, the assessment of electrolyte balance in the heart failure patient, and the lipid workup for the patient with suspected coronary artery disease are important diagnostic tests. The purpose of this chapter is to provide a brief overview of specific laboratory tests and demonstrate their application to the cardiac patient population.

ELECTROLYTES

Sodium, potassium, and calcium are the key ions in the depolarization and repolarization process. An explanation of cardiac electrophysiology is found in chapter 8.

Sodium

Sodium (135–145 mEq/L) is the most abundant cation in the body. Its primary systemic functions include maintenance of osmotic pressure, acid-base balance, and transmission of nerve impulses. In the heart, sodium is the key extracellular electrolyte in the electrical depolarization of cardiac cells. Sodium is regulated by the kidneys. As sodium ions are reabsorbed in the kidneys, water molecules follow; consequently, sodium ion concentration directly affects extracellular fluid (blood) volume. When a patient experiences low cardiac output, glomerular filtration decreases and more sodium is reabsorbed in the renal tubules. The increase in serum sodium results in water retention and an increase in blood volume. Conversely, when excessive sodium has been excreted, there will be too little water and hypovolemia may occur. This may happen during aggressive diuresis of the patient. Wide vacillations in blood volume levels increase the workload on the heart and can result in ischemia or heart failure.

Several factors affect sodium reabsorption in the kidneys. Increased sodium reabsorption is usually caused by renal hypoperfusion secondary to hypovolemia, decreased cardiac output, increased aldosterone secretion, and certain drugs. Decreased sodium reabsorption is usually caused by increased glomerular filtration secondary to hypervolemia, increased cardiac output, decreased aldosterone secretion, secretion of ADH, and diuretics.[1,2]

Patients with congestive heart failure and/or hypertension may have difficulty maintaining a normal serum sodium level. These conditions result in decreased blood flow to the kidneys, signaling them to retain sodium and water. The added blood volume further stresses the heart, and forward flow from the heart to the tissues is impaired. This results in a further decrease in flow to the kidneys and subsequent additional sodium reabsorption and water retention. This cycle is complicated by the use of diuretics, which usually aid in sodium excretion. Also, renal insufficiency can result in increased sodium reabsorption.[2]

Hypernatremia

Hypernatremia (serum sodium >145 mEq/L) exists when the ratio of sodium ions to water molecules is increased. In the cardiac patient this is likely to result from dehydration when excessive diuresis has occurred. Dehydration may also be due to deficient water intake or may occur in severe protracted diarrhea or vomiting. Patients with diabetes insipidus and uncontrolled diabetes mellitus with osmotic diuresis may also suffer from dehydration and subsequent hypernatremia.

The clinical presentation of hypernatremia is consistent with that of dehydration. The patient will have dry mucous membranes, a loss of skin turgor, and an initial elevated body temperature. Hypotension may occur with or without postural changes. A compensatory tachycardia may occur. The patient may complain of thirst, oliguria or anuria, weight loss, muscle cramps, and constipation. Concurrent laboratory values include increased hematocrit, BUN, serum osmolality, and urine osmolality. The urine specific gravity will be abnormally high. Early neurologic signs such as fatigue and lethargy may progress to coma and seizures at serum sodium levels greater than 160 mEq/L.[3]

Treatment for the hypernatremic patient is designed to normalize the ratio of sodium to water by replacing water. Intravenous fluids that replace water without adding sodium are administered until the serum sodium or serum osmolality is within normal limits. Measurement of intake and output and daily weights should be done. In the patient with heart failure, fluid replacement must be done judiciously so as not to exacerbate the failure.

Hyponatremia

Hyponatremia (serum sodium < 135 mEq/L) exists when there is a disproportionate amount of water in relation to sodium. This can occur from overhydration or from excessive sodium loss. With respect to cardiac patients, hyponatremia will most likely occur in the patient with untreated heart failure or in patients who are given certain diuretics or other drugs that waste sodium. In addition, hyponatremia may occur from water loss due to diarrhea, vomiting, excessive sweating, diabetic acidosis, or diuretics.[2,3]

The clinical presentation of the hyponatremic patient will depend on the etiology. For the patient who has water excess, signs and symptoms will be consistent with those of water intoxication. Physical findings may include headache, weight gain, decreased hematocrit and BUN, low serum osmolality, and mental status changes ranging from confusion to seizures. For the patient who has lost sodium in excess of water, the following signs and symptoms may be noted: headache, weakness, weight loss, poor skin turgor, abdominal cramps and nausea, decreased urinary sodium, and mental status changes ranging from malaise to coma.[3]

Treatment for hyponatremia is etiology driven. For water intoxication, fluid restriction and diuretic therapy are necessary. For combined sodium and water loss, liberalization of dietary sodium as well as intravenous replacement with normal or hypertonic saline are suggested.[4,5]

Careful monitoring for fluid intolerance, renal function, and mental status changes should be done.

Potassium

Potassium (3.5–5.5 mEq/L) is the major cation of intracellular fluid. Ninety percent of the body's potassium is concentrated within the cell. Potassium is primarily regulated by the kidneys. Potassium has an important role in nerve conduction, muscle cell (especially cardiac) depolarization and repolarization, acid-base balance, and maintenance of osmotic pressure.

Because potassium is primarily intracellular, serum concentrations are small and there is a very narrow normal range. Imbalances in serum potassium have serious, often critical consequences.

Hyperkalemia

The most common cause of hyperkalemia (serum potassium > 5.5 mEq/L) is renal insufficiency or renal failure in which adequate excretion of potassium does not occur. This is often the case in chronic heart failure patients with poor renal function. Another common cause of hyperkalemia is overmedication with potassium chloride supplements or overuse of dietary potassium. Medications such as ACE inhibitors may be associated with hyperkalemia. Occasionally hyperkalemia is caused by extensive tissue damage where potassium is released into the bloodstream.[1,3]

Regardless of the cause, hyperkalemia alters myocardial cell electrophysiology. The increase in extracellular potassium effectively reduces the potassium ion gradient across the cell membrane and thereby reduces the resting membrane potential. As a result, phase 0 of the action potential is reduced, thereby slowing conduction, and phase 3 is accelerated, resulting in a quicker repolarization. This can result in bradycardia and moderate to severe conduction abnormalities in the heart.[6]

The clinical presentation of hyperkalemia includes complaints of numbness of the extremities, abdominal cramping, diarrhea, and mental confusion or a sensation of not feeling "right." On the ECG, tall, peaked T waves will appear. If left untreated, the patient will eventually develop prolonged PR interval with bradycardia, flattened P wave, and a widened QRS complex. This may be associated with hypotension and will eventually progress to asystole[6] (see chapter 2).

Treatment for hyperkalemia is aimed at moving potassium out of the extracellular fluid as quickly as possible. Intravenous glucose and insulin is given to temporarily drive potassium into the cells. This intervention must be followed up with oral or rectal Kayexalate and sorbitol. Kayexalate exchanges potassium for sodium at a 1:1 ratio in the bowel, and sorbitol produces an osmotic diarrhea to eliminate the potassium. If these interventions are unsuccessful, dialysis may be necessary. Throughout treatment for hyperkalemia, the electrocardiogram and the serum potassium level should be closely monitored.

Hypokalemia

The most common cause of decreased potassium in cardiac patients is aggressive use of diuretics. These agents often cause potassium wasting in the kidneys. Other problems, such as liver disease, metabolic alkalosis, and severe nausea and vomiting, can contribute to decreased serum potassium levels.

Hypokalemia (serum potassium < 3.5 mEq/L) is very dangerous and is especially problematic for people with ischemic heart disease, heart failure or those with preexisting ventricular arrhythmias. Cardiac cell resting membrane potential becomes less negative and both pacemaker and nonpacemaker cells develop increased excitability. This can result in significant arrhythmias. If the patient is concurrently receiving digitalis, the digitalis will compete with the available potassium for cell membrane binding sites and may result in digitalis toxicity.[4,6]

Patients with decreased potassium may complain of anorexia, nausea and vomiting, and muscle weakness. The electrocardiogram depicts the progression of abnormal repolarization. The T wave decreases in amplitude and the U wave increases in amplitude. The prolonged repolarization period increases the risk of ventricular tachyarrhythmias.[7]

Treatment of the patient with hypokalemia centers on replacing potassium. Initially, oral potassium supplements are supplied if possible. When potassium levels are dangerously low, slow intravenous potassium should be administered. The electrocardiogram and serum potassium levels should be monitored closely. It may be advisable to reduce the dose of digitalis until the serum potassium is within normal limits. In the patient with chronic heart failure or cardiomyopathy where long-term diuretics are used and in whom dietary absorption of magnesium may be impaired, it is prudent to add magnesium supplements to the regimen.

Calcium

Most of the body's calcium (98–99%) is stored in the bones and teeth.[3] The rest of the calcium is divided into ionized calcium and protein-bound calcium. Only the protein-bound calcium be used by the body for such purposes as muscle contraction, cardiac function, transmission of nerve impulses, and blood clotting. Serum calcium (8.5–10.5 mg/dL) is regulated by the parathyroid gland. Renal excretion and intestinal absorption of calcium also play a role in maintaining calcium balance.[4]

Calcium regulation is essential for two reasons. It is a necessary component for the actin-myosin interaction that causes muscle fiber contraction. It is also responsible for prolonging the action potential and decreasing the threshold potential of the cardiac electrical cells.

Hypercalcemia

The most common cause of increased calcium is excessive release of bone stores. This may be due to primary hyperparathyroidism, immobility, metastatic carcinoma, hypophosphatemia, or thyrotoxicosis.[3,4] Excessive calcium or vitamin D intake can also result in increased calcium levels. Finally, altered tubular reabsorption of calcium may occur from chronic diuretic use. This is the most likely cause of increased calcium in the cardiac patient.

Hypercalcemia (serum calcium > 10.5 mg/dL) reduces the action potential and the threshold potential, making the cardiac cells more receptive to arrhythmias. Digitalis toxicity is also more likely in hypercalcemic states.

Patients with hypercalcemia may experience neuromuscular weakness, subtle personality changes, and gastrointestinal symptoms. Shortening of the ST and QT segments on the electrocardiogram also occurs.[7] Renal calculi with subsequent flank pain may be present. Untreated, hypercalcemia can progress to lethargy and eventual coma. Heart failure may be precipitated or exacerbated by the forceful contractions and additional workload on the heart.

Treatment of hypercalcemia is usually done by flushing calcium out of the kidneys.[1,2] Oral phosphate absorbs calcium from the intestine. Mithramycin therapy increases bone uptake of calcium. Throughout treatment, the patient should be observed for heart failure, neurological changes, and electrocardiographic abnormalities.

Hypocalcemia

Hypocalcemia (serum calcium level < 8.5 mg/dL) in the cardiac patient is most likely caused by dietary deficiencies or malabsorption of vitamin D or calcium. This is particularly true in chronically ill patients with CHF. Other causes of decreased calcium include excessive loss of calcium due to diarrhea or diuretic use and hypoparathyroidism or hyperphosphatemia, which can prevent calcium from being absorbed in the intestine. Excessive phosphorous binds with calcium and precipitates in the tissues.

Hypocalcemia prolongs the action potential and increases the threshold potential in myocardial cells. This increases the risk of ventricular tachyarrhythmias and may enhance the toxic effects of digitalis. Electrocardiographic changes include prolonged ST and QT intervals.[7]

Clinical findings in hypocalcemia include musculoskeletal cramps, tetany leading to seizures, and carpopedal spasm.[3,4,5] Pathological fractures may occur. The slower and less forceful contraction of the heart results in decreased cardiac output. Other signs include laryngeal stridor, decreased prothrombin time, and positive Chvostek's and Trousseau's signs (muscle spasms). Treatment of hypocalcemia is aimed at increasing the serum calcium level. This can be done with oral or intravenous calcium, depending upon the severity of the patient's clinical presentation. If the cause of hyocalcemia is vitamin D deficiency, appropriate supplementation is provided. Monitoring for neuromuscular and electrocardiographic changes is essential throughout treatment. Digitalis should be used with caution in hypocalcemic patients.

Phosphorus

Eighty-five percent of the body's phosphorous content (3.0–4.5 mg/dL) is combined with calcium in the bone. The rest is located within the cells. Phosphate is responsible for bone construction, glucose and lipid metabolism, acid-base balance, and energy storage and transfer.[4,5]

When caring for the cardiac patient with a phosphorus imbalance, the most important thing to remember is that phosphorus has an inverse relationship to calcium. Just like calcium, phosphorus is controlled by the parathyroid gland and regulated in the kidneys. Consequently, when serum calcium levels increase, the kidneys excrete phosphorus and vice versa.

Hyperphosphatemia

Cathartic and cytotoxic medications have unusually high levels of phosphorus and may result in hyperphosphatemia (serum phosphate level > 4.5 mg/dL). The most common treatment for hyperphosphatemia is administration of aluminum hydroxide gels that bind to phosphate in the gut. In the patient with normal kidneys, acetazolamide may be given to promote urinary excretion of phosphate.[3,5]

Hypophosphatemia

Hypophosphatemia (serum phosphate level < 3.0 mg/dL) may be caused by excessive glucose administration without sufficient phosphate (such as during chronic hyperalimentation) because glucose requires phosphate to be metabolized. Loss of phosphates in the urine leads to Fanconi's syndrome, which eventually results in osteomalacia.[8] Fanconi syndrome is a group of transport defects in the proximal renal tubule that result in a number of amino acid, mineral, and electrolyte disturbances including hypophosphatemia and hypercalciuria. It is associated with dwarfism and rickets along with a variety of inherited systemic diseases. Absence of phosphates in red blood cells may precipitate hemolytic anemia. Chronic alcoholics may develop Zieve syndrome, which is a severe intravascular hemolysis due to long-term hypophosphatemia.[8] Treatment for hypophosphatemia is aimed at treating the underlying etiology.

Magnesium

Magnesium (1.5–2.5 mEq/L) is an abundant electrolyte that is intimately involved with calcium absorption and metabolism. It is necessary in the metabolism of adenosine triphosphate as a source of energy. Consequently, it plays a role in carbohydrate metabolism, protein synthesis, nucleic acid synthesis, and muscular contraction.[9] Magnesium also helps regulate neuromuscular activity and is a vital component in blood clotting.[3,5] It may be involved in the generation and/or prevention of arrhythmias.[7] A study of AMI patients showed a modest decrease in mortality in patients who received a magnesium infusion during the perinfarction period.[10] Magnesium is regulated by the kidneys.

Hypermagnesemia

Hypermagnesemia (serum magnesium level > 2.5 mEq/L) has three primary causes. It may be caused by decreased excretion due to renal insufficiency or failure, excessive intake of magnesium-containing medications, or metabolic acidosis.

The clinical presentation for hypermagnesemia includes lethargy and diminished neuromuscular activity. At levels above 6 mEq/L, respiratory depression leading to apnea and bradycardia leading to asystole may occur.[4,7]

The primary goal in treating hypermagnesemia is to alleviate the underlying cause. If the patient is symptomatic, however, emergent interventions, such as dialysis for the patient with renal failure and diuretic administration for the patient with normal kidneys, should be done. Calcium gluconate administration may be helpful as well. Electrocardiographic and neuromuscular monitoring are essential throughout treatment.

Hypomagnesemia

Although there are several possible causes of hypomagnesemia (serum magnesium level < 1.5 mEq/L), such as decreased intestinal absorption, alkalosis, and excessive adrenal corticoid secretion, the most common cause in the cardiac patient is renal loss from diuretic administration. Hypomagnesemia often occurs concurrently with hypokalemia, which is also frequently caused by diuretic use. Magnesium plays an essential role in maintaining potassium stores and thus should be monitored closely in patients on diuretics.

The clinical presentation of the patient with hypomagnesemia ranges from subtle to overt. There may be mental status changes from mild lethargy to coma. Anorexia and nausea may be present and the patient may have tremors or tetany.[3,4] Electrocardiographic changes include flat or inverted T waves, ST segment depression, and a prolonged QT interval.[7] This can predispose the patient to a life-threatening ventricular arrhythmia.[4,7]

Hypomagnesemia is treated with an intravenous infusion of magnesium sulfate.[11] Therapy is guided by the severity of the deficit. When there is concurrent hypokalemia, it is recommended that the hypomagnesemia be treated first. As with hypermagnesemia, electrocardiographic and neuromuscular monitoring are essential.

Chloride

Chloride (95–105 mEq/L) is an anion that is mostly found in extracellular spaces. It helps to maintain cellular integrity via osmotic pressure and to maintain acid-base and water balance. Chloride has a strong affinity for sodium and potassium and is usually absorbed or excreted with them.

Hyperchloridemia

Hyperchloridemia (serum chloride > 105 mEq/L) occurs in a variety of conditions including dehydration, Cushing's syndrome, hyperventilation, eclampsia, anemia, and cardiac decompensation. The treatment for hyperchloridemia centers around treating the underlying cause.

Hypochloridemia

Most often, hypochloridemia (serum chloride < 95 mEq/L) occurs in concert with hyponatremia or hypokalemia. Chlorothiazide diuretics, used in the treatment of heart failure and hypertension commonly cause wasting of chloride. Metabolic alkalosis with hypokalemia requires chloride replacement in addition to potassium replacement.

CARDIAC ENZYMES

Creatine kinase (50–180 IU/L)
MB Isoenzyme (< 3% IU/L or 0%)

Creatine kinase (CK) is an enzyme found in the heart, skeletal muscle and brain. It consists of three isoenzymes: MM, found in the skeletal muscles; MB, found in the cardiac muscles; and BB, found in brain tissue.[6] Damage to any of these tissues causes the release of CK into the serum. The isoenzymes are then used to further differentiate the damaged tissue. Due to the exclusivity of the MB isoenzymes presence in the cardiac muscle, serum MB elevations greater than 3% are definitive in the diagnosis of myocardial infarction.[6] In the post–cardiac surgery patient, MB elevations greater than 7% indicate myocardial infarction.

After cardiac tissue injury, CK and MB isoenzymes will be released into the blood at a predictable rate. Within 2 to 5 hours, serum levels will rise above the normal limits, indicating tissue destruction.[4–6] A peak of 5 to 15 times the baseline is reached within 24 hours, the levels will return to normal within 2 to 3 days. If the CK continues to rise after the 24-hour point, it is assumed that ongoing injury is occurring and immediate intervention is necessary.[6]

One disadvantage of CK-MB is that it is not particularly sensitive to micro infarcts, which are associated with unstable angina and poor outcomes. Another disadvantage of CK-MB is that rapid and early detection of infarct is not possible because often there is no significant rise in CK-MB until 4 to 5 hours after symptom onset. Further, the isoenzyme measurement takes time to perform, often delaying a definitive diagnosis even longer.

Recent research has shown that the protein which helps to regulate heart muscle contraction can be isolated in the serum and is a sensitive indicator of myocardial injury. The Troponin protein actually consists of three separate proteins, Troponin I, T, and C, each with a different function.[12]

Following myocardial infarction or injury, Troponin T rises in the serum and correlates with the amount of tissue damaged. Troponin T is measurable in the serum within 4 hours of symptom onset, peaks at about 72 hours, and remains detectable in the blood for up to 14 days, providing a diagnostic advantage for patients who have delayed seeking treatment for their symptoms.

A bedside assay recently has been developed to detect Troponin T in the blood. This test is inexpensive and provides results within minutes, allowing for rapid triage of patients with AMI or unstable angina. It also helps to reduce observation time for patients with non-cardiac chest pain. Through early detection and rapid treatment of cardiac events, while at the same time reducing the use of resources for patients with non-cardiac symptoms, many millions of dollars in health care costs can be saved annually.[12]

Lactic Acid Dehydrogenase (63–155 U)
LDH1 (25–40%)
LDH2 (35–46%)

Lactic acid dehydrogenase (LDH) is an intracellular enzyme that is found in many tissues in the body, including the kidney, heart, and skeletal muscles. Destruction of tissue causes release of LDH into the bloodstream.

Since serum LDH elevations are nonspecific, this test may be used to confirm a suspected myocardial infarction in the patient who has elevated CK or in the patient who seeks medical attention after the CK level has returned to normal. LDH elevation begins within 6 to 12 hours after cardiac cell death. It peaks at 2 to 8 times normal in 3 to 4 days and returns to normal within 14 days.[5,6]

Isoenzymes LDH1 and LDH2 are found in the heart. In the normal patient, the ratio of LDH1 to LDH2 is 1:2. In the patient with acute myocardial infarction, that ratio is reversed. This reversal occurs between 48 hours and 7 days after the infarction; the ratio then slowly returns to normal. Serum elevations may also indicate myocardial cell death. However, since these isoenzymes are also present in the kidney and red blood cells, serum elevations must be correlated with other diagnostic data.[3,6]

Serum Glutamic-Oxaloacetic Transaminase (0–36 IU/L)

Serum glutamic-oxaloacetic transaminase (SGOT) is another enzyme that is abundant in intracellular tissue such as the heart, liver, skeletal muscles, and kidney. Cardiac tissue damage will be reflected in serum SGOT levels. The initial elevation occurs about 6 hours after infarction. The peak of 2 to 15 times normal is reached in 24 to 48 hours. The level returns to normal in 3 to 4 days. However, since serum SGOT elevation may be due to cellular damage in numerous organs, this test may only be useful in confirming CK elevations.

RENAL FUNCTION TESTS

Blood Urea Nitrogen/Creatinine

Blood urea nitrogen (BUN) and creatinine primarily reflect renal function. BUN is an end product of protein catabolism that is formed in the liver and excreted in the urine. Creatinine is a by-product in the metabolism of creatine phosphate, which provides energy.[1,2] When kidney function is impaired, neither BUN nor creatinine can be sufficiently excreted and serum levels rise.

In the cardiac patient, serum BUN/creatinine (10–15 mg/100mL/ 0.6–1.7 mg/dL) is used to assess renal function and overall hydration. An elevated BUN and creatinine indicate that renal function is impaired due to decreased renal perfusion or chemotoxic effects. Cardiac medications, especially diuretics and ACE inhibitors, may cause elevations in BUN and creatinine reflecting impaired renal function. With respect to fluid status, a decreased BUN with a normal creatinine indicates dehydration. On the other hand, an increased BUN with a normal creatinine indicates overhydration.

Following cardiac catheterization, certain patients may experience a rapid rise in BUN/creatinine. This is usually the result of acute renal tubular necrosis (ATN) following the contrast injection. Patients at risk for ATN include the elderly, those with diabetes mellitus, and those who are dehydrated. Good hydration prior to and after the catheterization and close observation of urine output immediately following the procedure are helpful. Patients may require diuresis if they do not void in sufficient quantity within 2 hours following the procedure. Nonionic contrast may be used in high-risk patients to decrease the possibility of acute renal tubular necrosis.

HEMATOLOGY TESTS

The cellular components of blood include red blood cells (erythrocytes), white blood cells (leukocytes), and platelets (thrombocytes). Each of these cells will be considered separately in relation to their normal and abnormal values with particular consideration given to the cardiac patient.

Erythrocytes

Men: 4.2–5.4 million/mm³
Women: 3.6–5.0 million/mm³

Erythrocytes, or red blood cells (RBCs), are produced in the bone marrow in response to erythropoietin stimulation. Their primary function is to carry oxygen to body cells. Oxygen binds reversibly with the hemoglobin portion of the RBC, allowing oxygen to be transported from the lungs to the tissues. The red blood cells occupy approximately 40% to 50% of the blood volume. This measurement is called the hematocrit. It should be noted that in addition to differences in normal values based on sex and age, racial differences also exist. Blacks have hemoglobin levels approximately 1 gm/dL lower than whites.[13]

Anemia

Men: less than 4.2 million/mm³
Women: less than 3.6 million/mm³

Anemia refers to a decrease in the erythrocytes or in hemoglobin concentration. Anemias may be classified in several ways. First, there may be deficient factors for RBC production or maturation. Factors required for RBC development include vitamin B_{12}, folic acid, and iron. Second, there may be bone marrow suppression, which may occur with toxic chemical agents, infections, immunologic and neoplastic disease, and radiation. Third, blood cells may be formed normally but lost from the circulation by either hemorrhage or hemolysis (intravascular destruction). Kidney failure also results in anemia.

The patient with cardiac disease may be prone to anemia from intravascular destruction secondary to drug-induced hemolysis (e.g. quinidine and methyldopa), traumatic hemolysis secondary to prosthetic heart valves (rare, but possible if the valve rocks or is functionally impaired), or increased RBC sequestration in the spleen secondary to chronic congestive heart failure. Patients in intensive care are also prone to anemia resulting from repeated blood drawing for laboratory tests. Anemia of any cause produces a stress on the cardiovascular system, requiring compensation to maintain adequate oxygen delivery to vital organs and tissues.

Compensation for acute blood loss in the presence of anemia involves several changes. The cardiovascular system responds immediately with vasoconstriction, increased heart rate, and increased cardiac output. Attempts to maintain blood volume by increasing plasma volume result in decreased blood viscosity. While these attempts to minimize further blood loss, restore blood volume, and maintain tissue oxygenation are beneficial at first, they are undesirable for long-term compensation. The tachycardia increases the heart's oxygen demand at a time of limited supply. In fact, the development of anemia may unmask symptoms of ischemic heart disease, including palpitations, dyspnea, angina, and congestive heart failure. Therefore, anemia may have serious consequences for the patient with coronary artery disease.

At the cellular level, the hemoglobin releases oxygen to the tissues depending upon blood flow, hemoglobin concentration, the arterial partial pressure of oxygen (PaO_2), the difference between the PO_2 and the venous partial pressure of oxygen (PvO_2), and the influence of four factors that affect how tightly "stuck" the oxygen is to the hemoglobin carrier. These factors include carbon dioxide level, hydrogen ion concentration, temperature, and a chemical known as 2,3-diphosphoglycerate (2,3-DPG).[13] An increase in any of these elements will decrease the affinity of oxygen for hemoglobin and promote oxygen unloading to the tissues.[12] This is known as a "shift to the right" of the oxyhemoglobin dissociation curve. Such a shift would be reflected in an arterial blood gas sample as a drop in the oxygen saturation (e.g. more oxygen released to the tissues). Decreased concentrations of the intracellular factors would result in a "shift to the left"[13] (Figure 3.1).

FIGURE 3.1

The oxyhemoglobin curve illustrating the effects of temperature, PCO_2, and pH on oxygen saturation and PO_2.

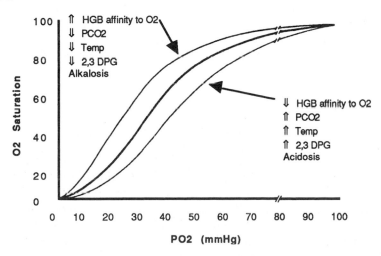

Other cellular compensatory mechanisms for acute blood loss include increased RBC production and release by the bone marrow. Following acute blood loss, erythropoietin levels rise within 6 hours and reticulocytosis (increased number of young RBCs in the blood) is seen in 24 hours.

Because these compensatory mechanisms may be inadequate or detrimental to the cardiac patient, correction of the anemia is essential. Therapy is directed at the responsible underlying mechanism. Transfusions may be necessary for rapid replacement of blood volume when compensation attempts are ineffective or undesirable. The nurse should exercise caution when administering blood to a patient with congestive heart failure since rapid volume replacement can exacerbate angina or heart failure.

Red Blood Cell Indices

Mean corpuscular volume: 87–103 µm/RBC
Mean corpuscular hemoglobin concentration: 32–36%
Mean corpuscular hemoglobin: 27–32 pg

Red blood cell indices are used to define the size and hemoglobin content of the erythrocyte and thus to differentiate anemias. *Mean corpuscular volume* (MCV) refers to the volume occupied by a single red blood cell. Erythrocytes with a MCV greater than normal would be considered macrocytic, while erythrocytes with a MCV less than normal would be considered microcytic. *Mean corpuscular hemoglobin concentration* (MCHC) indicates the average concentration of hemoglobin in the red blood cells. This test is commonly used to differentiate anemias and evaluate the effectiveness of anemia treatments. It is the most accurate of the RBC indices because it is based on the level of hemoglobin and the hematocrit, which are the two most accurate hematological calculations.[13] *Mean corpuscular hemoglobin* (MCH) refers to the average weight of hemoglobin in the red blood cell. This test may be used to differentiate macrocytic from microcytic anemia, but it is less accurate than the MCHC because it is based on the counting of RBCs.[13]

Polycythemia

Men: greater than 5.4 million
Women: greater than 5.6 million

Polycythemia refers to an excess of RBCs or, more specifically, an increased hematocrit, and may occur as a primary or secondary disorder. *Primary polycythemia* (polycythemia vera) is an abnormal overproduction of RBCs as well as white blood cells and platelets by the bone marrow. The cause of this chronic bone marrow abnormality is unknown. It most commonly occurs in middle-aged men and is often associated with thrombotic or hemorrhagic complications.[9]

Secondary polycythemia refers to increased RBC production in response to tissue hypoxia. Erythropoietin is released in response to hypoxia. Therefore, secondary polycythemia may occur in patients with chronic low arterial oxygen saturation, such as those persons living at high altitudes, those with chronic lung disease and chronic hypoxemia, or those with right-to-left intracardiac shunts. (In contrast, patients with polycythemia vera have normal arterial oxygen saturations). The increased red cell production improves the oxygen-carrying capacity. However, the increased RBC mass is detrimental because of the resulting increased viscosity of the blood.[13]

Polycythemia creates serious cardiovascular problems related to the hyperviscosity, including sluggish venous circulation, thrombosis, myocardial infarction, and embolization. The hypervolemia may also precipitate heart failure.[13] Therapy is directed at decreasing viscosity and/or circulating volume to improve flow through vessels. Secondary polycythemia may be treated by increasing the arterial oxygen saturation.

It should be noted that the hematocrit can be increased in the dehydrated patient secondary to hemoconcentration. Restoring intravascular fluid volume will result in a more accurate hematocrit value.

Erythrocyte Sedimentation Rate

Men: 0–15 mm/h
Women: 0–20 mm/h
Child: 0–10 mm/h

Another laboratory test involving red blood cells is the *erythrocyte sedimentation rate* (ESR). The ESR measures the settling of RBCs in a tube over a specific period of time. It may be used to help detect obscure inflammatory conditions. In normal blood there is a relatively slower settling of red cells, while in many inflammatory diseases the red cell settling will be increased. The faster the settling of red cells, the higher the ESR. However, it is a nonspecific test that may be normal despite the presence of disease. Altered plasma proteins will also affect the ESR. For example, in multiple myeloma the ESR tends to be markedly increased.[2,3] Normal value ranges depend on the laboratory technique used.

The ESR may be abnormal in various cardiac conditions. In acute myocardial infarction the ESR may remain elevated for several weeks in response to the tissue necrosis. The ESR is also typically elevated with active rheumatic fever and infective endocarditis and may be used to follow the course of these illnesses.[3,4] In infective endocarditis the ESR is elevated in more than 90% of cases. The ESR is not increased in angina pectoris and is low in congestive heart failure.

Leukocytes

Leukocytes (normal: 5000–10,000/mm^3), or white blood cells (WBCs), are produced in the bone marrow and lymphatic tissue and use the blood stream for transportation to their site of function.There are five different types of WBCs. The absolute number as well as percentage of total WBCs are determined by the differential cell count. Neutrophils, basophils, and eosinophils contain granules in their cytoplasm and are referred to as *granulocytes*, while lymphocytes and monocytes do not have granules. Each of these cells has a special function, thus the differential may provide greater information about the cause and course of an illness than the WBC count alone. On the other hand, some have suggested that the differential cell count may be unnecessary if the diagnosis is clinically apparent and if therapy will not be affected. This may be particularly true in uncomplicated coronary artery disease.

Polymorphonuclear neutrophils (neutrophils, PMNs, or polys) are the most numerous circulating WBCs. They provide the body's first line of defense through the process of phagocytosis. Therefore, during infection and tissue damage, the total WBC count and neutrophil count are increased. The bone marrow also responds by increasing the release of immature WBCs. This is called a "shift to the left." The phrase originates from earlier laboratory texts that diagrammed the maturation of WBCs, with the youngest cells at the left and progressing to the more mature cells at the right.[8] A shift to the left identifies the body's response to infection or stress. Recent interest has also focused on the predictive value of elevated WBCs for increased morbidity and mortality from coronary events.

Eosinophils are phagocytic cells which are associated with allergy, antigen-antibody reactions, and immune responses. *Basophils* release histamine and heparin and play a role in allergic, anaphylactic, and inflammatory reactions. *Lymphocytes* function in immune reactions and antibody production against foreign substances. They are particularly active in humoral immunity, as is seen in transplant rejection. *Monocytes* remove cellular debris following infection and inflammation to prepare the tissues for healing. While a complete discussion of each of the cellular components and functions is beyond the scope of this text, abnormalities that may be related to the cardiac patient are listed in Table 3.1.[14]

Platelets

Thrombocytes, or platelets (normal: 150,000–400,000/mm^3), are required for normal hemostasis, a major protective function of the body. At the time of trauma, platelets adhere to the damaged endothelium and form a platelet plug, thereby producing a mechanical barrier to stop blood loss. They then release several substances (e.g. thromboxane A$_2$,

TABLE 3.1

Significance of the Differential to the Cardiac Patient

Cell Type	Normal Values*	Abnormality	Possible Cause in Cardiac Patients
Neutrophils	2.0–7.7 (40–75%)	Neutrophilia	Acute physical and emotional stress. Endocarditis, acute rheumatic fever. Drug reaction. Heparin, epinephrine, digitalis, corticosteroids. Tissue destruction (MI).
		Neutropenia	Overwhelming infection. Drug induced: quinidine, indomethacin, procainamide, thiazides
Eosinophils	0.04–0.4 (1–6%)	Eosinophilia	Allergic diseases. Hypereosinophilic syndrome.
		Eosinopenia	Congestive heart failure. Stress. Drugs: ACTH, epinephrine. Severe infections.
Basophils	0.01–0.1 (0–1%)	Basophilia	Polycythemia vera. Allergic reactions.
		Basopenia	Because few basophils are normal, low levels are not specific for any disease.
Monocytes	0.2–0.8 (2–10%)	Monocytosis	Subacute bacterial endocarditis. Recovery from acute infection. Hematolic disease. Malignancy.
Lymphocytes	1.5–4.0 (20–45%)	Lymphocytosis	Infectious diseases: infectious lymphocytosis, toxoplasmosis
		Lymphocytopenia	Steroids. Severe debilitating illness (congestive heart failure).

* Normal values from Dacie & Lewis, 1991; Widmann, 1983.

serotonin, adenosine diphosphate) that cause further platelet aggregation and activate the clotting mechanisms. Circulating fibrinogen then surrounds and infiltrates the platelet plug. Thrombin converts fibrinogen to fibrin, forming an insoluble fibrin network to stabilize the clot. Major blood loss is prevented from small vessels primarily by this mechanism.

Thrombocytopenia refers to a low platelet count. The causes of platelet deficiency include decreased production, increased destruction (caused by quinidine, digoxin, heparin, methyldopa, and other drugs), or sequestration in the spleen as occurs in splenomegaly. The platelet count at which abnormal bleeding occurs is variable. Platelet counts less than $80,000/mm^3$ can result in abnormal bleeding in some patients; others do not bleed with counts of $20,000/mm^3$. Platelets also maintain capillary integrity; therefore petechiae resulting from minimal trauma to blood vessels is a hallmark of thrombocytopenia. The spleen normally contains approximately 25% of the platelets.[15]

The normal actions of platelets are of great concern to the clinician treating cardiac patients. Platelet aggregation and thrombus formation is a common substrate for coronary occlusion in myocardial infarction.[16] Platelet aggregation may also play a role in determining the size of an AMI. Patients with congestive heart failure are also at risk for thromboembolism, which may be related to platelet dysfunction. Drugs that inhibit platelet function are part of the standard treatment for unstable angina, myocardial infarction, and the prevention of postangioplasty restenosis.[17,18] For example, in the postangioplasty patient aspirin interferes with the production of thromboxane A_2, thereby inhibiting platelet aggregation on the vessel wall that may impair coronary blood flow.[19] Multiple studies have shown that one aspirin tablet per day can significantly decrease the incidence of MI and death in patients with unstable angina and reduce mortality during acute myocardial infarction.[20,21] Effective daily doses may be as low as 50 mg/d. This lower dose inhibits aggregation but does not impair the fibrinolytic capacity of blood vessel walls. The anticoagulant effect of aspirin persists for as long as five days after a single dose of 300 mg.[22] New platelet-inhibiting drugs are also being researched, but aspirin is most frequently used because of its low cost, low toxicity rate and safety in administration. One recently approved drug for use as an antiplatelet agent is ticlopidine (Ticlid), which has shown success in preventing thrombosis in intracoronary stents, coronary artery bypass grafts, and during extracorporeal circulation.[23,24]

An entirely new group of anti-aggregation agents has been undergoing clinical trials. The direct thrombin inhibitors such as hirudin and hirulog interfere with clotting factors V, VIII, and XIII, and have a powerful inhibitory effect on thrombin formation.[25] A large clinical trial of c7E3 (Reopro), the monoclonal antibody to the platelet glycoprotein (GP) IIb/IIIa receptor, demonstrated improvement in the incidence of ischemic complications following high-risk coronary angioplasty.[26] There is an increased risk of bleeding episodes when these drugs are used, and researchers continue to evaluate other compounds with these chemical properties.

PROTHROMBIN (PT) AND PARTIAL THROMBOPLASTIN TIME (PTT)

Normal PTT: 30–45 sec
Normal PT: 11–16%

While platelets are responsible for initiating the clotting process, formation of a strong, effective clot requires the activity of a complex series of steps referred to as the coagulation cascade (Figure 3.2). In this cascade, activation of one clotting factor triggers a series of steps resulting in activation of other clotting factors. The final result is the generation of thrombin, which then converts fibrinogen to fibrin. Two coagulation pathways have been described: the intrinsic and extrinsic systems.

FIGURE 3.2

The coagulation cascade. The intrinsic and extrinsic pathways lead to the combination of phospholipids, calcium, factors X and V to convert prothrombin to thrombin. This causes the conversion of fibrinogen into the fibrin strands that make up the blood clot.

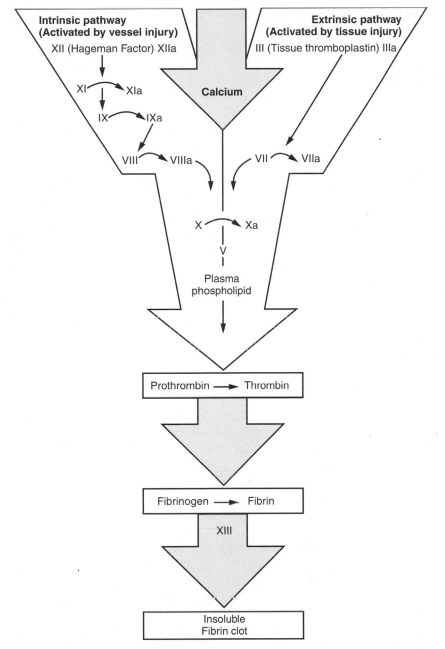

From Porth C, *Pathophysiology: Concepts of Altered Health States*. Philadelphia: JB Lippincott; 1982. Used by permission.

Intrinsic Pathway

The intrinsic pathway refers to coagulation initiated by factor XII, which is activated upon contact with a negatively charged surface (e.g. damaged endothelium). This in turn triggers a series of reactions ultimately resulting in the activation of factor X, which is responsible for the release of thrombin from prothrombin.[27] Its activity is measured by the partial thromboplastin time (PTT). A modification of the PTT is called the activated partial thromboplastin time (APTT), which has a normal value of 35–45 seconds. All clotting factors with the exception of factor VII are reflected in the PTT. Causes of prolonged PTT include vitamin K deficiency, liver disease, disseminated intravascular coagulation (DIC), or the presence of anticoagulants.

Extrinsic Pathway

The extrinsic pathway refers to coagulation initiated by the reaction of factor VII with tissue thromboplastin, which then activates factor X. Note that both the intrinsic and extrinsic systems result in the activation of factor X.[27] The extrinsic pathway is evaluated by the prothrombin time (PT). The normal PT may vary among laboratory controls.

The PT will be prolonged if factors of the extrinsic pathway are deficient. A deficiency of factor VII will prolong the PT but not the PTT. Both the PT and PTT will be prolonged with deficiencies of factor X, factor V, prothrombin, or fibrinogen. Liver disease is the most common cause of a prolonged PT.

Many patients with cardiovascular disease are prone to intravascular thrombosis. Examples of high-risk patients include those with atrial fibrillation, acute myocardial infarction, valvular heart disease, and peripheral vascular disease. Patients with prolonged immobility, low cardiac output states, and congestive heart failure are also at risk.

Anticoagulants may be used to prevent or treat the development of venous or arterial thrombi. Heparin will decrease the incidence of venous thrombosis and pulmonary embolus and is therefore recommended in the setting of AMI.[28] Heparin (given intravenously or subcutaneously) and warfarin (given orally) are the most commonly used anticoagulants. Heparin interferes with thrombin formation as well as with the conversion of fibrinogen to fibrin. Heparin therapy is monitored using the PTT or ACT. The therapeutic range for the PTT is 1.5 to 2.5 times control.

Warfarin acts indirectly by interfering with the formation of vitamin K–dependent clotting factors, and is therefore antagonized by vitamin K. Oral anticoagulants are used long-term in patients with atrial fibrillation, rheumatic heart disease, or prosthetic valves, and occasionally during recovery from AMI. Deep vein thrombosis and pulmonary embolism may also be treated with long-term anticoagulation. The suggested optimal therapeutic range for the PT is considered to be 1.5 to 2.5 times control. Recently this range has been challenged as being excessive, with the recommended therapeutic range of 1.2 to 1.5 times control.[29] Levels of 1.5 to 2.0 times control may be appropriate for patients with prosthetic valves or recurrent systemic emboli. Patient Education Box 3.1 summarizes instructions for patients on anticoagulants.

PATIENT EDUCATION BOX 3.1

Anticoagulation Therapy

Your doctor has prescribed a drug to help prevent blood clot formation in your body. You may experience increased bleeding while you are taking this drug. The following information is provided for your safety.

WHILE YOU ARE TAKING THE DRUG

You may experience an increase in minor bleeding, including nose bleeds, bleeding gums, and easy bruising. Small amounts of bleeding from your stomach or bowels may result in black stools. Any bright red blood from your stomach or rectum should be reported to your doctor immediately. Try to minimize trauma to your skin and mouth to help prevent bleeding. Wear shoes or slippers as much as possible and use gloves when gardening. Use a soft bristle toothbrush and a gentle stroke when brushing your teeth.

Many over-the-counter drugs can interfere with this drug. No medications should be started or stopped without the approval of your physician. It is particularly important not to start any new medication without telling the prescribing physician that you are on blood thinner medication. Remember that alcohol is a drug that may interfere with your medication.

You should also note that vitamin K, found in green, leafy vegetables, may alter the effect of the medication. It is okay to regularly include these foods in your diet, but large increases or decreases are not recommended.

Take your medication on time and keep appointments for regular lab tests to monitor the level of medication in your blood.

Medical alert identification and information should be carried at all times in case of an emergency.

If you require any surgery while you are taking this drug, be sure to tell your surgeon or doctor that you are taking a blood thinner (anticoagulant).

International Normalized Ratio

The International Normalized Ratio (INR) is the most accurate method of assessing the adequacy of Coumadin therapy. It is based on the PT ratio and the International Sensitivity Index (ISI). The ISI is a value that is determined by the thromboplastin reagent used by the individual laboratory. This makes the PT accurate to the laboratory's methodology and instrumentation.

ARTERIAL AND MIXED VENOUS BLOOD GASES

Arterial blood gases are obtained in an effort to assess oxygenation, ventilation, and acid-base balance. Mixed venous blood gases aid in determining oxygen consumption and cardiac output. Together, they add considerable information to the cardiovascular assessment.

Normal values for arterial and mixed venous blood gases are listed in Table 3.2. The PaO_2 (arterial partial pressure of oxygen) measures the amount of oxygen dissolved in the plasma. However, dissolved oxygen alone does not contribute significantly to tissue oxygenation: Oxygen must be carried by the hemoglobin to be used by the tissues. Most of the oxygen (97–98%) binds with the hemoglobin within the red blood cells. The remaining oxygen is carried in solution.

The oxyhemoglobin dissociation curve represents the relationship between PaO_2 and hemoglobin saturation (Figure 3.1). The flat portion of the curve shows that increasing the PaO_2 above 60 mmHg does little to increase saturation. The steep portion of the curve shows that once the PaO_2 is less than 60 mmHg, even small changes in PaO_2 result in large hemoglobin desaturation changes. In other words, there is a reserve for oxygen delivery: If the PaO_2 falls from 90 mm Hg to 60 mmHg, the saturation falls minimally, maintaining tissue oxygen delivery. The oxyhemoglobin dissociation curve can be used to estimate hemoglobin saturation and is reliable provided the hemoglobin, temperature, and pH are all normal. The curve is altered, or "shifted," when these parameters vary. Hemoglobin saturation can also be measured directly by some blood

TABLE 3.2

Arterial and Mixed Venous Blood Gas Values

	Arterial	Mixed Venous
PO_2 (mm Hg)	80–100	30–40
Saturation (%)	95–100	75
PCO_2	35–45	41–51
pH	7.35–7.45	7.31–7.41

gas machines. Direct measurement is the most accurate technique for determining oxyhemoglobin levels.

Patients with cardiac disorders may have lower arterial oxygen tensions and may need oxygen therapy. One common cause of impaired oxygenation is interstitial and alveolar fluid that interferes with ventilation of perfused lung units.[30] This can result from left ventricular failure and pulmonary congestion associated with acute myocardial infarction or cardiomyopathy. A fall in cardiac output can also cause hypoxemia. A right-to-left intracardiac shunt, which may be seen in septal rupture following infarction, will mix desaturated (right-sided, venous) blood with arterial blood, reducing the PaO_2 and oxyhemoglobin saturation. While oxygen therapy should improve the PaO_2 in the patient with a ventilation-perfusion abnormality, it will have little effect in the patient with an intracardiac shunt. Oxygen therapy is routinely used in acute myocardial infarction to avoid or treat hypoxemia that may develop.[30] It should also be noted that the patient with anemia may have a normal PaO_2 and hemoglobin saturation, but the decreased hemoglobin level will significantly impair oxygen delivery to the tissues.[31]

The $PaCO_2$ (arterial partial pressure of carbon dioxide) is a reflection of tissue carbon dioxide production and lung elimination. Ventilation is normally maintained at a level sufficient to eliminate CO_2 produced by the tissues. When the $PaCO_2$ is elevated, the patient is said to be *hypoventilating*, as alveolar ventilation is inadequate to maintain a normal $PaCO_2$. When the $PaCO_2$ is below normal, the patient is *hyperventilating*, since alveolar ventilation is in excess of that required to maintain a normal $PaCO_2$. Therefore, the $PaCO_2$ reflects adequacy of ventilation.

The acutely ill cardiac patient may hyperventilate because of pain, fear, or anxiety. In addition, early pulmonary edema and pulmonary emboli stimulate lung receptors and produce a strong stimulus to breathe, often resulting in tachypnea and hyperventilation. Hypoventilation can occur in severe pulmonary edema with alveolar flooding, or secondary to oversedation with respiratory depressants such as morphine sulphate. The acuteness of these changes will be reflected in the arterial pH.[32]

Acid-Base Balance

The arterial pH represents the body's acid-base balance. An increase in acids (H+) or decrease in bases (HCO_3^-) will result in acidosis, or a low pH. The loss of acids or an excess of base will result in alkalosis, or an elevated pH above 7.45. Hypoventilation (elevated $PaCO_2$) results in respiratory acidosis, while hyperventilation (decreased $PaCO_2$) results in respiratory alkalosis. Metabolic acid-base derangements which alter the arterial pH are listed in Table 3.3.

Metabolic derangements can alter the pH in the cardiac patient. A decreased cardiac output insufficient to meet tissue oxygen needs will

TABLE 3.3

Causes of Metabolic Acid-Base Derangements

Metabolic Acidosis	Mechanism	Metabolic Alkalosis	Mechanism
Diarrhea, fistula	Intestinal bicarbonate loss	Diuretics	Excess H^+ loss; excess bicarbonate reabsorption
Kidney disease	Excess acids; bicarbonate loss	Excess ingestion of alkaline drugs	Excess sodium bicarbonate; antacids
Diabetic ketoacidosis	Excess keto acids	Gastric loss (vomiting, suction)	H^+ loss
Acetazolamide (Diamox) therapy	Bicarbonate loss	Excess aldosterone	Renal H^+ secretion
Lactic acidosis	Excess H^+ production		

result in anaerobic metabolism with the production of lactic acidosis. Also, cyanide toxicity from nitroprusside administration, while rare, can result in metabolic acidosis. Metabolic alkalosis can result from overaggressive bicarbonate administration (e.g. during cardiac arrest). Prolonged diuretic therapy may cause chloride loss with bicarbonate retention, also resulting in metabolic alkalosis.[32] For these reasons, the patient's arterial blood gases must be interpreted along with the history, physical examination findings, and other laboratory data.

Mixed venous oxygen saturation ($S\bar{v}O_2$) is used to estimate the adequacy of tissue oxygenation. A special pulmonary artery catheter measures the oxygen saturation of venous blood as it returns to the heart. A blood sample is obtained from the distal port of the catheter to assure adequate mixing of venous blood. (Blood sampled from peripheral or central venous catheters would reflect local or regional differences in oxygen consumption.) If the $S\bar{v}O_2$ decreases, then either the oxygen consumption has increased or oxygen delivery to the tissues has fallen. When oxygen delivery decreases (e.g. because of a decreased cardiac output) the tissues extract more oxygen from the blood because the blood is flowing more slowly. This will decrease the mixed venous oxygen content. Therefore, if the arterial oxygen content is adequate, and the tissue oxygen consumption has not changed, a decreased mixed venous oxygen content could imply that flow has decreased or that there has been a drop in cardiac output. Clinical correlation and close observation of the patient would be required.

LIPID PROFILE

Among the many risk factors identified for the development of atherosclerosis, one of the most clearly and repeatedly documented is the association between blood lipids (specifically, blood cholesterol) and coronary artery disease (CAD). The lipid profile measures levels of cholesterol, triglycerides, and lipoproteins. Lipoproteins are protein molecules that combine with and transport normally insoluble lipids such as cholesterol and triglycerides. These lipoproteins are called very-low-density lipoproteins (VLDLs), low-density lipoproteins (LDLs), and high-density lipoproteins (HDLs). Their values are considered together in determining risk for atherosclerotic heart disease.

Cholesterol

Cholesterol (normal: < 200 mg/dL, or < 5.2 mmol/L) is the most abundant steroid in the body, and is found in high concentrations in brain and nervous tissue. It is necessary for cell membrane formation and hormone synthesis, but may harmfully accumulate in arterial walls where it is atherogenic. There is a direct relationship between increased plasma cholesterol levels and the severity of atherosclerosis. This relationship is continuous and graded, not limited to the upper cholesterol limits. In general, the higher the cholesterol level the greater the risk of CAD.

Cholesterol levels vary with age, sex, diet, geographic location, race, activity level, and stress level. In patients with no risk factors or coronary disease, cholesterol levels should be less than 220 mg/dL. In patients with known coronary disease or with two or more risk factors, the cholesterol level should be between 180 and 200 mg/dL.

Low-Density Lipoproteins

The risk of CAD is related to the lipoprotein system as well as to the cholesterol level. The low-density lipoprotein (LDL) is the major carrier of cholesterol, conveying approximately two-thirds of cholesterol. LDL (normal: 62–160 mg/dL) carries cholesterol into the cell where it is deposited after the carrier protein is degraded. This results in deposits of cholesterol throughout the body, including the arterial vessel walls. LDL is primarily removed by LDL receptors on liver cells. Because of the relationship between LDL and cholesterol, higher LDL levels are associated with an increased incidence of atherosclerosis and CAD.[34] This relationship is clear in patients with abnormalities in LDL metabolism. In familial hypercholesterolemia, genetic LDL receptor abnormalities result in elevated LDL cholesterol levels, premature severe atherosclerosis, and CAD. Excess dietary intake of cholesterol and saturated fats also results in elevated LDL. Factors that lower LDL cholesterol include weight loss, decreased saturated animal fat consumption, and decreased cholesterol intake.[35]

Treatment of hyperlipoproteinemias begins with dietary restriction of total lipids and cholesterol as well as reduction or elimination of other cardiac risk factors. If interventions (diet, lifestyle changes, medications) are successful in lowering the cholesterol level, the CAD risk also decreases. Patients should be placed on diets low in cholesterol and saturated fats. Usually a 6-month trial of dietary restrictions is tried; however, if this is unsuccessful, drug therapy should be used.[36,37] Because diet will affect the lipoprotein levels, patients should fast for 12 hours and avoid alcohol for 24 hours prior to the study. Water is allowed.

High Density Lipoproteins

High density lipoproteins (HDL) provide a protective function by removing cholesterol and returning it to the liver for elimination. HDL (normal: Men—44 mg/dL; Women—55 mg/dL) may also play a role in inhibiting cellular uptake of LDL. HDL levels have an inverse relationship with CAD: the higher the HDL, the lower the cardiovascular risk. Increased HDL levels are associated with regular physical exercise and moderate alcohol consumption. Decreased HDL levels, which would adversely affect the LDL/HDL ratio, are seen in patients with risk factors such as smoking, diabetes, sedentary behavior, and obesity.

Antihypertensive agents also have an effect on cholesterol levels. Thiazide diuretics, beta-blockers, reserpine, and methyldopa lower HDL cholesterol. Alpha-blockers appear to offer benefits including lower total cholesterol and elevated HDL cholesterol.

Triglycerides

Triglycerides (normal: 40–150 mg/dL) are lipids composed of glycerol and three fatty acids. They are used as an energy source, stored in adipose tissue, and carried by VLDLs. VLDLs are degraded to an intermediate form (IDLs) and then to LDLs. While cholesterol and triglycerides may vary independently, many factors that affect cholesterol levels may similarly affect triglycerides. In fact, borderline hypertriglyceridemics frequently have exogenous factors such as alcohol use, diabetes, hypothyroidism, obesity, or renal disease. Triglyceride levels correlate positively with LDL levels and inversely with HDL levels. Hypertriglyceridemia is associated with hypercoagulability and reduced fibrinolytic capacity in post–myocardial infarction patients.[38]

Homocysteine

Some patients suffer acute coronary events fairly early in life (under age 55) and have a very low risk profile for coronary disease. Recent research has identified elevated levels of homocysteine in the blood of patients who fit the low profile for risk, but had suffered an AMI. Homocysteine is a break-down product of methionine, an essential amino acid. Patients with high serum levels of homocysteine also had low levels of erythrocyte folate and vitamin B_{12}.[39] It is unclear exactly how to lower a patient's risk relative to high levels of homocysteine, but this is an area of active research.

ANTISTREPTOLYSIN TITER

Group A β-hemolytic streptococci produce substances that have enzymatic as well as antigenic properties. Streptolysin O is a hemolysin produced by group A streptococci that stimulates antibody production. The antibody formed is called antistreptolysin O (ASO). The antibody does not have protective effects, but its existence indicates a recent streptococcal infection.[8] Active streptococcal infections can often be cultured in the blood. When the organism cannot be cultured (as when the patient is convalescing) the ASO titer will detect the infection or poststreptococcal insult. The test measures the highest serum dilution at which there is no further hemolysis. Significant findings include a single serum titer of greater than 250 or a fourfold rise between two specimens. The elevations are greatest during the first 2 months after onset of symptoms.[8]

Streptococci may cause scarlet fever, bacterial endocarditis, rheumatic fever, and poststreptococcal glomerulonephritis. Ninety percent of patients with rheumatic fever will have increased ASO titers during the first 3 weeks after the onset of illness. The course of the disease can also be monitored by the ASO, as the ASO gradually decreases over the first few months following an infection. False-positive results may be caused by elevated β-lipoprotein levels. Antibiotic and corticosteroid therapy will inhibit the ASO response.

CARDIAC TRANSPLANTATION

Cardiac transplantation continues to grow as a therapeutic option for patients with end-stage cardiac disease. Advanced immunosuppression with cyclosporine and other agents and highly effective antirejection surveillance have improved transplant outcomes considerably in the past decade. Success also depends on donor-recipient compatibility. Currently, survival rates for cardiac transplant patients are 80% to 90% at 1 year and 70% to 80% at 5 years.[40]

Donor-recipient matching is evaluated by ABO blood group compatibility, HLA screening, and lymphocyte crossmatching. The ABO system is characterized by the presence or absence of antigens A and B on red blood cell membranes. Anti-A and anti-B antibodies are present in serum lacking the corresponding antigens. The antigen-antibody reaction that occurs with mismatched blood results in intravascular hemolysis and serious complications.[41] Therefore, ABO compatibility is one requirement for donor-recipient matching

The second major histocompatability system is the HLA system. HLA refers to antigenic substances found on many cells. The HLA antigens are genetically determined and located on chromosome 6. While screening for HLA-A, HLA-B, and HLA-C antigens is generally done, matching is not predictive of success. Matching of HLA-D and HLA-DR, however, strongly correlates with survival after transplant.[42] Mismatching of the HLA antigen may be associated with increased coronary atherosclerosis in the transplanted heart.[42]

The most important factor in graft survival may be the white blood cell or lymphocyte crossmatch. This assay tests for the presence of cytotoxic antibodies in the recipient that react with donor lymphocytes. A positive crossmatch is considered a contraindication to transplant since immediate rejection will occur.[40,43] A negative lymphocyte crossmatch means there is a lack of cytotoxic effect of the recipient's serum on donor lymphocytes.

Immunologic rejection is a significant problem in organ transplantation. The goal of pretransplant testing is to select the most compatible match between donor and recipient. Graft rejection can result in graft failure. Therefore, heart transplant recipients will require lifelong immunosuppressive therapy and monitoring.[44] Advances in donor-recipient matching, immunosuppression, and early recognition of rejection should continue to improve heart transplant outcome.[45]

References

1. Fischbach FT. *A Manual of Laboratory Diagnostic Tests*. 4th ed. Philadelphia: JB Lippincott; 1992.
2. Kee JL, Tang HL. *Laboratory and Diagnostic Tests with Nursing Implications*. 3rd ed. Norwalk, Conn.: Appleton Lange; 1990.
3. Ravel R. *Clinical Laboratory Medicine: Clinical Application of Laboratory Data*. 5th ed. Chicago: Yearbook Medical Publishers; 1989.
4. Tilkian A, Tilkian S, Conover M. *Clinical Implications of Laboratory Tests*. 4th ed. St. Louis: CV Mosby; 1987.
5. Bishop M, Duben-Engelkirk J, Fody E. *Clinical Chemistry. Principles, Procedures, Correlations*. 2nd ed. JB Lippincott; 1992.
6. Woods S, Laurent-Bopp, D. Laboratory tests using blood and urine. In: Under hill S, Woods S, Froelicher E, et al., eds. *Cardiac Nursing*. Philadelphia: JB Lippincott; 1989.
7. Felder L. The effect of electrolyte imbalances on the cardiovascular system. In: Underhill S, Woods S, Froelicher E, et al., eds. *Cardiac Nursing*. Philadelphia: JB Lippincott; 1989.
8. Widmann F. *Clinical Interpretation of Laboratory Tests*. 9th ed. Philadelphia: FA Davis; 1983.
9. Porth C. *Pathophysiology*. 3rd ed. Philadelphia: JB Lippincott; 1990.
10. Woods KL, Fletcher S, Roffe C, Haider Y. Intravenous magnesium sulphate in suspected acute myocardial infarction: Results of the second Leicester

Intravenous Magnesium Intervention Trial (LIMIT-2). *Lancet*. 1992;339: 1553–1558.

11. Goodman L, Gilman A. *The Pharmacological Basis of Therapeutics*. 8th ed. New York: Macmillan; 1990.

12. Muller-Bardorff M, Freitag H, Scheffold T, et al. Development and characterization of a rapid assay for bedside determination of cardiac troponin T. *Circulation*. 1995;92:2869–2875.

13. Shapiro MF, Greenfield S. The complete blood count and leukocyte differential count: An approach to their rational application. *Ann Int Med*. 1987; 106:65–74.

14. Dacie J, Lewis S. *Practical Haematology*. 7th ed. New York: Churchill Livingstone; 1991.

15. Sivarajan ES, Christopherson DJ. Anticoagulant antithrombotic and platelet modifying drugs. In: Underhill S, Woods S, Froelicher E, et al., eds. *Cardiac Nursing*, Philadelphia: JB Lippincott; 1989.

16. Braunwald E., ed. *Heart disease: A Textbook of Cardiovascular Medicine*. 4th ed. Philadelphia: WB Saunders; 1992.

17. Sarin S, Shami SK, Cheatle TR, et al. When do vascular surgeons prescribe antiplatelet therapy? Current attitudes. *Eur J Vasc Surg*. 1993;7:6–13.

18. Verstraete M. Risk factors, interventions and therapeutic agents in the prevention of atherosclerosis-related ischaemic diseases. *Drugs*. 1991; 42(suppl 5):22–38.

19. Chen Z, Xu Y, Yu Q, et al. Secondary prevention of myocardial reinfarction with low dose aspirin. *Chin Med Sci J*. 1991;6:141–144.

20. de Gaetano G. Aspirin as an antithrombotic drug: From the aggregometer to clinical trials. *Verh K Acad Geneeskd Belg*. 1990;52:459–473.

21. Lekstrom JA, Bell WR. Aspirin in the prevention of thrombosis. *Medicine (Baltimore)*. 1991;70:161–178.

22. McAnally LE, Corn CR, Hamilton SF. Aspirin for the prevention of vascular death in women. *Ann Pharmacother*. 1992;26:1530–1534.

23. Haynes RB, Sandler RS, Larson EB, Pater JL, Yatsu FM. A critical appraisal of ticlopidine, a new antiplatelet agent. Effectiveness and clinical indications for prophylaxis of atherosclerotic events. *Arch Intern Med*. 1992; 152:1376–1380.

24. Ito MK, Smith AR, Lee ML. Ticlopidine: A new platelet aggregation inhibitor. *Clin Pharm*. 1992;11:603–617.

25. Lefkovits J, Topol EJ. Direct thrombin inhibitors in acute coronary syndromes and coronary angioplasty. In: Topol EJ, Serruys PW, eds. *Current Review of Interventional Cardiology*. 2nd ed. Philadelphia: Current Medicine; 1995.

26. The EPIC investigators: Evaluation of a chimeric monoclonal antibody c7e3 Fab fragment directed against the platelet glycoprotein IIb/IIIa receptor for preventing ischemic complications of high risk angioplasty. *N Engl J Med*. 1994;330:956–961.

27. Berne R, Levy M. *Physiology*. 3rd ed. St. Louis: CV Mosby, 1993.

28. Chow MS, Wu TS, Chan CL. The controversy of heparin therapy as an adjunct to thrombolysis in acute myocardial infarction. *DICP*. 1991;25:613–616.

29. Hirsch J, Deykin D, Poller L. Therapeutic range for oral anticoagulant therapy. *Chest*. 1986;89:suppl 11S–15S.

30. Fulmer J, Snider G. American College of Chest Physicians National Heart, Lung, and Blood Institute Conference on Oxygen Therapy. *Heart and Lung*. 1984;13:550–562.

31. Dantzker D. *Cardiopulmonary Critical Care*. 2nd ed. Philadelphia: WB Saunders; 1991.

32. Griffin JP, D'Arcy PF. *A Manual of Adverse Drug Interactions*. 4th ed. Bristol, England: Wright & Sons; 1988.
33. Jones D, Dunbar C, Jirovec M. *Medical Surgical Nursing: A conceptual approach*. 2nd ed. New York: McGraw-Hill; 1982.
34. Andersen P. Hypercoagulability and reduced fibrinolysis in hyperlipidemia: Relationship to the metabolic cardiovascular syndrome: *J Cardiovasc Pharmacol*. 1992;20(suppl 8):S29–S31.
35. Aronow WS. Cardiac risk factors: Still important in the elderly. *Geriatrics*. 1990;45:71–74, 79–80.
36. Gotto AM. Overview of current issues in management of dyslipidemia. *Am J Cardiol*. 1993;71:3B–8B.
37. Peters WL. Hyperlipidemia. What to do when life-style changes aren't enough. *Postgrad Med*. 1991;90:213–217,220–224.
38. Vogt HB. Hyperlipoproteinemias: Part III. When to treat. *S D J Med*. 1991; 44:97–100.
39. Israelsson B, Brattstrom LE, Hultberg BL. Homocysteine and myocardial infarction. *Atherosclerosis*. 1988;71:227–233.
40. Olson LJ, Rodeheffer RJ. Management of patients after cardiac transplantation. *Mayo Clin Proc*. 1992;67:775–784.
41. Lancaster L. Immunogenetic basis of tissue and organ transplant and rejection. *Crit Care Nurs Clin*. 1992;4:1–24.
42. Winters GL. The pathology of heart allograft rejection. *Arch Pathol Lab Med*. 1991;115:266–272.
43. Bigley N. *Immunologic Fundamentals*. Chicago: Yearbook Medical Publishers; 1975.
44. Duquesnot RJ, Cramer DV. Immunologic mechanisms of cardiac transplant rejection. *Cardiovasc Clin*. 1990;20:87–103.
45. Valantine HA. Long-term management and results in heart transplant recipients. *Cardiol Clin*. 1990;8:141–148.

4

ECHOCARDIOGRAPHY

COLLEEN M. CORTE

GLOSSARY

Acoustic Window   Area of precordium from which ultrasound waves can be transmitted directly to the heart without striking the ribs or lungs, as bone and air are poor mediums for ultrasound transmission.

Four-Chamber View   Term used to describe the plane of view that allows visualization of all four chambers of the heart simultaneously. It can be achieved with the transducer in the parasternal, apical, and subcostal positions.

Frequency   The number of complete oscillations per second a vibrating sound wave makes about a baseline. The unit of measurement is cycles per second (cps) or Hertz (Hz).

Long-Axis View   The plane of view that allows visualization of the heart longitudinally from base to apex.

Phonocardiogram   Noninvasive cardiac diagnostic test that graphically displays auscultatory events of the heart.

Resolution   The ability to distinguish between structures within the heart.

Short-Axis View   The plane of view that is directly perpendicular to the long axis, or the cross-section view.

Transducer   Device that transmits ultrasound waves to body structures and transforms the sound waves it receives back into electrical signals that can be displayed on an oscilloscope.

Ultrasound   Sound waves of a frequency range above that which can be detected by the human ear (20,000 Hz). Echocardiography employs ultrasound in the range of 1.6 to 7.5 million Hertz (MHz).

Echocardiography (echo) is a noninvasive ultrasonic imaging technique used to visualize the heart. Echo had its earliest beginnings as sonar in World War II. It was first used in America in 1956 in the analysis of mitral valve stenosis. Since then, echo has made a tremendous impact on cardiac diagnosis by providing a means to accurately diagnose and guide therapy for problems with the structure, function, and motion of the heart and great vessels. Prior to the advent of echocardiography, there were no comprehensive diagnostic tests that were noninvasive in nature. If the results of the clinical examination, electrocardiogram, and chest x-ray were inconclusive, the patient required cardiac catheterization and/or angiography.

The different ultrasound examination methods yield valuable information regarding the heart's structural relationships, chamber sizes, wall motions, and valvular functions. The results often dictate whether or not invasive procedures need to be done or surgery performed. In many cases echocardiography provides the definitive diagnosis.[1]

The procedure itself involves the transmission of ultrasound waves to the heart and the reception of the "echoes" that are reflected back from the various structures within the heart. Since most of the structures within the heart can be visualized with echocardiography, it is used to diagnose many pathologic conditions.

Echocardiography has greatly reduced the necessity of using invasive diagnostic procedures for patients with valvular disease, left ventricular dysfunction, and congenital heart disease.[2] It is also useful in the detection of thrombi and the assessment of prognosis after AMI. In addition, echocardiography is used to diagnose pericardial effusion, pericardial tamponade, atrial and ventricular septal defects, atrial myxoma, hypertrophic cardiomyopathy, pulmonary hypertension, and congenital defects.[3]

Echocardiography is painless, widely applicable, and, as already noted, generally noninvasive. Consequently, there are no inherent risks involved. In addition, the cost is much less than other invasive studies. All of these factors make echocardiography an ideal cardiac diagnostic tool.[4]

PRINCIPLES OF ULTRASOUND

In order to understand the theory behind echocardiography, a basic knowledge of the principles of sound and sound wave propagation is helpful. Sound is a form of mechanical energy resulting from the vibration of an object within a suitable medium. The vibrations cause alternating high and low pressure zones in the medium, represented graphically as oscillations about a baseline. Frequency is determined by the number of complete oscillations per second and is referred to as cycles per second (cps) or Hertz (Hz).

The normal human ear can detect sound in the frequency range of 20 to 20,000 Hz.[5] *Ultrasound* is defined as sound in the frequency range over 20,000 Hz or above that detected by the normal human ear. In echocardiography, ultrasound waves are transmitted to the heart in the frequency range of 1.6 to 7.5 million Hz (MHz).[2]

As the sound waves travel through the chest wall, they strike the different structures within the heart. The pericardium, ventricular wall, blood, and heart valves, for instance, each have different densities. When sound waves meet tissues with different densities, they are reflected back in different ways. This reflection allows adjacent structures to be identified as separate entities. This ability to differentiate adjacent structures is called *resolution*.

Resolution is a critical factor in echocardiography. It is vitally important to be able to distinguish different structures of the heart. Frequency plays a major role in resolution. As the frequency increases, the resolution improves. However, with an increase in frequency, the tissue penetration decreases. Since the various structures within the heart are at different depths in the chest wall, a balance between resolution and tissue penetration is necessary. The object is to maximize the amount of useful information from the study. This is frequently accomplished by "zeroing in" on those structures of interest and sacrificing those of lesser importance.

The time that it requires for the echoes to return to the transducer dictates how far the structure in question is from the transducer. The deeper the structure is in the chest wall, the longer it will take for the echoes to return. One of the most critical factors in the performance and interpretation of an echocardiogram is a sound knowledge of cardiac anatomy.

EQUIPMENT

The echo machine is a self-contained unit that consists of a TV monitor at the top; a transducer for transmitting and receiving the ultrasound pulse; instrumentation for initiating, modifying, and storing the impulse; and a strip chart recorder. Although the examination is usually performed in the echo lab, the unit is portable and can be taken to the patient's bedside.

The TV monitor is used for display purposes. There are several basic modes of display, including A-mode, B-mode, M-mode, Doppler, two-dimensional, and three-dimensional echoes. The *A-mode* is amplitude modulated. This is an antiquated format in which the echoes are displayed as spikes. The stronger the signals are on an A-mode presentation, the taller the spikes are. The *B-mode* format is brightness modulated. The echoes are displayed as dots that get brighter as the signals intensify. Both of these formats are stationary, which limits their usefulness for cardiac studies since the heart is such a dynamic organ. However, by adding the dimension of time to the B-mode presentation, the structures in the heart can be visualized in motion as a series of moving dots. This format is called *M-mode*. M-mode and the remaining modes of display are discussed in detail later in this chapter.

The transducer is an instrument that is used both to transmit ultrasound impulses to the heart and then to receive the echoes that are reflected back. It functions as a transmitter less than 1% of the time and as a receiver more than 99% of the time.[6] Very simply, the transducer actually converts one form of energy into another. While in the transmitting cycle it converts electrical energy into mechanical (sound) energy, and while in the receiving cycle it converts sound waves into electrical impulses that can be recorded.[6]

The strip chart recorder uses light-sensitive paper to run a continuous strip of the graphic images being displayed. The ECG is also displayed on the strip as a point of reference for the timing of cardiac events. In two-dimensional and Doppler studies, a video tape is inserted into the machine prior to the echocardiogram for easy storage and retrieval of information.

EXAMINATION TECHNIQUES

Patient Considerations

At the beginning of the procedure the patient is instructed to lie supine with the head elevated slightly, or on the left side, depending upon the requirements of the exam. ECG leads are placed on the patient and the ECG is displayed on the monitor. The transducer is then placed on the chest after a generous application of conducting gel, which allows air-free contact between the transducer and the skin and also allows the transducer to slide easily across the chest.

There are no risks associated with the procedure and it usually lasts approximately 30 to 60 minutes. The only discomfort the patient may experience is due to the pressure of the hand-held transducer on the chest wall.

Transducer Positions

There are several standard transducer positions on the chest wall (Figure 4.1). The various structures in the heart can be visualized from each of these positions. The standard transducer positions are (1) apical, (2) left parasternal, (3) subcostal, (4) suprasternal notch, (5) right parasternal, and (6) supraclavicular. Many factors play a role in the choosing of

FIGURE 4.1

Transducer positions on the chest wall. **A:** The suprasternal angle, which is directed inferoposteriorly and gives a view of the great vessels. **B:** The parasternal angle, which is directed posteriorly and gives a view of the long and short axes. **C:** The apical angle, which is directed superiorly and rightward to give four-chamber and two-chamber views of the heart. **D:** The subcostal view, which is directed superiorly and leftward to demonstrate four-chamber and short-axis views of the heart.

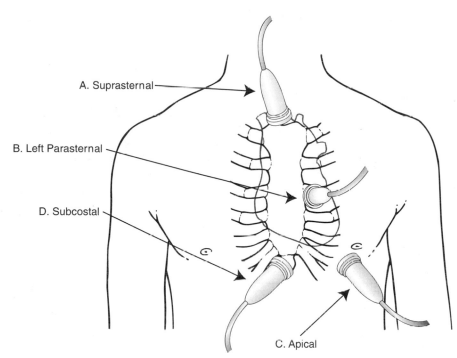

(Adapted from: Come P. *Diagnostic Cardiology: Noninvasive Imaging Techniques.* Philadelphia: JB Lippincott; 1985: 241. Used with permission.)

transducer positions. Depending upon the configuration of the chest wall, the ability of the patient to cooperate with positioning, and whether or not the patient has hyperinflated lungs, one position may be chosen over another. Usually, several transducer positions are used during one study. The *left parasternal* approach allows visualization of all valves and chambers. The *subcostal* approach is helpful in patients with hyperinflated lungs because their precordial "acoustic window" (area on the precordium through which ultrasound travels freely) frequently disappears. (Air is a poor medium for ultrasound transmission. In patients with overexpanded lungs the parasternal approach is avoided as the ultrasound beam would be aimed at the air-filled lungs.[2]) The *apical* approach is helpful for evaluation of mitral and aortic valve prostheses.[2] The *suprasternal notch* approach allows evaluation of the great vessels.[2] Patients with right-sided displacement of the heart, as in dextrocardia, or with conditions where the configuration of the chest is altered, as it is in Marfan's syndrome, can sometimes be examined with right-sided transducer positions.[2] Echocardiographic techniques vary and a great deal of skill is required on the part of the technician to produce a high-quality recording.

M-MODE ECHOCARDIOGRAM

The M-mode echocardiogram presents a unidimensional or "icepick" view of the heart. The technique involves a narrow ultrasonic beam aimed directly perpendicular to the structure(s) in question. Sound impulses are transmitted at a rate of approximately 1000 cps.[7] The returning echoes are then recorded over time on the strip chart recorder. The echoes at the top of the strip represent the structures that the ultrasound beam meets first (i.e., chest wall). Moving vertically down the strip, the deeper structures are visualized. Viewing the recording horizontally allows comparison of the structures as they move over time. Since motion is being recorded over time, the technique is referred to as the time-motion mode, abbreviated as M-mode (Figure 4.2).

FIGURE 4.2

Schematic M-mode echocardiogram. Apex-to-base scan showing various intracardiac measurements and structures. The anterior mitral valve leaflet is labeled **A** through **F**. RVWT = right ventricular wall thickness; RVD$_d$ = right ventricular dimension, end-diastole; LVD$_s$ = left ventricular dimension, end-systole; Ch = chordae tendinae; En = endocardium; Ep = epicardium; P = pericardium; VST = ventricular septal thickness; PWT = posterior wall thickness; AoV = aortic valve; Ao = aorta; LA = left atrium.

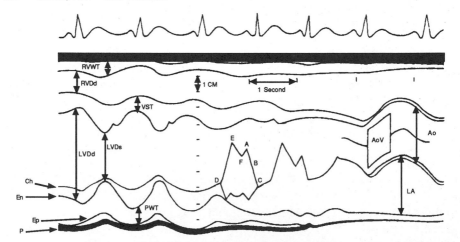

(From: Schlant RC, Alexander RW. *Hurst's The Heart, Arteries and Veins.* 8th ed. New York: McGraw-Hill; 1994:383. Used with permission.)

For the M-mode exam, the patient usually lies in the left lateral decubitus position. Occasionally, the patient is asked to lie supine. The left parasternal transducer position is used and the transducer is placed perpendicular to the chest wall. With this positioning, the mitral valve is easily visualized. The mitral valve has a characteristic shape in patients with normal sinus rhythm (Figure 4.3). In diastole, when the mitral valve is open, the anterior leaflet resembles an *M*. The smaller posterior leaflet is a mirror image of the anterior leaflet, and thus has a *W* shape. Because it is so easily recognized, the mitral valve is used as a landmark during the entire M-mode exam[2] (Figure 4.4).

FIGURE 4.3

An M-mode echocardiogram of a normal mitral valve. The anterior leaflet (AL) opens with passive filling of the left ventricle to point *E* and begins to gradually close until the force of atrial contraction forces it open (*A*) again. The smaller posterior leaflet (PL) is recorded as a mirror image of the anterior leaflet. The leaflets come together at *C*, the onset of systole.

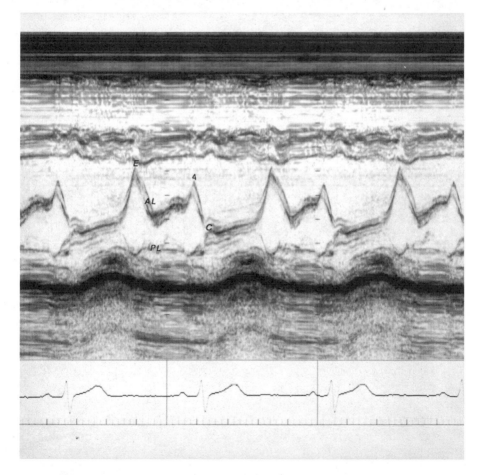

FIGURE 4.4

M-mode echocardiogram from a 24-year-old male with an apical systolic murmur. Mid- to late-systolic prolapse of both mitral leaflets is demonstrated.

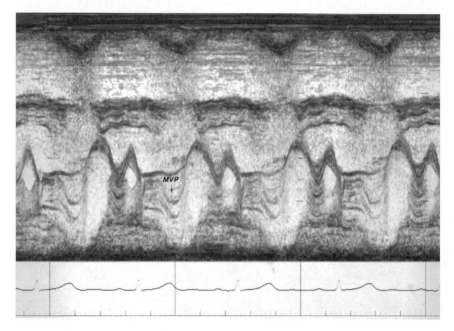

Stenosis is a condition in which the orifice of the valve is narrowed due to thickening and fusion of the valve leaflets, which impedes blood flow through the valve. *Regurgitation* is a condition in which the valve is unable to close completely, permitting backward flow of blood through the valve. Some of the causes of valvular heart disease include rheumatic fever, infective endocarditis, congenital malformations, and papillary muscle dysfunction.

The most common form of valve disease is mitral valve disease (Figure 4.5). It can be congenital or acquired and the symptoms generally depend on the severity of the lesion. Mitral stenosis is easily detected by an M-mode echo, as is mitral valve prolapse, a condition in which one or both leaflets of the mitral valve balloon back into the left atrium during systole, causing mitral regurgitation. Both mitral regurgitation and mitral stenosis can be mild or severe. If left untreated, pulmonary edema can ensue. Endocarditis and dysfunction of the chordae tendineae and papillary muscles can also be visualized from this position.

By changing the angle of the transducer in the parasternal position, the other structures in the heart can be visualized. When the transducer is angled superiorly and medially, the left atrium, aortic root, and aortic valve can be seen. The aortic valve has a characteristic boxlike shape during systole (Figure 4.6). Aortic stenosis, aortic regurgitation, and the

FIGURE 4.5

Schematic M-mode echocardiographic patterns of the mitral valve. The anterior leaflet is designated by letters *A* to *F* (AL = anterior leaflet, PL = posterior leaflet). Elevated left ventricular end-diastolic pressure (LVEDP) is characterized by a notch on the closing slope called the B notch (arrow). The double diamond configuration of the mitral valve in diastole and slight hammocking of the leaflets in systole is characteristic of LV dysfunction. Mitral regurgitation (MR) may show fluttering of the valve. In MR due to rheumatic disease, the leaflets may resemble a ski slope. Flutter waves may be seen on the leaflets in patients with atrial flutter.

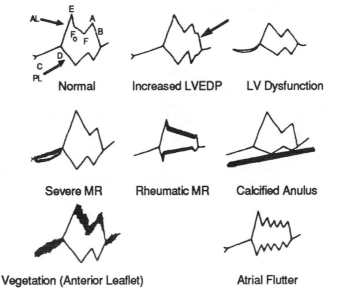

(Adapted from: Schlant RC, Alexander RW. *Hurst's The Heart, Arteries and Veins.* 8th ed. New York: McGraw-Hill; 1994:400. Used with permission.)

dimensions of the left atrium can be determined from this view. Aortic stenosis is a serious condition that frequently leads to sudden death. It is associated with angina, syncope, and left ventricular failure (Figure 4.7). Aortic valve disease often occurs in combination with mitral valve disease.

The right ventricle, interventricular septum, and left ventricle can be seen by angling the transducer inferiorly and laterally. Left ventricular function can be assessed based on the left ventricular dimensions at end-diastole and end-systole. The disorders that can be determined from this vantage point are dilated and hypertrophic cardiomyopathy, left ventricular hypertrophy, and pericardial effusion and tamponade. Echocardiography is the diagnostic procedure of choice for pericardial effusion and tamponade, life-threatening conditions that require immediate and accurate diagnosis and treatment. It is also used to guide the needle in pericardiocentesis—the treatment employed for both effusion and tamponade.

FIGURE 4.6

M-mode echocardiogram through the chest wall (CW), right ventricular outflow tract (RVOT), aortic root (AOR), and left atrium (LA). Normal systolic opening of the aortic valve cusps (AO) is demonstrated.

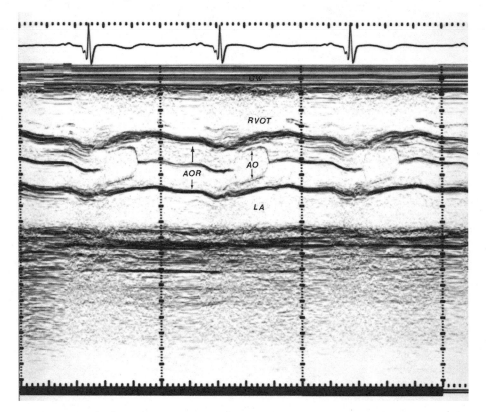

The tricuspid valve and the pulmonic valve are more difficult to visualize on M-mode exam than the other valves.[3] Tricuspid stenosis and regurgitation can be detected if the valve is visualized well enough. Tricuspid disease is relatively rare and is usually seen with aortic and/or mitral valve disease. Diseases of the pulmonic valve are more common. Both pulmonic stenosis and pulmonary insufficiency can be detected with M-mode echocardiography.

If the M-mode exam is accurately performed and interpreted it yields precise measurements in the small area in which the sound beam passes. Due to the fact that the sampling rate (rate at which sound impulses are transmitted) is so high, it is extremely accurate in determining wall thickness, chamber size, and precise timing of cardiac events.

The limitations associated with M-mode echocardiograms are a lack of spatial orientation (the ability to ascertain position with respect to surrounding structures) and inability to assess shape. Since this tech-

FIGURE 4.7

Schematic M-mode echocardiographic patterns of the aortic valve. Flail leaflet, aortic regurgitation, vegetations, and fibrosis are illustrated.

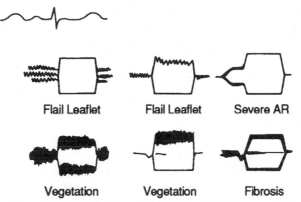

(Adapted from: Schlant RC, Alexander RW. *Hurst's The Heart, Arteries and Veins*. 8th ed. New York: McGraw-Hill; 1994:401. Used with permission.)

nique only permits visualization of the heart along the narrow pathway of the ultrasound beam, no inferences about shape and relationships between structures can be made.

TWO-DIMENSIONAL ECHOCARDIOGRAM

Two-dimensional or cross-sectional echocardiography was introduced in 1975 and has become a widely used technique for cardiac imaging. In this form of echocardiography, a large section of the heart can be viewed at one time as the ultrasound beam rapidly sweeps across the heart in a single plane. The resulting fan-shaped image yields valuable information about the size, shape, and relationship of all cardiac structures.

Two-dimensional (2-D) echocardiograms permit views of the heart in three different imaging planes (Figure 4.8). The long-axis view is the plane that divides the heart into two sagittal sections from the base to the apex. The short-axis view is the plane directly perpendicular to the long axis. The four-chamber view is the plane dividing the heart into two equal sections, with all four chambers exposed in each section.

The apical, parasternal, subcostal, and suprasternal notch transducer positions are all used in 2-D echocardiography. By angling the transducer from any given position, several imaging planes can be viewed. The long axis can be viewed from the parasternal and apical transducer positions. The short axis can be seen from the parasternal and subcostal transducer positions. All four chambers can be visualized from the apical and

FIGURE 4.8

Tomographic planes. The long axis planes run from the apex to the base at 90°
angles. The short axis plane is perpendicular to the long axis planes.

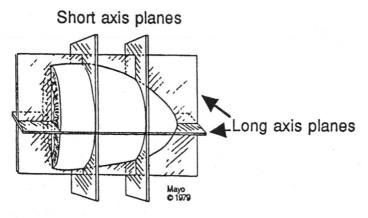

(Adapted from Seward JB, Tajik AJ. Two dimensional echocardiography. *Med Clin
North Am*. 1980;64:177. Used with permission.)

subcostal transducer positions (Figure 4.9).[8] Generally, at least one optimal view in each of the imaging planes is recorded.

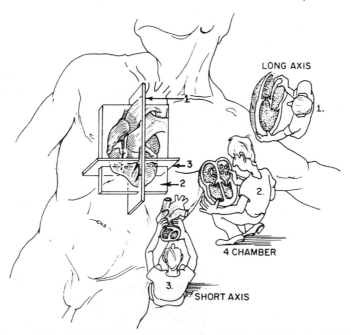

(From: Seward JB, Tajik AJ. Two dimensional echocardiography. *Med Clin North
Am*. 1980;64:177. Used with permission.)

Obtaining the 2-D Echocardiogram

As in the M-mode examination, the patient lies in the left lateral decubitus position. The transducer is placed on the chest after the coupling gel is applied, and a sweeping wave of ultrasound is transmitted into the heart tissue. The electronic circuitry within the echo machine then analyzes the time delay and direction of the reflected echoes. The resulting image is fan shaped and lies along the plane in which the ultrasound beam was directed. The image reveals detailed information about size, shape, and relationship of all the structures within the plane being imaged (Figure 4.10).

The procedure usually begins with a parasternal long-axis view. From this vantage point, the left side of the heart can be visualized. Aortic and mitral valve disease can be detected, as can problems with the outflow of blood from the left ventricle. The dimensions of the left ventricle and left atrium as well as wall motion of the left ventricle can be assessed. Left atrial myxoma (tumors) or thrombi within the left atrium can also be visualized from the parasternal long axis.

By rotating the transducer, the parasternal short axis can be seen. This permits visualization of the apex, papillary muscles, chordae tendineae, mitral valve, aortic valve, and the great vessels.

Next, the transducer is moved to the apical position. The apical transducer position is especially helpful in patients with dilated hearts or apical aneurysms[8] (Figure 4.11). From this position, all four chambers and the interventricular septum can be visualized, allowing evaluation of wall motion, chamber size, septal defects, prosthetic valve function, cardiac tumors, and an estimation of left ventricular volumes[8] (Figure 4.12). Aneurysms and congenital abnormalities can also be diagnosed from this viewpoint.

The subcostal position is used in patients with chronic obstructive pulmonary disease (COPD) and in patients with low diaphragms because the parasternal acoustic window is usually abolished. Although the images are frequently not of good quality, they may be the only obtainable images in these patients. It is possible to examine the heart in the four-chamber and short-axis views from this position. The subcostal view is most useful for detecting and localizing atrial and ventricular septal defects.[8]

Finally, the transducer is placed suprasternally. Suprasternal views allow good visualization of the aortic arch and pulmonary artery.[2]

FIGURE 4.9

Four-chamber view with the long-axis, short-axis and four-chamber tomographic planes. In the long-axis view, the observer can see the heart as it would appear if sliced from apex to base, anteriorly to posteriorly (plane 1). In the four-chamber view, the observer visualizes the image as if the heart were cut by plane 2 and the top half removed. The short-axis view visualizes the heart as if it were cut by plane 3 and the lower segment removed.

FIGURE 4.10

Injected two-dimensional four-chamber echo. (**A**) Preinjection. Dilated right ventricle (RV) and right atrium (RA); normal left ventricle (LV) and left atrium (LA). (**B**) Postinjection. A 20-cc bolus of saline via peripheral vein that demonstrates opacification of the RA and RV.

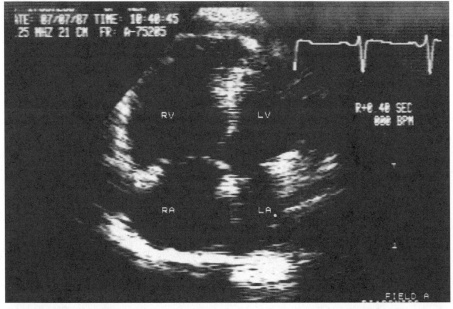

A

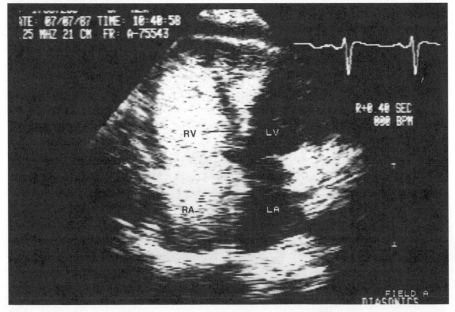

B

FIGURE 4.11

A two-dimensional (2-D) image using the four-chamber viewing angle. RV = right ventricle; LV = left ventricle; RA = right atrium; LA = left atrium; TV = tricuspid valve; MV = mitral valve.

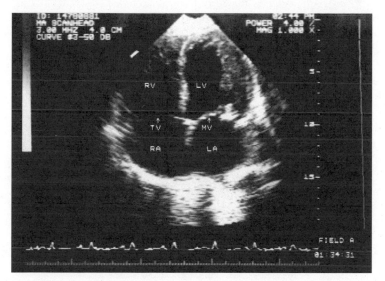

  The 2-D echocardiogram has the distinct advantage over M-mode in that it offers information about the shape of certain cardiac structures and about their relationship to one another. Indeed, some experts hail 2-D echo as second only to cardiac catheterization in its ability to provide detailed information about the structure and function of the heart. 2-D echo also is used to determine prognosis after AMI by detecting both septal and apical dysfunction in the postinfarction period.[1,9]

DOPPLER ECHOCARDIOGRAM

Doppler echocardiography has developed into an invaluable noninvasive cardiac diagnostic tool. The technique is a supplement to the M-mode and two-dimensional exams and offers enormous potential in the analysis of the character and direction of blood flow. Basically, it is an analysis of the echoes produced from moving targets such as red blood cells.

  The Doppler principle explains that the sound transmitted from a moving source changes in frequency depending upon its direction relative to the observer. For example, the whistle on an approaching freight train appears to have a higher pitch as it approaches and a lower pitch as it passes by and moves away. The reason for this is that the sound waves are compressed as the train approaches, which results in an increase in frequency (cycles per second). When the train is moving away the sound waves are stretched out (frequency is decreased), with the resultant low-

FIGURE 4.12

Two-dimensional apical four-chamber view from a patient with cardiac tampon-ade. This diastolic frame shows a large pericardial effusion (PE) that completely surrounds the heart. The right ventricular cavity is virtually nonexistent. There is both right ventricular wall collapse (large arrows) and right atrial wall collapse (small arrows) consistent with tamponade. LV = left ventricle.

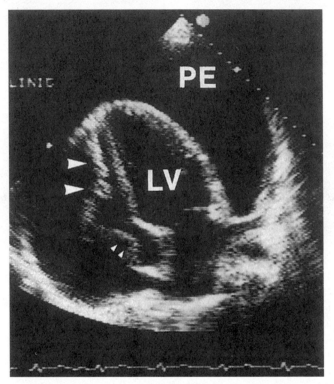

(From: Schlant RC, Alexander, RW. *Hurst's The Heart, Arteries and Veins*, 8th ed. New York: McGraw-Hill; 1994:402. Used with permission.)

ering of the perceived pitch of the train whistle. This change in frequency is called the Doppler shift. The information obtained with Doppler echocardiogram is dependent upon the acquisition and analysis of this frequency change—the Doppler shift.

In Doppler echocardiograms, ultrasound is transmitted to the heart and backscattered signals are received by the transducer. Changes in direction and frequency of the backscattered signal indicate direction and velocity of blood flow with respect to the transducer.

Because they focus so well on blood flow, Doppler echocardio-grams are very useful in determining the origin of heart murmurs, locating intracardiac and extracardiac shunts, assessing the presence and severity of valvular regurgitation and stenosis, and evaluating the patency of coronary bypass grafts.[10] Doppler echocardiography is also the only non-invasive procedure proven to be effective in the assessment of prosthetic valve function. Cardiac output can be calculated if the cross-sectional area of the valve and the flow velocity across the valve is measured during the Doppler study. Doppler is also a good noninvasive method for determining intracardiac pressures and pressure gradients within the heart and great vessels.[10,11]

In the Doppler study, the transducer is placed on the chest wall, most commonly in the apical and suprasternal notch positions.[11] The ultrasound beam is directed exactly parallel to the area of blood flow being studied, in contrast to the perpendicular placement of the ultrasound beam in the other methods of echocardiography.

There are two forms of Doppler ultrasound transmission. The continuous wave system detects backscattered signals all along the ultrasound beam and has poor depth resolution. It is best suited to analysis of a single vessel or valve.[2] On the other hand, the pulsed system only detects backscattered signals from the area being studied and is capable of good depth resolution, making it ideal for evaluating blood flow at specific areas in the heart.[2]

A small area of the ultrasound beam from which returning echoes are examined is known as the *sample volume*. The sample volume is an area of interest that can be selected in different parts in the heart. The sample volume is marked off on the screen as a tiny rectangular box. The depth of the sample volume can also be adjusted so that only the areas within the designated depth will be evaluated. This method is called "range-gating",[11] and it allows a very specific area of the blood flow to be assessed (Figures 4.13 and 4.14).

The sample volume is strategically placed depending upon the particular problem being evaluated. In suspected valvular regurgitation, the sample volume is placed in the chamber proximal to the valve so it can detect signals from the regurgitant blood flow into that chamber. If valvular stenosis is suspected, the sample volume is placed in the chamber distal to the valve so that backscattered signals can be detected from the turbulent flow into that chamber.

If shunting (blood flow from a high-pressure chamber into a low-pressure chamber) is suspected, the sample volume is placed in the low-pressure chamber where the turbulent blood will flow and backscattered signals will be emitted. The goal is to detect peak flow velocities and maximum Doppler shifts.[10]

A special Doppler system called multigated pulsed Doppler permits assessment of backscattered signals from several precise points on the Doppler beam simultaneously.[10] The returning backscattered signals are displayed on the monitor. Positive deflections depict flow toward the transducer; negative deflections depict flow away from the transducer. The display is then written onto a strip chart recorder for analysis and diagnosis (Figures 4.13 and 4.14).

FIGURE 4.13

(A) Pulsed Doppler echocardiogram of the mitral valve. The sample volume (SV) assesses the flow from the left atrium (LA) to the left ventricle (LV) through the mitral valve. This is a 2-D apical four-chamber view. (B) Note the flow moves toward the transducer, hence the upward deflections on the spectral tracing.

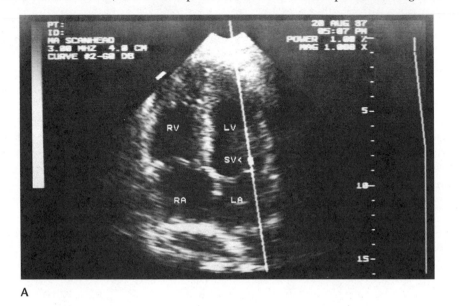

A

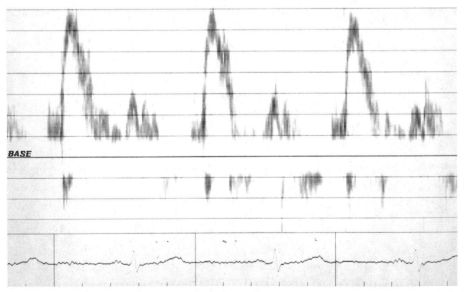

B

FIGURE 4.14

(A) Pulsed Doppler echocardiogram using a sample volume proximal to the aortic valve to record left ventricular outflow. (B) Movement of blood is away from the transducer and the spectral tracing reflects this as a negative deflection.

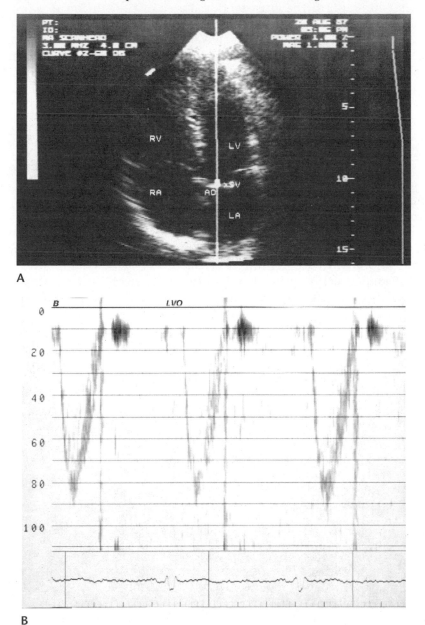

Doppler echo has proven useful for the noninvasive measurement of ejection fraction and cardiac output. Studies have shown that it correlates well with the reference standard thermodilution method of measuring cardiac output.[13,14] The Doppler measurement of ejection fraction is a function of the cross-sectional area of the aortic valve (mitral valve area if the patient has aortic valve disease) and the flow velocity across the valve. First, the aortic valve area is measured from the trailing edge of the anterior cusp to the leading edge of the posterior aortic cusp. The cross-sectional area is measured several times and averaged. Next, the Doppler sample volume is placed in the middle of the left ventricular outflow proximal to the aortic valve leaflets. A 2-D echo is then obtained by angling the ultrasound beam to obtain the best flow velocity. Cardiac output can then be determined by multiplying the ejection fraction by the heart rate.

In addition to the broad clinical applications previously discussed, Doppler echo is the exclusive diagnostic test for many functional deficits of the heart. It is the only noninvasive diagnostic test capable of estimating the severity of aortic stenosis.[10] It is also very helpful in evaluating stenosis and regurgitation of other valves that are difficult to assess with M-mode or two-dimensional echocardiograms.[10] The ability to provide noninvasive determinations of blood velocity and pressures makes Doppler echo an invaluable tool in diagnostic cardiology, especially in the ongoing assessment and treatment of congestive heart failure. See Figure 4.15 for a sample critical pathway that can be modified for use with the patient with congestive heart failure.

COLOR DOPPLER

Doppler color flow imaging allows visual representation of blood flowing through the heart. Technically speaking, it is a form of pulsed wave Doppler in which blood flow is analyzed at multiple points (sample volumes) along the Doppler beam simultaneously. The different directions and velocities of blood flow are characterized by the computer as different colors. For example, blood flow toward the transducer is represented by the color red, while flow away from the transducer is represented by the color blue. The velocity of blood flow is indicated by the intensity of the color. Also, turbulent blood flow is characterized by a mixture of green with the above colors to produce a mosaiclike pattern.

The resulting color images are superimposed on a two-dimensional image, thus giving the appearance of blood flowing through the cardiac anatomy and making it much easier to detect flow abnormalities, especially in the presence of unusual and unexpected jet flows (flow patterns). On the monitor, there are several different colors, each representing different characteristics of blood flow in the specific chamber being visualized. This is extremely helpful in the evaluation of shunts, valvular stenosis and regurgitation, prosthetic valve leaks, and in the assessment of diastolic filling.[15,16]

Doppler color flow imaging offers the distinct advantage of allowing the immediate visualization of the extent and direction of regurgitant blood flow as opposed to mapping out the extent of regurgitation little by little by moving the sample volume. Estimates of the severity of the valvular regurgitation can then be made based on the length and width of the regurgitant jet flow.[17]

Doppler color flow imaging is also useful in the evaluation of multivalvular heart disease.[17] For instance, in patients with combined mitral stenosis and aortic insufficiency, there are two abnormal jet flows in the left ventricle during diastole. Color Doppler provides a spatially oriented color picture of both jet flows.

Ejection fraction can also be measured accurately by color Doppler.[17] To do this, a 2-D echo is performed with the color sector placed over the left ventricle. This technique is especially useful because the blood pool can be distinguished from the borders of the left ventricular wall.[17]

CONTRAST ECHOCARDIOGRAM

Contrast echocardiography was once widely used to assess intracardiac structures, especially the tricuspid and pulmonic valves. Its most important use was in the diagnosis of congenital heart disease. It is now used to enhance Doppler signals in certain patients. The procedure involves the injection of a contrast agent into a central or peripheral vessel while a simultaneous conventional or color Doppler echocardiogram is performed.

Two contrast agents commonly used are saline and 5% dextrose in water. Prior to injection the contrast solution is agitated to create microbubbles within the syringe. The microbubbles in the contrast produce dense echoes that enhance Doppler signals. This allows for assessment of flow patterns[2] (Figure 4-16). The actual contrast portion of the study begins when the solution is rapidly injected intravenously. Direct injection into a cardiac chamber during cardiac catheterization can also be performed. The microbubbles disappear after traversing a capillary bed.[18]

Contrast Doppler echocardiography has been particularly useful in the evaluation of tricuspid incompetence and in the measurement of systolic and pulmonary artery pressure. Blood flow in patients with congenital heart disease can also be evaluated with this method of echocardiography. By observing the contrast material in the blood along with a simultaneous echocardiogram, various congenital anomalies and abnormal flow patterns such as those seen in atrial septal defect, ventricular septal defect, and patent ductus arteriosus can be detected.[18]

FIGURE 4.15

Critical pathway for the congestive heart failure patient.

Collaborative Problems	Nursing Diagnoses	Expected LOS
• SOB	• Activity intolerance	
• Edema	• Self-care deficit	**Admission Date**
• Increased fatigue	• Decreased tissue perfusion r/t decreased cardiac output	
• Pain	• Potential for decreased oxygenation r/t impaired gas exchange	**Discharge Date**
• Anxiety		

Day of Admission	Day 1	Day 2	Day of Discharge
MEDICAL CARE			
Assessment	**Assessment**	**Assessment**	**Assessment**
• Include allergies, health hx	• Assess change from baseline	→	• Assure labs WNL
• Physical exam, labs, ECG			
Medical orders	**Medical orders**	**Medical orders**	**Medical orders**
• Diet: low Na	→	→	• D/C IV
• Fluid restriction (consider)	→	→	
• IV access	→	→	• Write prescriptions, F/U appointments
• Consider PA catheter	• Adjust prn	→	
• Diuretics, ACE inhibitors, Digoxin	• Adjust prn	→	
• K⁺ supplements	• Monitor prn	→	
• Labs (esp. K⁺), ECG	• Adjust prn	→	
• Order patients routine meds	→	→	• D/C monitor, D/C to home
• Determine ICU or Telemetry bed	• Transfer to telemetry bed when stable	→	
• Wt. qd, I&O	• Evaluate test results		
• Order ECHO, MUGA			

MULTIDISCIPLINARY TEAM CARE

Patient and Family Education • About CHF, treatment • Importance of meds, Na+ and fluid limitations, weighing self qd • Diagnostic tests to be ordered: ECHO, MUGA, or others • Signs of electrolyte imbalance	**Patient and Family Education** • Reinforce teaching • Review meds, side effects, and actions • Teach about test results • Review action plan for pt if signs of K+ imbalance	**Patient and Family Education** • Teach patient to weigh self q a.m. • Patient to call MD if wt gain or loss > 3 lbs/d or 5 lbs/wk	**Patient and Family Education** • Importance of attending F/U appointments Consider longterm ambulatory care, potassium monitoring
Discharge planning • Assess need for social work, rehab, dietary, home care, referrals	**Discharge planning** →	**Discharge planning**	**Discharge planning** Make final arrangements for F/U care .
NURSING **Assessment** • Health hx • Vital signs, telemetry, heart sounds, lung sounds, coping • Assess for SOB, edema, fatigue, activity to erance • Wt. • labs (esp K+)	**Assessment** • q 2–4hr and prn • q 2–4hr and prn • q day • prn	**Assessment** →	**Assessment** • Assure WNL • Assure absent • Teach patient to weigh self at same time q day • Assure WNL
Nursing Orders • Maintain fluid and NaCl restriction as ordered • Administer meds • I&O • Telemetry monitoring as ordered • Prepare for ECHO or MUGA • Activity as tol	**Nursing Orders** • Teach patient to keep fluid I&O record → → • Obtain test results →	**Nursing Orders** →	**Nursing Orders** • Teach patient to monitor at home • Provide medication schedule • Teach patient to monitor at home • D/C telemetry • D/C to home

FIGURE 4.16

Four-chamber apical view after the injection of contrast in a patient with an angiographically proven aneurysm of the membraneous ventricular septum. The ventricular septal aneurysm is well delineated by the contrast opacification of the right heart chambers. RV = right ventricle; RA = right atrium; LV = left atrium; AN = aneurysm; LA = left atrium.

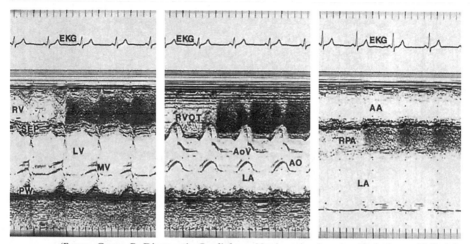

(From: Come P. *Diagnostic Cardiology: Noninvasive Imaging Techniques.* Philadelphia: JB Lippincott;1985:284. Used with permission.)

STRESS ECHOCARDIOGRAPHY

Stress echocardiography is a relatively new but widely used functional diagnostic test that is useful in identifying the extent and location of coronary artery disease. It is often used for preoperative clearance and to determine the need for further testing (e.g. cardiac catheterization). Because of its high degree of sensitivity and specificity, stress echo can be used to accurately predict the number and location of significant (> 50%) stenotic coronary lesions.[19] Studies have shown that the results correlate well with coronary angiography.[19,20]

There are two types of stress echoes. One is the treadmill echo, which combines the standard 2-D echo and the treadmill stress test. In this test, a baseline ECG, blood pressure, and 2-D echo of the heart are obtained. Then the patient runs or walks on the treadmill while the ECG and blood pressure are continually monitored. At peak stress (which is decided by the patient and/or the physician), the exercise is stopped and a 2-D echo is obtained within 60 seconds. A poststress echo is done after the patient's heart rate and blood pressure have returned to baseline, and comparisons are made.

The other type of stress echo is the dobutamine echo, in which a 2-D echo is recorded while the patient receives a stepwise infusion of dobutamine. Dobutamine causes a relative ischemia by increasing the heart rate and the myocardial wall tension, thereby increasing the myocardial oxygen demand. Such "pharmacologic" stress is used for patients who are unable to exercise to the degree necessary for assessment of left ventricular function. An advantage of the dobutamine echo is the elimination of respiratory artifact that is often present with actual physical exercise.

The dobutamine echo is similar to a treadmill stress echo in that an ECG, blood pressure, and baseline 2-D echo are obtained prior to the infusion. Then the patient is given a brief infusion of dobutamine starting with a low dose (5 mcg/kg/min) and progressing to a high dose (30–40 mcg/kg/min). The dobutamine is increased by 5 to 10 mcg/kg/min every 3 minutes until the peak dose is reached. The high dose of dobutamine is necessary to produce a myocardial oxygen demand out of proportion to supply and thus procure diagnostically useful data. An ECG, blood pressure, and 2-D echo are obtained with every increase in dosage. The infusion is terminated if the patient experiences angina, severe arrhythmias, or 1 mm ST segment depression on the ECG.[19]

The results of either the treadmill or dobutamine echo are interpreted by comparing the baseline echocardiograms with those at peak exercise (or low-dose and high-dose dobutamine), and those postexercise (postinfusion). An abnormal stress response is seen as a decrease in ventricular wall thickening or wall motion with exercise or dobutamine.

There are many benefits associated with the stress echocardiogram: It is safe and well tolerated, it is inexpensive and portable, it can be used on any patient, and it has a high diagnostic yield. The stress echo also has an advantage over submaximal exercise electrocardiography, which gives similar prognostic information but is not as sensitive for coronary artery disease.[19]

TRANSESOPHAGEAL ECHOCARDIOGRAPHY

Transesophageal echocardiography (TEE) entails the acquisition of a cross-sectional image of the heart via a transducer on the end of a gastroscope in the esophagus (Figure 4.17). Because of the close proximity of the esophagus to the heart, a high-frequency transducer is used, providing high-quality, high-resolution images. It is helpful for patients with chronic obstructive pulmonary disease and/or skeletal deformities in whom visualization with routine echocardiographic techniques is often impossible because the ultrasonic beam cannot penetrate bones or air-filled lungs. The transesophageal study can also be performed with Doppler to enhance its utility.[21]

Transesophageal echo is used to assess the functioning of prosthetic valves, to examine the heart for endocarditis, and to evaluate

FIGURE 4.17

Transesophageal echocardiogram (TEE) probe. The probe is placed into the esophagus after the throat is anesthetized and is advanced to various locations in order to view the intracardiac structures.

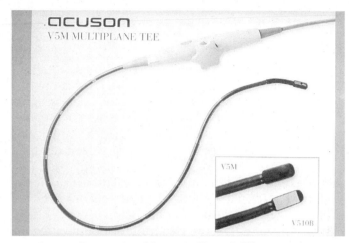

(Courtesy Acuson Corporation, Mountain View, Calif.)

valvular regurgitation and congenital abnormalities (Figure 4.18). It can be used to examine the aorta for dissections. Surgeons have used TEE intraoperatively to assist in removing air from the heart before closing and to help evaluate repairs of congenital defects.[21,22] In addition, it has been widely used intraoperatively to monitor left ventricular wall motion.[23]

Recently, TEE has measured ejection fraction in selected patients. The technique involves measuring the aortic valve diameter from an esophageal level with the transesophageal probe. Maximal flow across the aortic valve can be obtained by manipulating the probe. Ejection fraction is a function of aortic valve cross-sectional area and flow velocity across the valve. Cardiac output can then be calculated by multiplying the stroke volume by the heart rate.

The advantage of TEE over the traditional thermodilution method of cardiac output measurement is that TEE does not require right heart catheterization. The limitations associated with this new technique include technical difficulties that may result in poor image quality. Also, in some patients a sufficient transgastric window cannot be obtained.

Current research efforts in TEE include evaluating coronary artery lesions and determining viability of cardiac tissue. Biplane (two-dimensional) and multiplane probes have been developed to allow multiple views and three-dimensional reconstruction of cardiac images.[23]

FIGURE 4.18

Transesophageal echocardiogram of a prosthetic aortic valve. Resolution is excellent—even the sutures can be visualized.

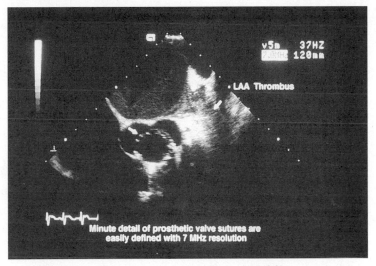

(Courtesy Acuson Corporation, Mountain View, Calif.)

INTRACORONARY ECHOCARDIOGRAPHY

This still-developing technique incorporates an ultrasonic transducer within the tip of a 4.9 or 5 French intracardiac catheter. The transducer probe rotates at 1800 rpm and employs a mirror to reflect the echo wave perpendicular to the long axis of the catheter. This allows the visualization of sequential short-axis views of the coronary artery.

Intracoronary echo allows for examination of all three layers of the arterial wall and for the assessment of the atherosclerotic lesions within the vessel. Calcified areas of plaque can be distinguished from soft plaque by their brightness. The major use of intracoronary echo at this time is in the assessment of complications such as coronary dissection during percutaneous coronary transluminal angioplasty (PTCA). See chapter 7 for additional information.

PATIENT PREPARATION FOR THE ECHOCARDIOGRAM

As with most procedures, patients do best when they understand what the echo procedure is and what they need to do to make it successful. An explanation of the specific type of echocardiogram and the pertinent manipulations that accompany it is generally much appreciated (see Patient Education Box 4.1).

PATIENT EDUCATION BOX 4.1

Echocardiogram

The purpose of an echocardiogram is to examine the size and function of your heart muscles and valves. It is painless and lasts about 30 to 90 minutes.

BEFORE THE PROCEDURE

There is no special preparation for a regular echocardiogram. If you are having a contrast or dobutamine stress echocardiogram, a needle will be placed in your vein before the test so that medication may be given.

If you are having a transesophageal echo (TEE), you must not take anything by mouth for 8 hours before the test. Unless instructed otherwise, however, you should take your medicines with a small sip of water.

DURING THE PROCEDURE

The test is usually done in a quiet, dimly lit room.

You will lie on your back with your head slightly elevated or on your left side during the procedure.

Your heartbeat will be monitored on an ECG during the test.

The technician will place a lubricated device called a transducer on your chest. It sends ultrasound waves to your heart. The ultrasound waves are harmless. They bounce back to the transducer and are seen on a screen housed in the echo machine. These waves describe the walls of the heart and the heart valves.

If you are having a contrast or stress echocardiogram, the technician will inject solution or medication into the needle that was put in before the test. If you are having a TEE, the transducer is placed into your mouth and you will be asked to swallow as it is advanced into your esophagus. You will be given medicine to make this easy and comfortable.

If you are having a stress echocardiogram, you will notice your heart rate increases during the exam. You may feel like resting for a short time after the test.

AFTER THE PROCEDURE

For a regular echo, you may resume your usual activities and medications as soon as the test is finished.

For a TEE, you will be instructed to wait until you can swallow easily and you are wide awake before you resume any food or fluids.

Your doctor will be able to discuss the results of your echo shortly after the procedure. Together you can plan any further treatments or procedures.

No physical preparation is necessary prior to an M-mode, two-dimensional, or Doppler echocardiogram. However, patients should expect that the study will be done in a dimly lit room, and they will need to lie supine or on the left side throughout the procedure. The study will take approximately 30 to 90 minutes, depending on the type of echocardiogram being done.

Patients having a contrast or dobutamine echocardiogram should expect that an intravenous needle will be inserted for injection of a contrast solution or medication. Although complications are infrequent, patients having a dobutamine echo may experience palpitations, arrhythmias, or angina with the infusion of dobutamine. If the symptoms are severe, they can be reversed with the use of short-acting beta-blockers.

Preparing patients for a TEE includes withholding food and fluids for 8 hours prior to the test. Patients will be sedated and have their throats anesthetized, which will impair the gag reflex for a period of time following the study. There may be a mild sore throat for a short time after the test. Patients may resume their usual diets and fluids as soon as a normal gag reflex returns.

PHONOCARDIOGRAPHY

Phonocardiography is a procedure that graphically depicts heart sounds and murmurs on a strip chart recorder. It has been used since the early 1900s to visually display the vibrations emanating from the heart and great vessels during different phases of the cardiac cycle.[3] Since the availability of Doppler echocardiography, phonocardiography is used less often.

Phonocardiograms are used to confirm the clinical diagnosis of specific valvular disease; precisely time cardiac events; and make possible the distinguishing of extra sounds, splitting of sounds, and identification and classification of murmurs. It should be noted, however, that the phonocardiogram will not make cardiac events audible, but rather will display them *visually*, permitting precise timing and correct diagnosis[3] (Figures 4.19 and 4.20).

The human ear can detect sound vibrations in the range of 20 to 20,000 Hz; and since most heart sounds are in the 20 to 500 Hz range, they are audible. However, since the human ear can hear more easily in the high-frequency range, some of the sounds go undetected or are difficult to interpret. Very low-pitched sounds produced within the chest are not detected as sound but rather as palpable vibration. During the course of the phonocardiogram, certain frequency ranges can be filtered out or amplified in order to zero in on specific sounds.

FIGURE 4.19

Phonocardiogram and carotid pulse tracing (CPT). The ECG is monitored on lead II (LII) with the phono tracing obtained from the left sternal border. S_1 = first heart sound; S_2 = second heart sound.

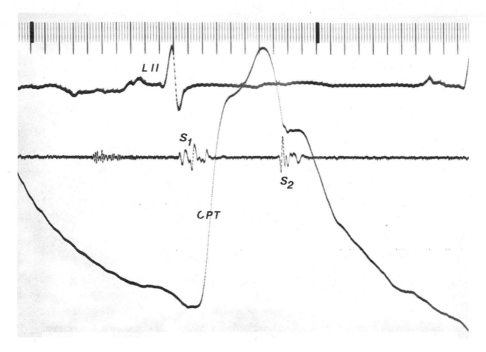

Technique of Phonocardiography

After the patient is connected to the phonocardiography machine, the microphones are placed on the chest over the base and apex of the heart, and the sound recording is done. An M-mode echocardiogram can be done at the same time so that a comparison between auscultatory events and valve movements can be made.

Pharmacologic agents and physiologic measures are often used to bring about and/or accentuate heart sounds and murmurs. When the patient is asked to speed or slow his breathing pattern in order to make certain murmurs more evident, the inspiratory and expiratory cycles are marked off manually by the technician to provide a point of reference.

Patient Preparation

No physical preparation is necessary for a phonocardiogram. The procedure should be explained to the patient. It should be stressed that extreme quiet is necessary during the procedure. Also, patients should be told that they may be given medication or asked to alter their

FIGURE 4.20

Phonocardiogram from a 60-year-old male with aortic stenosis. Demonstrates the crescendo-decrescendo murmur during systole (SM). The ECG is monitored in lead II (LII).

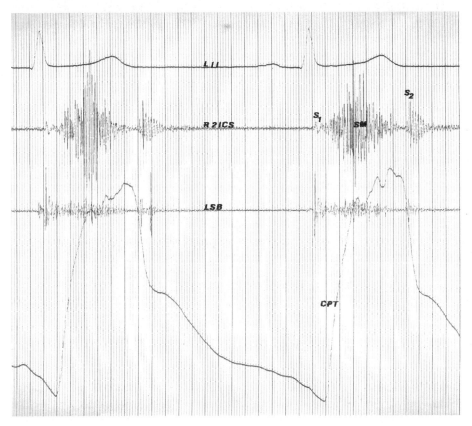

breathing pattern during the procedure to enhance heart sounds or murmurs.

NORMAL HEART SOUNDS

Physical assessment remains a clinically important diagnostic tool in the evaluation of heart sounds and murmurs. Cardiac auscultation is perhaps one of the most challenging aspects of physical assessment. Heart sounds are transient vibrations thought to be secondary to sudden tension on the valve leaflets. Heart sounds originating from each particular valve are usually recorded best from their respective auscultatory areas on the chest.

There are several factors that influence auscultation of the heart. A quiet environment is of fundamental importance in the detection of most cardiac sounds, especially those of high frequency that might otherwise go unnoticed.

Proper use of a good quality stethoscope is also important. Although the stethoscope does not accentuate heart sounds, it does have a limited ability to filter out unwanted sounds and allow the examiner to focus in on a specific range of heart sounds. Desirable characteristics of a stethoscope include proper-fitting earpieces, tubing length of approximately 10 to 12 inches, double tubing (separate or encased), and a chest piece with a diaphragm and a bell. The diaphragm is used for listening to high-pitched sounds and should be held firmly on the chest wall. The bell is used for listening to low-pitched sounds and should be held with the lightest pressure necessary to maintain skin contact. Firm pressure on the bell filters out the low-pitched sounds it is designed to detect.

First Heart Sound

The first heart sound, S_1, occurs at the onset of systole. The sound itself is relatively high pitched and originates from vibrations produced after the closure of the mitral and tricuspid valves. The mitral valve component is louder than the tricuspid valve component due to the higher pressure on the left side of the heart. The mitral valve also closes a fraction of a second sooner than the tricuspid valve.

The S_1 is heard best over the apex of the heart. Occasionally both components of S_1 (M_1 = mitral valve component; T_1 = tricuspid valve component) can be heard by placing the diaphragm of the stethoscope over the tricuspid area. This is called normal splitting of S_1.

Many factors can have an effect on the intensity of S_1. The S_1 is loudest when the mitral valve closes rapidly and when the mitral valve leaflets are widely separated at end-diastole.[27,28] Some conditions that cause an increase in the intensity of S_1 are tachycardia, rapid atrioventricular conduction (short PR interval), and hyperdynamic states such as exercise and fever that increase the force of contraction of the left ventricle. Mitral stenosis without calcification of valve leaflets is also associated with a loud S_1. The intensity of S_1 decreases when the atrioventricular conduction is slow (long PR interval) because the mitral valve is already partially closed at end-diastole. Decreased left ventricular contractility and mitral stenosis with calcification of valve leaflets are also associated with a soft S_1.

First heart sounds can vary in intensity and duration when the atria and ventricles are asynchronous, as in complete heart block, atrial fibrillation, and ventricular tachycardia. This is because leaflet separation and rate of closure in the mitral valve vary with each beat.

It is sometimes difficult to differentiate S_1 from S_2 (see next section) during rapid heart rates—that is, as systole and diastole approach equal duration. It is helpful to bear in mind that S_1 is consistent with the apical impulse and just precedes the carotid impulse.

Second Heart Sound

The second heart sound, S_2, occurs at the onset of diastole. The origin of the second sound is due to vibrations produced after closure of the aortic and pulmonic valves. The S_2 is a high-pitched sound that is loudest at the base of the heart. The aortic valve component is louder than the pulmonic valve component and the aortic valve normally closes just before the pulmonic valve. This separation is augmented during active inspiration as pulmonic valve closure is delayed due to increased venous return to the right side of the heart. This normal splitting of the components of S_2 (A_2 = aortic component; P_2 = pulmonic component) is usually easily identifiable with the phonocardiogram and is frequently audible with the stethoscope.[5] The components of the second heart sound are heard best over the pulmonic area with the diaphragm of the stethoscope. Erb's point is an area on the chest where many murmurs of aortic and pulmonic origin are transmitted (Figure 4.21).

The S_2 can also be abnormally split and is then termed *paradoxical (reversed) splitting*. It is heard characteristically during inspiration, with P_2 occurring before A_2. The most common cause of paradoxical splitting is left bundle branch block.

Wide splitting of S_2 occurs in situations where right ventricular systole is delayed, as in right bundle branch block, pulmonic stenosis, and left ventricular pacing. It is actually an accentuation of normal splitting. Wide splitting is most pronounced in inspiration and often present in expiration.

Fixed splitting is manifested by wide splitting throughout the respiratory cycle with no change between inspiration and expiration. It occurs most commonly with atrial septal defect.

The intensity of S_2 can vary as well. Increased intensity of A_2 is indicative of arterial hypertension. Aortic stenosis causes a decreased intensity of A_2. Similarly, pulmonary hypertension causes the P_2 to increase in intensity whereas pulmonic stenosis causes the P_2 to decrease in intensity.

EXTRA HEART SOUNDS

Third Heart Sound

The third heart sound, S_3, is an early diastolic sound. The sound is generated from vibrations produced during rapid filling of the ventricles in patients with ventricular dysfunction and overfilled ventricles (as in congestive heart failure). It can also be a normal variant in individuals

FIGURE 4.21

Auscultatory areas on the chest.

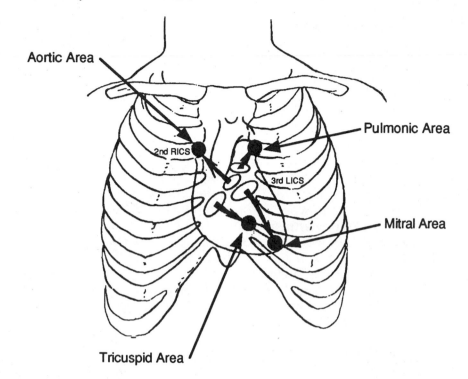

up to 30 years of age. It is a low-frequency pitch that often can be detected on phonocardiogram when it cannot be heard at the bedside.[5] For purposes of specific timing, it occurs approximately 0.15 second after A_2.[5] The S_3 can be augmented in the left lateral decubitus position and in conditions where the venous return is increased. It is heard best at the apex with the bell. An S_3 may also be heard over the lower left sternal border in patients with right ventricular failure.

Fourth Heart Sound

The fourth heart sound, S_4, is a low-pitched, presystolic sound. It is secondary to a forceful atrial contraction into a ventricle that has decreased compliance. Chronic ischemia, ventricular hypertrophy, cardiomyopathy, and idiopathic hypertrophic subaortic stenosis are some of the conditions in which an S_4 may be heard. The S_4 is also easily detectable on the phonocardiogram. It occurs prior to the S_1, and for timing purposes, about 0.14 second after the onset of the P wave.[5] Like the S_3, it can be heard best at the apex in the left lateral decubitus position with the bell.

Summation Gallop

The summation gallop is the triple sound complex that is heard during a tachycardia in individuals that have both an S_3 and an S_4. These two sounds fuse together at high heart rates to form a diastolic sound. This happens because atrial contraction and rapid ventricular filling occur simultaneously with rapid heart rates.

Ejection Clicks

Ejection clicks are high-frequency sounds that can immediately follow S_1. They are frequently heard in pulmonary and systemic hypertension. Aortic ejection clicks are heard in aortic stenosis, aortic insufficiency, and aortic dilatation.[25] These sounds are heard best at the apex.[5] Pulmonary ejection clicks are heard in pulmonary stenosis and pulmonary hypertension and are heard best in the pulmonic area.[5,25] Because of the timing of ejection clicks relative to the cardiac cycle, they can be mistaken for a split S_1. The distinction can be made based on the location in which the "double sound" is heard. The split S_1 is best heard over the tricuspid area.

Clicks that occur in mid- to late-systole are related to the billowing of a mitral valve leaflet in mitral valve prolapse. Sometimes more than one click will be present. It is believed that these sounds are due to the chordae being pulled taut suddenly during systole when the mitral valve billows back into the left atrium. The intensity and timing of a mid- or late-systolic click may vary with changes in position and with respiration. It is most easily detected with the diaphragm at the apex of the heart.[26]

Opening Snap

Opening snaps are high-pitched sounds that occur upon opening of a stenosed mitral or tricuspid valve. The sound is thought to occur as a result of sudden tension on the partially open valve leaflets very early in diastole. Opening snaps closely follow A_2 and are heard best at their respective auscultatory areas with the diaphragm[5] (Figure 4.22).

Pericardial Friction Rub

A pericardial friction rub is a high-pitched, grating sound resembling the characteristic sound heard when using sandpaper. Some people compare it to the sound produced when a lock of hair is held in front of the ear and rubbed between the fingers. It occurs in pericarditis and may have as many as three distinct components. The pericardial friction rub is usually heard best with the diaphragm at the right and left sternal border. It may be accentuated with the patient sitting up and leaning forward while holding his or her breath in exhalation.

FIGURE 4.22

Heart sounds and the cardiac cycle. Extra heart sounds are graphically depicted as they would appear in the cardiac cycle. Always be aware of the effect of splitting and timing on heart sounds: S_1 = first heart sound; S_2 = second heart sound; S_3 = third heart sound; S_4 = fourth heart sound; E = ejection click (early systolic); M = ejection click (mid systolic); L = ejection click (late systolic); OS = opening snap.

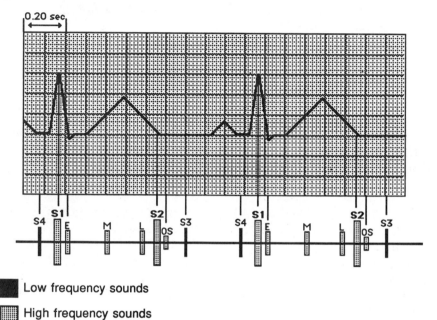

Low frequency sounds

High frequency sounds

MURMURS

Murmurs are auscultatory events that have a longer duration than heart sounds. On the phonocardiogram they are recorded as a series of vibrations[5] (Figure 4.23).

Murmurs occur because of turbulent blood flow that results from flow through stenotic or regurgitant valves, increased velocity of blood flow, decreased blood viscosity (e.g. anemia), flow into a dilated chamber, shunting of blood from a high-pressure chamber into a low-pressure chamber, or increased cardiac output (e.g. fever or exercise). Murmurs may occur in any part of the cardiac cycle and may be normal in some individuals. Often, however, they represent a specific dysfunction within the heart.

Murmurs are evaluated according to their timing in the cardiac cycle, location, and intensity. The intensity of a murmur is objectively rated on a six-point grading scale:

Grade 1	a very faint murmur that seems to fade in and out
Grade 2	a soft but easily detectable murmur
Grade 3	a moderately loud murmur
Grade 4	a loud murmur that is associated with a thrill (palpable vibration)
Grade 5	a very loud palpable murmur that is audible with the stethoscope partly off the chest wall
Grade 6	a very loud palpable murmur that is audible with the stethoscope held off the chest wall

FIGURE 4.23

Murmurs. Graphic representations of how the indicated murmurs would appear on a phonocardiographic recording. This list is not all inclusive and variations in timing within the cardiac cycle can be found among both systolic and diastolic murmurs (i.e., murmurs may be early, middle, or late in occurrence). Often, certain murmurs will begin with a click or opening snap. In addition, the prefixes *pan-* or *holo-* are applied to those murmurs that persist throughout systole or diastole (e.g the holosystolic murmur of mitral insufficiency). Systolic murmurs are often described as producing a harsh or blowing sound (especially the pansystolic regurgitant murmur of mitral insufficiency); diastolic murmurs may assume a rumbling quality. More than one murmur may also occur, producing a combination of sounds.

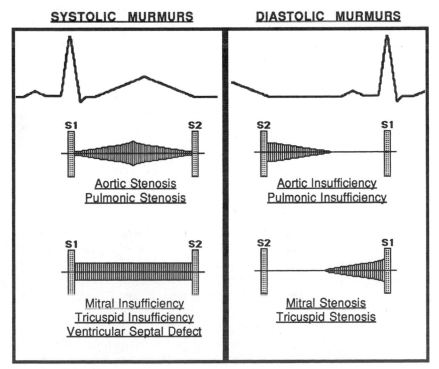

Heart murmurs are also classified as harsh, rough, blowing, rumbling, musical, or machinerylike. They may be high, medium, or low pitched, and they may be localized or radiate along the precordium. Finally, murmurs may be classified according to their intensity and may be diagrammed with a specific shape that represents that intensity. For instance, they may be diamond shaped (crescendo-decrescendo), progressively increase in intensity (crescendo), progressively decrease in intensity (decrescendo), or remain the same intensity throughout the duration of the murmur.

Systolic Murmurs

Systolic murmurs may be classified as flow murmurs, ejection murmurs, or regurgitant murmurs. *Ejection murmurs* occur as blood flows forward through the semilunar valves during systole. *Regurgitant murmurs* occur as blood flows backward through an incompetent atrioventricular valve during systole.

Flow Murmurs

Flow murmurs occur as a result of physiologic changes associated with increased cardiac output, such as those consistent with tachycardia and anemia, and fluid overload. They are the most common type of murmur and are not indicative of any type of heart disease.[26] Flow murmurs are usually heard best at the base of the heart with the diaphragm.

Pathologic Ejection Murmurs

These murmurs are due to stenosis of the aortic or pulmonic valves. Aortic stenosis is the most common cause. The murmur of aortic stenosis is harsh and crescendo-decrescendo in nature. It is audible with the diaphragm in the aortic area and may radiate down the left sternal border or up into the carotid arteries.

Regurgitant (Pansystolic) Murmurs

Systolic regurgitant murmurs characteristically have a more even intensity and often last throughout systole (i.e., they are "pansystolic"). Pansystolic murmurs often obscure the first and second heart sounds. Mitral regurgitation represents the most common type of pansystolic murmur, which usually has a blowing quality. It is heard best with the diaphragm at the apex and may radiate to the axilla. In individuals with mitral valve prolapse, a late systolic mitral regurgitant murmur may be present.

Blood flow from the left ventricle into the right ventricle in ventricular septal defect will also produce a pansystolic murmur. This is usually a loud murmur with an associated thrill that may be audible over most of the anterior precordium. Tricuspid regurgitation, although un-common, is another cause of pansystolic murmurs.

Diastolic Murmurs

Diastolic murmurs always indicate some type of pathology. They are frequently of shorter duration than systolic murmurs and, therefore, are sometimes mistaken for extra sounds. The most common diastolic murmurs are those of mitral stenosis and aortic insufficiency (regurgitation). Other causes are tricuspid stenosis and pulmonary insufficiency. Diastolic murmurs are classified as either mid or early.

The murmur of mitral stenosis is often difficult to hear. It is a low-pitched, mid-diastolic rumbling murmur heard best at the apex with the bell of the stethoscope. It is usually very localized and often it will only be audible with the patient lying in the left lateral decubitus position.

The murmur of aortic insufficiency is a high-pitched, blowing, early-diastolic murmur that is heard best with the diaphragm in the aortic area and sometimes down the left sternal border. This murmur may be accentuated with the patient sitting up and leaning forward while holding his or her breath in exhalation. The Austin-Flint murmur is a mid-diastolic murmur found in patients with severe aortic insufficiency without mitral valve disease. The sound is produced by blood flow across a rapidly closing mitral valve. The murmur is usually pandiastolic and rarely accentuated just prior to systolic ejection.

At times, the sounds of a murmur can be heard throughout both systole and diastole. Such murmurs are called continuous murmurs and may reflect a single event (as occurs in patent ductus arteriosus) or may be the fusion of two or more events that must be differentiated. Accurate assessment in this circumstance is made by considering the location, intensity, and character of the murmur (Figure 4.23). For example, the patent ductus normally closes shortly after birth, so its appearance in an adult individual is uncommon. The machinerylike sound it produces is the result of turbulent blood flow between the aorta and the pulmonary artery and thus is best heard in the aortic or pulmonic region. However, the murmur combination of aortic stenosis and aortic insufficiency may be a real possibility in the older individual and is best appreciated in the aortic area or at the apex; these may be frequent radiation of the sound into the carotid arteries.

References

1. Dodek A. When echocardiography provides the final diagnosis. *Chest.* 1984;85:678–682.
2. Come P. *Diagnostic Cardiology: Noninvasive Imaging Techniques.* Philadelphia: JB Lippincott; 1985.

3. Xu M, McHaffie DJ. How is echocardiography used? An audit of 11,701 studies. *NZ Med J.* 1992;105:120–122.
4. Pasquale M. Echocardiography update: When to order which test. *Del Med J.* 1990;62:1209–1216.
5. Tavel M. *Clinical Phonocardiography and External Pulse Recording.* Chicago: Year Book Medical Publishers; 1985.
6. Felner J, Schlant R. *Echocardiography: A Teaching Atlas.* New York: Grune and Stratton; 1976.
7. Braunwald E. *Heart Disease: A Textbook of Cardiovascular Medicine.* 4th ed. Philadelphia: WB Saunders; 1992.
8. Roelandt J. *Cardiac Ultrasound.* New York; Churchill Livingstone; 1993.
9. Ritter SB. Two-dimensional doppler color flow mapping in congenital heart disease. *Clin Cardiol.* 1986;9:591–596.
10. Nanda NC. *Doppler Echocardiography.* 2nd ed. Philadelphia: Lea & Febiger; 1993.
11. Parisi, A. Doppler echocardiography: A perspective for the practitioner. *Cardiovasc Med.* March 1986;8–9.
12. Feigenbaum H. *Echocardiography.* 5th ed. Philadelphia: Lea and Febiger; 1994.
13. Sagar K, Wann S, Paulsen W, Romhilt D. Doppler echocardiographic evaluation of Hancock and Bjork-Shiley prosthetic valves. *J Am Coll Cardiol.* 1986;7:681–687.
14. Pai RG, Shah PM. Echocardiography and other noninvasive measurements of cardiac hemodynamics and ventricular function. *Curr Probl Cardiol.* 1995;20:681–770.
15. Roelandt J, ed. Colour-coded doppler flow imaging: What are the prospects? *Eur Heart J.* 1986;7:184–189.
16. Switzer D, Nanda N. Doppler color flow mapping. *Ultrasound Med Biol.* 1985; 11:403–416.
17. Roelandt J. *Color Doppler Flow Imaging and Other Advances in Doppler Echocardiography.* Boston: Martinus Nijhoff; 1986.
18. Meltzer RS. *Myocardial Contrast Two-Dimensional Echocardiography.* Boston: Kluwer Academic Publishers; 1989.
19. Pellikka PA, Roger VL, Oh JK, et al. Stress echocardiography Part II. Dobutamine stress echo: Techniques, implementation, clinical applications and correlations. *Mayo Clin Proc.* 1995;70:16–27.
20. Sawada SG, Segar DS, Ryan T, et. al. Echocardiographic detection of coronary artery disease during dobutamine infusion. *Circulation.* 1991;83:1605–1614.
21. Labovitz A. *Transesophageal Echocardiography: Basic Principles and Clinical Applications.* Philadelphia: Lea and Febiger; 1993.
22. Oka Y, Goldiner P. *Transesophageal Echocardiography.* Philadelphia: JB Lippincott; 1992.
23. Roelandt J. *Multiplane Transesophageal Echocardiography.* New York: Churchill Livingstone; 1996.
24. Bom N, Roelandt J. *Intravascular Ultrasound: Technique, Developments, Clinical Perspectives.* Boston: Kluwer Academic Publishers; 1989.
25. Abrams J. *Essentials of Cardiac Physical Diagnosis.* Philadelphia: Lea & Febiger; 1987.
26. Bates B. *A Guide to Physical Examination.* 5th ed. Philadelphia: JB Lippincott; 1991.

5

NUCLEAR MEDICINE STUDIES AND POSITRON EMISSION TOMOGRAPHY

EVAN PADGITT
EVA KLINE-ROGERS

GLOSSARY

Adenosine (Adenocard)   A naturally occurring nucleotide with powerful vasodilating properties, used in nuclear medicine scans to induce coronary artery dilation in patients who cannot exercise. Also used to counteract supraventricular tachycardias.

Akinetic   Without movement; in cardiology, usually refers to a part of the ventricular wall that is not moving as would be expected.

Antimyosin Antibodies   Antibodies to contractile proteins found in muscle cells. In nuclear medicine, antimyosin antibodies labeled with radioactive tracers bind to damaged myocardial cells, thereby aiding in the diagnosis of MI, transplant rejection, and myocarditis.

Bruce or Montoye Protocols   Procedures for cardiac stress tests in which the patient gradually increases exercise intensity. Used with exercise portion of nuclear medicine tests.

Bull's-Eye Chart   In SPECT imaging for thallium scans, a two-dimensional charting of the left ventricle myocardium, using concentric circles. Areas of poor thallium uptake show as darker zones. Allows for a more accurate estimation of how much myocardium is affected.

Coronary Angioplasty   Use of a balloon-tipped catheter to compress atherosclerotic plaque against the wall of a coronary artery, thus opening a stenotic artery and restoring blood flow to affected myocardium.

Dipyridamole (Persantine)   A potent vasodilator drug, used in nuclear medicine stress tests to dilate coronary arteries in patients unable to exercise. Acts by blocking reuptake of endogenous adenosine at receptor sites.

Dyskinetic   With inappropriate movement; in cardiology, refers to an area of ventricular wall that moves in the opposite direction of normal (such as outward during systole).

ECG Gating   In nuclear medicine tests, the synchronizing of scanning-camera imaging with a certain part of the cardiac cycle. The multiple images thereby obtained are pooled by computer processing to form a composite image of the heart.

Ejection Fraction   The percentage of blood introduced into a cardiac chamber (such as the ventricle) that is subsequently pumped out.

Equilibrium Studies   See *gated blood pool study.*

First-pass Studies   Nuclear medicine study of the heart in which high-speed scans are taken of the heart during the first pass of a bolus IV injection of radioactive tracer through the heart chambers.

Fixed Defects   In thallium scanning, portions of the myocardium that do not collect thallium, either in the initial exercise scan or in the subsequent resting scan. Presumed to be areas of myocardial infarction. Also called *permanent defects.*

Gated Blood Pool Study   Nuclear medicine scan in which a technetium tracer is tagged to red blood cells and distributed throughout the body's blood pool. As the blood circulates through the heart, gated images are made of heart function (see *gating*). Also known as *equilibrium study* or *MUGA.*

Gating   A computerized feature of nuclear medicine scans in which the imaging of each heartbeat is divided into a specified number of frames, or "gates," and the images from the corresponding frames of each heart cycle are combined into a composite film loop of one heartbeat.

Hypokinetic   Having diminished movement; in cardiology, refers to a ventricular wall that is moving less vigorously than normal.

Imaging   In nuclear medicine, composition of a picture by use of gamma-ray counter, or scintillation camera, which detects and localizes the radioactive tracer in the body.

Indium 111   Radioactive element used as a marker in antimyosin antibody scans.

Infarct Avid Scans   Nuclear medicine scans, such as those using technetium Tc 99m pyrophosphate, in which the tracer binds to infarcted myocardial tissue.

MUGA   Multiple gated acquisition; see *gated blood pool study.*

Permanent Defects   Synonym for "fixed defect"—see above.

Planar Imaging   Scanning technique in which pictures are taken through certain anatomical planes, or points of view. In thallium scans, it usually means three views—anterior, left anterior oblique, and left lateral.

Radionuclide   An atom that disintegrates with emission of electromagnetic radiation.

Radionuclide Ventriculography (RNVG) A nuclear medicine scan that uses a radioactive element to mark red blood cells, enabling outlining of the ventricles and analysis of their functioning.

Redistribution On thallium scans, the process by which thallium will only slowly fill in an ischemic area of myocardium. Thus, on initial (exercise) scan, the area takes up little or no thallium; over time, however, as thallium continues to move from the bloodstream into tissue, the area will show an increase in thallium level. When a two-part thallium scan shows redistribution, this indicates ischemia. Also called *reversible defects*.

Revascularization Restoration of blood supply to an affected area of myocardium—for example, by angioplasty or thrombolytic therapy.

Reversible Defects Synonym for *redistribution*—see above.

Scintillation Camera Imaging camera that detects gamma-ray emissions from nuclear medicine tracers.

Sensitivity The relative ability of a test to detect the desired disease entity when that condition is present. For instance, when a test has a sensitivity of 90%, the test will be positive for 90% of those who have the disease.

Single-Photon Emission Computerized Tomography (SPECT) Nuclear-imaging technique in which many slice scans are taken with a moving camera and reassembled by computer into detailed composite picture of the patient.

Sodium-Potassium Pump Cellular mechanism for active transport of certain substances across cell membranes. It is the means by which thallium enters myocardial cells.

Specificity The relative ability of a test to be positive only for the disease entity in question. For example, a specificity of 85% means that of all the people who test positive, some 85% really have the disease, while 15% do not (false-positives).

Stannous Pyrophosphate Tin compound used in radionuclide ventriculography to facilitate attachment of the technetium Tc 99m tracer to red blood cells.

Technetium Tc 99m Radioactive element used in a variety of nuclear medicine scans. Properties depend on the substance to which it is bound.

Technetium Tc 99m Pertechnate Used in first-pass and gated blood pool (MUGA) scans to mark red blood cells.

Technetium Tc 99m Pyrophosphate (Tc PYP) Infarct-avid tracer that binds to areas of myocardial infarction.

Technetium Tc 99m Sestamibi (Cardiolite) Marker which goes preferentially to healthy myocardial cells (as does thallium).

Technetium Tc 99m Teboroxime Similar to Technetium Tc 99m sestamibi but with much quicker uptake into cells and shorter half-life.

Thallium 201   Radioactive element used as a tracer in tests of myocardial viability. It has similar biological properties to potassium.

Thrombolytic Drugs   Pharmacologic agents (e.g. streptokinase, tissue plasminogen activator) used to dissolve blood clots, particularly in the setting of acute MI.

POSITRON-EMISSION TOMOGRAPHY

Nuclear scans such as thallium and MUGA imaging use radioactive gamma-emitting agents to study the function of the heart. Positron-emission tomography (PET) uses a different type of radioactive agent that allows observation of myocardial metabolism for the purpose of evaluating the myocardium's health and function. Although each test uses a different technique, both nuclear scans and PET study the myocardium using radioisotopes and so will be considered together in this chapter.

MYOCARDIAL SCANS

Nuclear medicine scans with tracers such as thallium-201 and the technetium agents are used to study the health and function of the myocardium. Unlike cardiac catheterization, which primarily looks at the anatomy of the coronary arteries, myocardial scans indicate the actual coronary blood supply to the heart muscle—a measure of its viability. Because the actual blood flow to regions of the heart muscle does not correspond well to blockages seen on cardiac catheterization, myocardial scans give the clinician important additional information on the presence and extent of ischemia and infarction.[1]

Thallium-201 Scans

The most commonly used agent for myocardial scans is thallium-201.[2] Thallium-201 is a radioactive isotope whose presence can be detected by an instrument called a scintillation camera. Because of its chemical resemblance to potassium, thallium-201 has similar biological properties. That is, when introduced into the body, thallium-201 behaves much as potassium would—including being actively transported into cells by the sodium-potassium pump.[1] Some 88% of thallium-201 "offered" to healthy myocardial cells is taken up by them.

The usefulness of thallium-201 for myocardial scans comes from its selective uptake by body cells, depending on their state of health. As is the case with potassium, thallium-201 injected into the bloodstream will be readily taken up by body cells that are healthy and have active transport across their cell membranes. However, where myocardial cells are ischemic due to restricted coronary artery flow, cell functions are damaged; thallium 201 will be taken up more slowly, and in smaller amounts. Infarcted tissue will not take up thallium at all. Therefore, regions of healthy myocardium will show high thallium content, with ischemic and infarcted areas showing little or no thallium count. It is this difference in regional thallium uptake that is the criterion for a "positive" thallium scan.[3,4]

Thallium-201 has a half-life of approximately 73 hours and will remain in circulation for some time. In spite of its slow uptake of thallium, a region with restricted blood flow (where cells are ischemic but still viable) may eventually "fill in" with thallium after several hours. This phenomenon is called *redistribution*, and the regions are said to have *transient* or *reversible defects*[1,2] (Figure 5.1). Areas that do not fill in with thallium on delayed scan are called *fixed* or *permanent defects* and are considered to be

FIGURE 5.1

Reversible thallium defect. Two views of the heart during initial thallium injection and after delay of 3 to 4 hours. The arrows in the left-hand images indicate perfusion defects in the septum and apex of the heart, which are slowly filled in by thallium before the delayed scan, seen on the right.

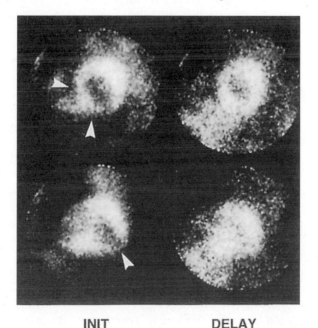

INIT   DELAY

From Miller DD, Burns RJ, Gill JB, Ruddy TD, et al. *Clinical Cardiac Imaging.* New York: McGraw-Hill; 1988, 32. Used with permission.

infarcted tissue. Because the distinction between infarct and ischemia is important, thallium tests normally include an initial scan, followed by a delayed scan some 3 to 4 hours later. Many centers employ a second, smaller injection of thallium just prior to the second, resting scan.[3,5]

Patients are asked to fast overnight prior to thallium testing, to prevent the increased blood flow to the digestive organs that may occur following a meal. (Increased visceral flow will decrease thallium delivery to the myocardium.) The patient should also refrain from eating between the first and second scans, unless this poses a hardship (for diabetics, for instance). Some researchers suggest withholding antianginal medications such as beta-blockers and nitrates, while others consider this unimportant.[1,3]

Role of Exercise

In the patient with coronary artery disease, the limited blood flow through a partly-stenosed vessel may be enough to supply the demands of the myocardium at rest. Diagnostic tests done in the resting state, including thallium scans, may not show any abnormalities.[3] However, ischemia may develop when the heart is exercised, because the partially blocked coronary artery may deliver insufficient blood to meet increased myocardial demand for oxygen, nutrients, and waste removal (Figure 5.2). In the normal heart, coronary blood flow increases up to two and a half times in response to exercise; in the stenosed artery, little or no increase in flow is possible, and the myocardium served by the vessel becomes ischemic.[6]

It is standard practice to perform a two-part thallium scan sequence, with exercise and rest components.[1] Patients who are physically able to exercise are put through a standard treadmill exercise routine of walking or jogging (such as the Bruce or Montoye protocols) with the goal of attaining 85% of maximal heart rate for their age. The patient is instructed to give his or her best effort, because *an adequate level of exercise is vital for an accurate test*. When the patient has reached the desired heart rate for the prescribed time, or when the patient states that he or she must soon stop due to exhaustion, the thallium dose is injected intravenously.[3] Ideally the patient will exercise for an additional minute to thoroughly circulate the thallium dose. (As indicated by the protocols, exercise is also stopped for ST segment changes, blood pressure above or below parameters, or arrhythmias.) The first scan is taken within 5 minutes of the end of exercise. The second, resting scan is then performed 3 to 4 hours after the exercise session to search for later areas of thallium fill-in (redistribution) consistent with ischemic myocardium.

The resting thallium scan alone is less sensitive in detecting coronary artery disease in a patient who has only activity- or exercise-related

FIGURE 5.2

Exercise-induced ischemia on a thallium scan. Thallium images and corresponding ECG tracings following exercise and after a 3 to 4 hour delay. The exercise ECG was inconclusive, although there was depression of the ST segments in both the delayed and exercise images. The exercise thallium image, however, shows a defect in thallium uptake (arrows), which resolved in the delayed image.

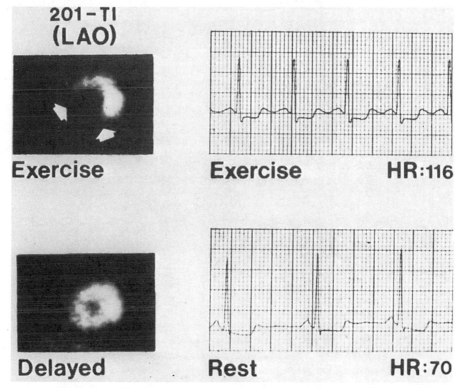

From: Iskandrian AS. *Nuclear Cardiac Imaging: Principles and Applications.* Philadelphia: F.A. Davis; 1987:166. Used with permission.

angina (Figure 5.3). Resting thallium scans are used primarily in cases where the patient is already having anginal symptoms at rest, or to determine the size of a recent or past myocardial infarction.[3]

Planar vs. SPECT Imaging

When clinical thallium-201 imaging came into use in 1975, the available equipment allowed the scintillation camera to be placed in the three most common anatomical planes for cardiac views—anterior (ANT), 45° left anterior oblique (45° LAO), and 70° LAO (also called left lateral or LAT).[1] Considerable training was needed to read these grainy, indistinct

FIGURE 5.3

Thallium images of exercise-induced ischemia. (Left) This patient had 70 percent occlusion of both left and right coronary arteries, and this is seen as widespread lack of thallium uptake just after exercise. (Right) Gradual "filling in" of thallium shows these defects to be reversible, or ischemic rather than infarct-related.

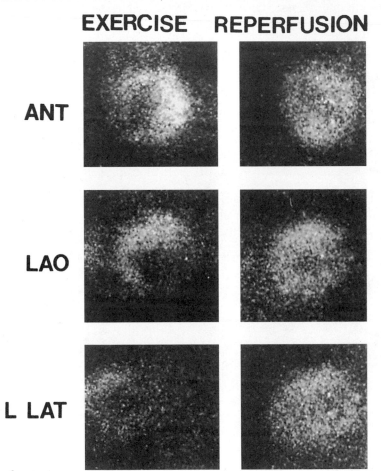

From: Gerson M. *Cardiac Nuclear Medicine.* 2nd ed. New York: McGraw-Hill; 1991:25. Used with permission.

images, and much depended upon the interpretation by the individual operator. In the 1980s, plotting and computer techniques were introduced to improve the detection of CAD with planar imaging (Figure 5.4).[7]

In spite of these improvements in planar imaging, new techniques were needed to more reliably assess the myocardium. In many centers, *single-photon emission computerized tomography* (SPECT) has superseded planar thallium imaging. SPECT combines scintillation photography with the computerized image reconstruction of traditional CAT scans to

FIGURE 5.4

Three standard views in planar thallium scans: anterior, left anterior oblique (LAO), and left lateral. The segments of the left ventricle seen in each view are diagrammed, and representative scan images shown.

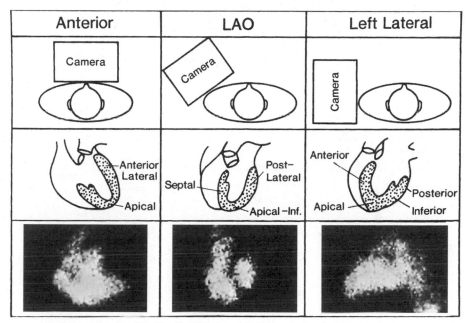

From: Gerson M. *Cardiac Nuclear Medicine.* 2nd ed. New York: McGraw-Hill; 1991:86. Used with permission.

improve thallium-scan images.[7] Instead of viewing the heart in only three planes, the SPECT camera is gradually rotated across the patient's chest in a 180° arc. Images are taken at every 4 to 6 degrees of arc, and these slices are reprocessed by a computer into a clearer picture of myocardial thallium distribution.[1]

SPECT data can be plotted onto a *bull's-eye chart*, an abstract representation of the left ventricle, with each region of the heart assigned a region of the circular plotting grid (Figure 5.5). The bull's-eye consolidates data from all the SPECT views into one chart and reduces the differences in interpretation seen among individual operators.[7]

Vasodilators and Thallium Imaging

A limitation in the use of thallium scans has been the inability of many patients to exercise to the level needed for accurate results— usually due to physical disability from medical conditions or aging. In recent years, however, the augmentation of the thallium test with certain vasodilator drugs has made possible useful thallium testing for those who

FIGURE 5.5

SPECT thallium bull's-eye chart. (**A**) Computer-generated report of stress and delayed thallium images in a 51-year-old man with a history of inferolateral myocardial infarction (MI) and new anginal symptoms. The old MI is seen as the inferior and lateral shadings that remain in the delayed scan (a fixed defect). Ischemia appears in the anterior and lateral regions as a *reversible* defect that disappears on the delayed scan. (**B**) Computer-generated adenosine thallium results on a 48-year-old woman with exertional chest pain. Image taken during adenosine "stress" shows inferior and septal thallium uptake that is gone by the time of the delayed scan. This is diagnostic for inferoseptal ischemia with stress.

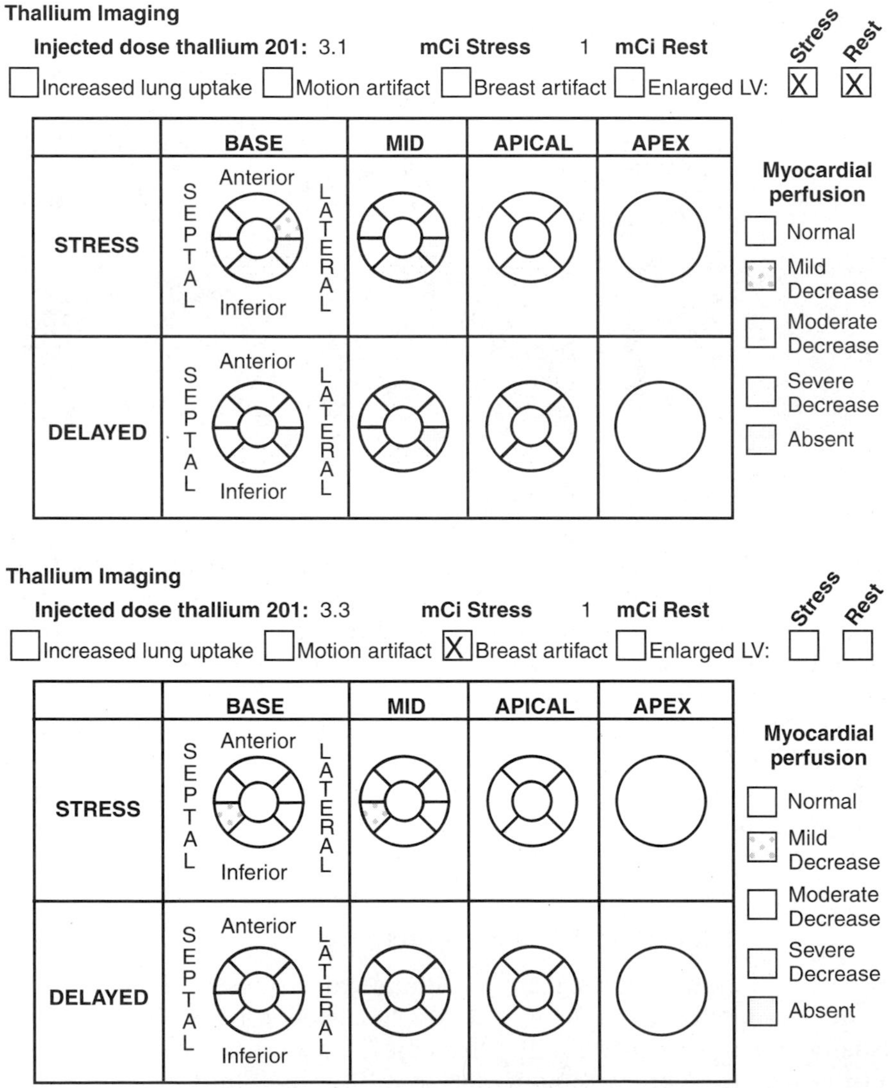

Courtesy Michigan Heart, P.C., Ann Arbor, Michigan.

cannot exercise.[1,2] Dipyridamole (Persantine) and adenosine (Adenocard) induce maximal dilation of the coronary artery beds, as occurs during exercise. Given just before thallium injection, these drugs simulate the "exercise effect" in which normal coronary vessels dilate to four times their normal size while stenosed vessels dilate much less. Along with the vasodilation, there is a reflex increase in heart rate. Ischemia that would normally be found only with exercise can thus be induced with dipyridamole or adenosine. Research suggests that the reliability of vasodilator thallium scans is comparable to that of exercise scans.[8,9]

Dipyridamole dilates arteries by blocking the cellular reuptake and breakdown of adenosine, a potent vasodilator produced by cells throughout the body.[8,10] Thus, while the dipyridamole acts, a greater than normal supply of adenosine is in circulation, causing vasodilation of the coronaries and other arteries. Intravenous dipyridamole works for 15 to 30 minutes.

The effects of dipyridamole are competitively blocked by aminophylline compounds (including theophylline) and by other xanthines such as caffeine; for this reason, all aminophylline/theophylline drugs are withheld for 36 hours before the scan, and all caffeine withheld for the prior 24 hours.[1,8] Patients taking oral dipyridamole should not take their medication the morning of the test. The use of dipyridamole is contraindicated in those with severe bronchospasm from asthma or COPD, as it may worsen these conditions (Figure 5.6).

The adverse effects of IV dipyridamole are usually related to vasodilation.[11] The most common are chest pain (20%), headache (12%), and dizziness (12%) as well as nausea, flushing, dyspnea, and palpitations. A 250 mg dose of IV aminophylline is recommended to alleviate these adverse effects.[1]

Adenosine, the actual vasodilating agent made more available through the action of dipyridamole, recently has been used directly as an adjunct for thallium studies (Figure 5.7). Its main advantage is its extremely short half-life (less than 10 sec), which limits its duration of action to 1 to 2 minutes.[1] A continuous infusion of 140 mcg/kg/min is delivered for 6 minutes. At the 3-minute mark, the thallium is injected.

Adenosine shares the same vasodilator side effects as dipyridamole. One study reported that 94% of patients experienced side effects, with 20% of the side effects rated as "severe."[8] However, due to adenosine's very short duration of action, no test had to be stopped, and all patients recovered quickly without aminophylline. As with dipyridamole, adenosine is contraindicated in bronchospastic patients; aminophylline and caffeine are likewise withheld before the test. An additional caution for adenosine—it may slow cardiac conduction, up to complete heart block.[1] The effect is generally transient; but any patient with existing second-degree or third-degree heart block or sick sinus syndrome might need a pacemaker in place if adenosine is to be used.[8]

FIGURE 5.6

Dipyridamole thallium scan. Three short-axis and one long-axis SPECT cross sections of the heart after (top) dipyridamole injection and (bottom) 4 hours later. The inferior wall shows reversible (ischemic) thallium defects that fill in the delayed images.

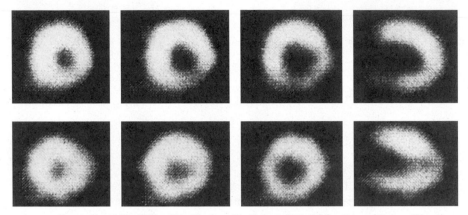

From: Zaret BL, Beller GA. *Nuclear Cardiology. State of the Art and Future Directions.* St. Louis: Mosby-Year Book; 1993:172. Used with permission.

Indications for Thallium Scanning

As a test of myocardial perfusion, thallium scanning is ideally suited for screening of suspected coronary artery disease (CAD), as well as for evaluating heart function in known CAD. It is also used, less commonly, to evaluate for other diseases that cause functional changes in the heart muscle.

Coronary Artery Disease Screening

The reliability of thallium scans in screening for CAD varies with the scan method. Planar thallium testing has a sensitivity for CAD of 80% to 85%, while SPECT imaging has a sensitivity of 90% to 97%.[3] SPECT is especially useful for detecting silent ischemia or mild CAD.[1,7] Adenosine thallium scans and exercise studies are similarly accurate. Accuracy in detecting CAD increases with the number of coronary arteries affected—for one-vessel disease, sensitivity in one study was 73%; for two-vessel disease, 90%; for three-vessel disease, 100%.[8,9]

Thallium screening for CAD is indicated when

- the patient has multiple risk factors;
- there is a difficult differential diagnosis of atypical chest pain;
- there are equivocal findings on a plain stress ECG;
- the patient has resting ECG abnormalities that make ruling out CAD difficult: bundle branch block, left ventricular hypertrophy, digoxin effect, Wolff-Parkinson-White syndrome.[2]

FIGURE 5.7

Adenosine thallium scan. In a format similar to that of Figure 5.6, a different patient undergoes "stress" with adenosine injection, showing reversible ischemia in the anteroseptal wall and apex.

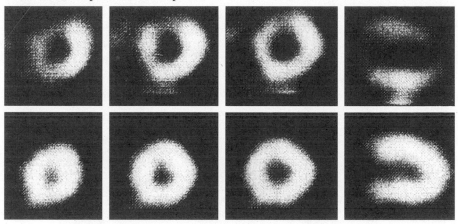

From: Zaret BL, Beller GA. *Nuclear Cardiology. State of the Art and Future Directions.* St. Louis: Mosby-Year Book; 1993:175. Used with permission.

Diagnosis of Acute MI

Thallium scans have proven to be highly accurate in detecting acute myocardial infarction (AMI), even within the first 24 hours. Detecting and sizing AMI is one of the few practical uses of resting thallium scans. Thallium scans have difficulty diagnosing apical and inferior MIs, though SPECT is somewhat better; transmural infarcts are easier to detect than non–Q wave infarcts.[1,2]

Assessing Prognosis and Significance of Known CAD/MI

Cardiac catheterization shows the anatomy of major coronary arteries and their blockages, but does not indicate how much blood flow is being delivered to a region of the heart muscle by the smaller, collateral blood vessels.[2] Thallium scans reveal the actual total blood flow to the heart muscle from all vessels, and thus show the true state of health of the myocardium.

Patients can be categorized into high-risk or low-risk categories based on presence and size of thallium redistribution: Those patients with areas of myocardium that show redistribution are at high risk because the areas are ischemic but not infarcted and may progress to an MI. Research has supported thallium redistribution as a significant predictor of risk—as good as or better than cardiac catheterization results and clinical observations.[12,13] Patients who need revascularization by coronary angioplasty or bypass can be identified based on redistribution findings.

Evaluating Results of Treatment Interventions

A thallium scan after medical therapy, coronary angioplasty, or surgical bypass will evaluate whether these treatments have reduced the area of ischemia.[3] Because reocclusion of the artery after angioplasty is a common problem, thallium scans can look for a resurgence of ischemia. In one study a positive thallium scan postangioplasty correlated with a high probability of reocclusion.[14] Assessing for myocardial reperfusion after use of thrombolytic drugs to dissolve clots in a coronary artery is another use for thallium[2] (Figures 5.8). While many patients have had myocardium salvaged by the use of thrombolytics, they may also be left with areas of ischemic tissue, where in earlier days an infarction would have occurred.[6] These patients are at risk for later MI from these ischemic zones, and can benefit from postthrombolytic thallium testing.

Evaluation of Cardiomyopathy

Thallium tests can assess the extent and degree of cardiomyopathy, especially of the ischemic type. However, the changes in myocardial cells in other types of cardiomyopathies (such as infiltrative or hypertrophic) may also cause a positive thallium scan. When the patient has a diagnosis of infiltrative disease—sarcoidosis, amyloidosis, or scleroderma— thallium scans can determine whether myocardium has been significantly affected.[2,15]

Diagnosis of Left Ventricular Aneurysm

Thallium scanning with SPECT techniques has been about 96% accurate in diagnosing left ventricular aneurysms in post-MI patients.[16]

Strengths and Limitations of Thallium Scans

Thallium scanning has shown high accuracy in detecting CAD. As a functional test of the myocardium's blood supply, it can be used to make a prognosis about as well as evaluate the effectiveness of medical and surgical interventions. The thallium scan is noninvasive, is performed with relative ease, and is generally well tolerated. The advent of adenosine and dipyridamole tests has allowed assessment of the large pool of patients unable to exercise adequately for standard stress scans.

However, the nuclear scanners are expensive, and personnel to operate them must be available. While the radiation dose is considered moderate (2–4 µCi), this must be considered a negative feature of thallium scans. Vasodilation effects of adenosine and dipyridamole, though brief, may be distressing for the patient.

Several health conditions can contribute to false-positive thallium tests, as can artifacts caused by natural and artificial noncardiac structures. These factors are listed in Table 5.1.

FIGURE 5.8

PTCA results assessed by thallium. The top images show preangioplasty (PTCA) perfusion defects in planar views after exercise. After angioplasty, the bottom images show marked improvement in the postexercise uptake of thallium.

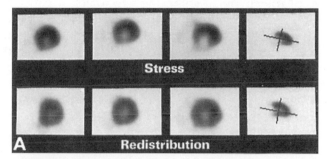

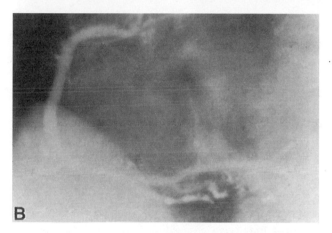

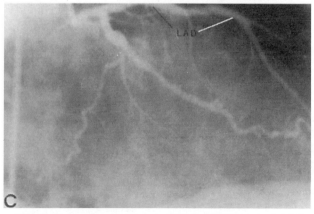

From: Elliott LP. *Cardiac Imaging in Infants. Children and Adults*. Philadelphia: JB Lippincott; 1991:189. Used with permission.

TECHNETIUM SCANS

Technetium (Tc 99m) is another radioactive tracer used in nuclear medicine scans of the myocardium. How it is used depends upon the biological properties of the chemical compound to which it is bonded. For instance, technetium Tc 99m pyrophosphate has been used for several years to detect and define areas of myocardial infarction because this particular tracer has an affinity for damaged cells. On the other hand, the technetium isonitriles such as technetium Tc 99m sestamibi can be used in a similar way to thallium because they also collect more readily in healthy cells than in damaged ones. These newer forms of technetium have several advantages over thallium, and may gradually replace thallium as the tracer of choice for myocardial scans.

Technetium Tc 99m Pyrophosphate

Technetium Tc 99m pyrophosphate (Tc-PYP) scans were first used to evaluate bony structures because of this tracer's tendency to bind with calcium. Since calcium was known to collect in irreversibly damaged myocardial cells, researchers in the 1970s employed this principle to create infarct avid scans with Tc-PYP.[16] Tc-PYP injected into a patient would collect in infarcted heart tissue, thus "lighting up" any area of recent heart attack. While Tc-PYP has useful properties in detecting MI, it also has significant limitations.

TABLE 5.1

Noncoronary Diseases That May Cause Positive Thallium Scans

- Cardiomyopathies (idiopathic, hypertrophic, other nonischemic)
- Valve diseases (e.g. aortic stenosis, mitral prolapse)
- Hypertension (and left ventricular hypertrophy)
- Idiopathic hypertrophic subaortic stenosis (IHSS)
- Sarcoidosis, amyloidosis (due to replacement of normal cells)
- Lymphoma; muscular dystrophy; diabetes

Artifacts and Other Problems During Thallium Scans

- Thallium uptake in lung (occurs in pulmonary hypertension; COPD)
- Thallium uptake in overlying breast and diaphragm tissue
- Obesity or thick chest wall muscles
- Breast implants
- Patient movement during scan
- Suboptimal exercise on stress portion
- Beta-blocker drugs (may make detection of ischemia more difficult)[2,16]

Infarct Scanning

Normally, Tc-PYP collects in bone but not in healthy myocardium. Tc-PYP will begin to collect measurably in irreversibly damaged myocardial cells about 12 hours after the beginning of infarction.[16] Peak concentration of Tc-PYP occurs at about 48 to 72 hours postinfarct, and detectible levels may continue for 7 to 10 days. Tc-PYP does not usually collect in infarcted tissue beyond this first 7- to 10-day period, and is therefore useful only in the acute phase and for a short time thereafter (Figures 5.9 and 5.10).

A Tc-PYP scan is primarily indicated when standard methods of diagnosing MI are unreliable. ECG diagnosis may be difficult in patients with non–Q wave MI or bundle branch block; cardiac enzyme levels may be already elevated after recent cardiac surgery or cardioversion. When used in the early phases, Tc-PYP scans have approximately 85% to 90% sensitivity for detecting MI. Tc-PYP with SPECT imaging can accurately size acute infarcts, including quite small areas of necrosis. Prolonged Tc-PYP uptake (after 7 to 10 days postinfarct) has been shown to correlate with ongoing cell death and reliably predicts increased risk of post-MI complications such as infarct extension and CHF.[16,17]

Limitations

Probably the biggest limitation of Tc-PYP scans is that deposition of the Tc-PYP in the infarcted tissue depends upon remaining regional blood flow to the infarcted area. Peak effectiveness of Tc-PYP requires a residual blood flow of at least 30% to 40% of normal to the infarcted area.[16] Since, by definition, infarction may occur when blood flow to a section of myocardium is totally blocked, this means that some infarcted areas may not receive any Tc-PYP, and therefore will not light up on the scan. Therefore, *a negative Tc-PYP scan does not prove there is no infarct.*

The affinity of Tc-PYP for calcium can lead to false-positive scans for MI due to uptake in other calcium-containing structures in and around the heart. These include calcified costochondral (rib) cartilages, heart valves, aorta, aneurysms, and inflammatory lesions. Other causes of damaged myocardial cells can also lead to false-positives—trauma, cardioversion, tumor, infection, and infiltrative diseases. Diffuse Tc-PYP uptake around the heart can be due to the circulating blood pool of tracer as it fills the ventricles.[16,17]

Procedure

Technetium pyrophosphate scanning is performed at rest and, because patients are suspected of AMI, must be done with close monitoring and trained personnel. Some centers use bedside cameras to perform

FIGURE 5.9

Technetium Tc 99m pyrophosphate infarct scan: Technetium Tc 99m pyrophospate is taken up preferentially by bone and by infarcted myocardium. The tracer is taken up by sternum and ribs, but also by the inferior myocardium (arrow), indicating an area of myocardial infarction.

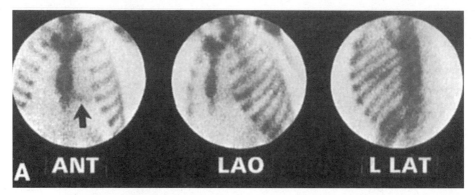

From: Elliott LP. *Cardiac Imaging in Infants, Children and Adults*. Philadelphia: JB Lippincott; 1991:196. Used with permission.)

Tc-PYP scans in the intensive care unit. Optimum time for the scan is from 48 to 72 hours after the suspected infarct or symptoms, although scans can be positive from 12 hours up to 7 to 10 days. There is no need to withhold food or medication. A single injection of 15 to 20 mCi of Tc-PYP is given, and the scan is performed 2 to 4 hours later.[16] A single scan session is required, lasting about 30 minutes. There is no special aftercare other than determining the patient's tolerance of the procedure.

Technetium Tc 99m Sestamibi

Although thallium has the widest use as a tracer for myocardial scans, studies of newer technetium compounds suggest that these agents are better than thallium in several ways.[1,18] Thallium has a long half-life (73 hours) and so must be given in small amounts, lest the radiation load for the patient be too great. This low tracer intensity leads to suboptimal images on the scan. The compound technetium Tc 99m sestamibi (Cardiolite) has higher energy intensity but a shorter half-life (6 hours), allowing higher-definition scan pictures with no greater patient risk than thallium.

FIGURE 5.10

Highly positive technetium infarct scan. Almost the entire myocardium has been highlighted by technetium Tc 99m pyrophosphate, indicating a massive infarct around all segments of the heart.

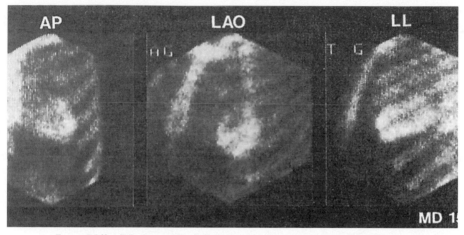

From: Miller DD, Burns RJ, Gill JB, Ruddy TD, et al. *Clinical Cardiac Imaging*. New York: McGraw-Hill; 1988:343. Used with permission.

Myocardial Scanning with Technetium Tc 99m Sestamibi

Like thallium, technetium Tc 99m sestamibi is distributed to myocardial cells in proportion to the blood supply they receive, and thus measures myocardial perfusion. The mechanism of technetium Tc 99m sestamibi transport into myocardial cells is not well understood, but it does not use the sodium-potassium pump. Technetium Tc 99m sestamibi binds to cell proteins, and washout from the cell is slower. Therefore, scanning can be done up to several hours after injection, if needed. Studies show good correlation between the results of thallium and Technetium Tc 99m sestamibi scans, with similar diagnostic and prognostic value (Figure 5.11).[1,18]

Procedure

Technetium Tc 99m sestamibi is used in much the same manner as thallium: with rest, exercise, and vasodilator–drug scans. Often the stress-then-rest scan sequence is reversed with technetium Tc 99m sestamibi, which due to its properties can be used in a rest-then-stress order—thus giving a "true" resting scan.[1] The patient receives up to 30 mCi of technetium Tc 99m sestamibi intravenously about 1 hour before the rest scan. Approximately 3 hours later 25 mCi is injected at peak stress; the second scan is performed 1 hour after the second injection.

Advantages of Technetium Tc 99m Sestamibi

Its provision of more detailed perfusion images has led technitium Tc 99m sestamibi to be chosen by some authors as the successor to thallium for myocardial scans.[4] The technetium agent also facilitates better SPECT performance and seems to allow better visualization of the right ventricle. An acutely infarcting patient can be given technetium Tc 99m sestamibi *before* reperfusion with thrombolysis; due to its slow washout, the technetium will mark the prethrombolytic state of the myocardium for the scan done *after* the artery is opened. A subsequent injection of technetium Tc 99m sestamibi will then light up the newly reperfused areas for comparison to the pretreatment state.[1,18]

FIGURE 5.11

Technetium Tc 99m sestamibi scan. Slice-image SPECT scans using technetium Tc 99m sestamibi. (Left) Images following tracer injection, in the emergency department, of a patient with acute anterior infarction. (Right) Images taken after the artery was reopened and perfusion restored (before discharge).

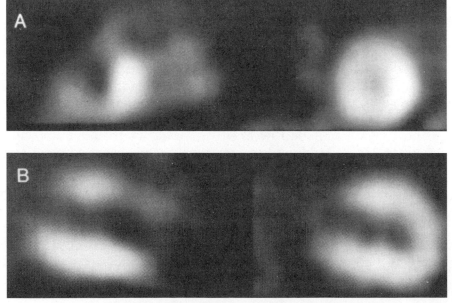

From: Gibbons RJ. Technetium 99m sestamibi in the assessment of acute myocardial infarction. *Semin Nucl Med.* 1991;21:213. Used with permission.

The higher-energy nature of technetium makes additional applications possible. Technetium Tc 99m sestamibi has been shown to be comparable to to the conventional technetium Tc 99m pertechnate agents for use in first-pass blood-pool imaging, and MUGA scans. Therefore, with the right scan equipment, an injection of technetium Tc 99m sestamibi can be used to evaluate both left ventricular function and myocardial perfusion—in effect combining the purposes of traditional thallium and MUGA scans in one test.

Technetium Tc 99m Teboroxime

Another technetium agent, technetium Tc 99m teboroxime (Cardiotec), has appeared attractive because it is both extracted by the myocardium very quickly and washed out rapidly, allowing for rapid scan results and a need for minimal time between rest and exercise scans.[1] Image quality is about the same as that of thallium. Technetium Tc 99m teboroxime does not stay in the myocardium long and thus makes SPECT imaging difficult.[18] Its widespread use may need to wait for development of faster scanning cameras.

ANTIMYOSIN MONOCLONAL ANTIBODY SCANS

A new technology being studied for myocardial imaging is the use of radio-labeled antibodies to the intracellular protein myosin. Myosin, along with the other contractile protein, actin, works to cause the contraction of each muscle cell. In the healthy myocardial cell, the cell membrane will block any antimyosin antibodies from entering and attaching to the myosin. However, an infarcted, necrotic myocardial cell loses its membrane integrity, thus allowing antimyosin antibodies to enter and latch onto the myosin proteins. Researchers artificially produce antimyosin antibodies and label them with a radioactive tracer such as indium 111. The injected antibodies will attach to necrotic cells, thus outlining the area of a myocardial infarction on a scan for the indium 111 (Figure 5.12). Sensitivity for detecting MI has been around 87%, with detection of smaller infarcts possible than with technetium Tc 99m pyrophospate scans.[3,19]

Antimyosin antibody imaging has shown promise in two other areas. First, the scan can detect cardiac transplant rejection with an accuracy similar to that of biopsy.[3,19] Antibody scans may eventually show superiority over biopsy alone, which samples only a small part of the myocardium (compared to the whole-myocardium scope of the scan). The antibody imaging is also sensitive in detecting myocarditis, or inflammation of the myocardium, which results in a diffuse uptake of antimyosin antibodies. Note that some false-positives can be caused by other conditions such as fibrosis.[3,19]

FIGURE 5.12

Antimyosin antibody scans of the myocardium. **(A)** Two views in a normal antimyosin antibody scan. The liver (lower left in each image) shows high uptake
of the tracer, but there is little or none in the heart (center of image). **(B)** Similar
views in a patient whose myocardium readily takes up antimyosin antibodies in
the anterior wall, indicating myocardial infarction. **(C)** Another antimyosin antibody scan, this time in a patient with inflammatory myocarditis. Note the diffuse
uptake throughout the entire heart.

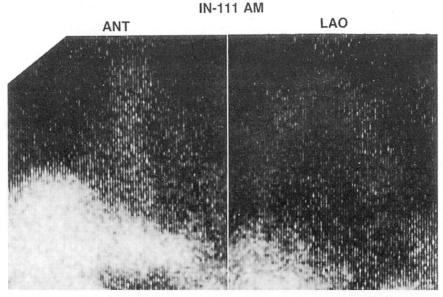

A

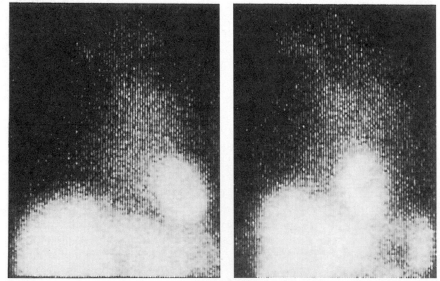

B

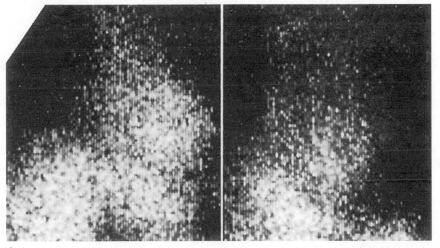

C

From: Miller DD, Burns RJ, Gill JB, Ruddy TD, et al. *Clinical Cardiac Imaging.* New York: McGraw-Hill; 1988:16–17. Used with permission.

Imaging is done using a standard scintillation camera, with either planar or SPECT technique. The antibody is cleared from the body within 24 to 48 hours. Theoretically, there can be adverse immune reactions in the host when the antimyosin antibodies are injected. Although further studies are needed, one study reported "no adverse responses" among its subjects.[3,19] A skin test for human antimurine antibodies may be performed before the antimyosin antibodies are injected, to screen for possible allergic response.

NURSING IMPLICATIONS OF MYOCARDIAL SCANS

The nurse plays an important role in preparing the patient for a nuclear medicine scan, ensuring patient safety and comfort as well as a useful diagnostic result. Some general principles apply to patient preparation and education for all of the scans, with some details particular to the type of test.

The patient may be anxious about the word *nuclear* or the use of radiation in the nuclear tracer. He or she should be reassured that the radiation exposure of most scans is about the same as a regular chest x-ray, and that the tracer is eliminated from the body in a few hours.[20] Pregnant women should probably not have nuclear scans due to unknown effects on the fetus. Patients unable to lie still on the scan table may have difficulty with this test.

Usually the patient is kept NPO for 3 or 4 hours before the scan, although some institutions will allow clear, noncaffeinated liquids or even a light breakfast if the test is to be later in the day.[20,21] As most scans require two sessions, these dietary restrictions should be maintained until the second scan is completed. Most but not all medications may be given as usual, but aminophylline/theophylline drugs, caffeine, and dipyridamole should be withheld before a scan using dipyridamole or adenosine; sometimes nitrates or beta-blocking drugs may be withheld for the preceding 24 to 48 hours. An intravenous line or heparin lock will be needed for all of the scans.

Patients undergoing an exercise test should be screened for their tolerance of the procedure. Those with a recent myocardial infarction, significant congestive heart failure, cardiomyopathy, or lung disease should not be doing a maximal stress test but may undergo a resting or possibly a submaximal (low-intensity) exercise routine.[20] Loose, comfortable clothing and nonskid shoes should be worn. Men may be asked to disrobe from the waist up, while women may wear a bra if it does not have metal underwire.

The patient undergoing an exercise thallium scan (see Patient Education Box 5.1) will have ECG monitor leads placed on the chest and a resting ECG taken. With the leads still in place, the patient then walks on a treadmill or pedals a stationary bicycle in a gradually escalating workload. Under the common Bruce protocols, the incline and/or speed of the treadmill is increased every 3 minutes.[20] Thallium is injected into the IV when the patient reaches a certain level of exercise, feels tired, or develops chest pain or other symptoms. (The injection is usually not felt, but some patients have brief flushing or dizziness.) If possible, the patient exercises for one more minute to circulate the tracer. Immediately, the patient is escorted to the scan table, where he or she lies with arms overhead for 10 to 40 minutes while a camera is rotated across the body taking pictures. It is important that the patient lie still.

The patient returns to the room or waiting area for 2 to 4 hours, still restricted to noncaffeinated liquids or perhaps a light snack. The IV remains in place.[20,21] On returning to the scan room, the patient has a similar scan session, but without the exercise. Many centers employ a second thallium injection just before the resting scan.

After the second scan session, patients may resume previous medicines, diet, and activities. They should be encouraged to drink plenty of liquids in the next few hours to aid in renal excretion of the tracer. No special precautions need be taken with the patient or their body fluids in regard to the thallium tracer.

In dipyridamole or adenosine thallium tests, the patient does not exercise but is first given either oral dipyridamole 20 to 40 minutes before the scan, IV dipyridamole 5 minutes before the scan, or IV adenosine at the time of the scan.[20,21] Flushing, nausea, and headache are common but will only last a few minutes; the patient is asked to endure these if he or she can. (Adenosine effects wear off in 5 minutes or so, and dipyridamole effects can be reversed with IV aminophylline.) The scan is then

PATIENT EDUCATION BOX 5.1

Thallium Scan

The purpose of the thallium scan is to determine how healthy your heart muscle is. This study will be done so that the best treatment for you can be prescribed. The study is done in two parts, each lasting about 1½ hours.

BEFORE THE TEST

Do not eat or drink anything after midnight the evening before the test unless instructed to do so by your doctor or nurse.

Take your medications as prescribed unless your doctor or nurse tells you otherwise. Certain medications may interfere with the test and thus you may be asked to not take them for a day prior to the procedure.

Wear comfortable, loose-fitting clothing. If you are to exercise, wear sneakers or rubber-soled walking shoes.

DURING THE TEST

You will be given an intravenous (IV) line in your hand or arm if one is not already in place. A slightly radioactive tracer, thallium, is then injected into the IV. The tracer makes the heart muscle visible to the special camera but does not cause harm to your body.

You will lie on a special table with your arms above you head while the pictures are taken. The camera rotates slowly around your chest.

If you are having an exercise study, you will be asked to walk on a treadmill for a few minutes. The speed and incline of the treadmill will be gradually increased. It is important to give your best effort.

If you are having an adenosine or dipyridamole thallium study, a drug will be given to you to increase your heart rate. This may cause a hot, flushed feeling and some nausea. These sensations will quickly pass. Report any unpleasant sensations to the doctor.

Be sure to tell the doctor, nurse, or technician if you have chest pain, shortness of breath, or dizziness.

AFTER THE FIRST PART OF THE TEST

You will be allowed to leave the test area until it is time to return for the second part of the scan, usually 3 to 4 hours later. It is important to avoid food, smoking, and caffeine until the second part of the test is done. You may drink juices and soft drinks that do not have caffeine.

AFTER THE TEST IS OVER

After the second part of the study, you may resume your usual activities, diet, and medications. Drink plenty of fluids for the next day or so, to help your body eliminate the tracer.

performed as noted above; after a 2- to 4-hour rest period, a follow-up scan without the adenosine or dipyridamole, is taken.

Technetium Tc 99m sestamibi and technetium Tc 99m teburoxime scans are similar to a thallium scan. However, the sequence of scans may be reversed: that is, the resting scan may be performed first, with the exercise scan done some hours later.[1] Adenosine and dipyridamole may be used, as described above. The technetium agents may allow for a faster scan, reducing the time the patient has to lie still on the table.

The technetium Tc 99m pyrophosphate infarct scan involves one scan done at rest; the IV injection is given at bedside 3 to 6 hours before the scan.[21] This is not done as an outpatient test, as the patient needing this scan is suspected of having an acute or recent myocardial infarction.

RADIONUCLIDE VENTRICULOGRAPHY

Radionuclide ventriculography (RNVG) uses radioactive labeling of the blood to study the working action of the heart. Whereas the myocardial scans test the relative health of the heart muscle, the RNVG scans measure the heart's *performance*—which, for the heart, means how strongly and efficiently the ventricles are pumping. A patient whose heart is pumping less vigorously than normal, or shows areas of abnormal muscle action, is likely to have ischemia, infarction, or other heart dysfunction. Radionuclide ventriculography can help diagnose coronary artery disease and cardiomyopathy, as well as provide data for prognosis.

There are two distinct tests that both employ RNVG: the first-pass scan and the gated blood pool imaging technique.[22] Both provide similar information about heart function, but each has practical considerations that may justify using one method over the other in certain situations. First-pass and gated blood pool studies may both be performed in the same scan session.

First-pass studies use a bolus of technetium-99m pertechnetate injected intravenously, immediately followed by rapid heart imaging as the tracer bolus makes its "first pass" through the heart. The heart chambers are thus well outlined through one or more cardiac cycles.[22]

In *gated blood pool imaging*, the patient's red blood cells are labeled with a technetium 99m tracer and the radioactive marker is allowed to distribute evenly throughout the "blood pool" before scanning begins. The gating technique is used to build a composite cinematic loop of a single heart cycle, with the cumulative data from many heartbeats formed into one set of images. Several terms have been used for the gated blood pool imaging scan; *MUGA* (multiple gated acquisition) is the most common, and will be used in this chapter to refer to all gated blood pool studies.[3,22]

Principles

Studying a heart in action is challenging because it is a moving target in which the object of interest, the cardiac cycle, takes place in 1 second or less. The first-pass and MUGA techniques are made possible by high-speed scintillation cameras that can take accurate radioactivity counts in a very short time (Figure 5.13). The patient's blood is labeled with radioactive contrast material so that the chambers of the heart can be outlined as the marked blood passes through. A fast series of images is then processed by a computer to form digital images of the heart at various points in the cardiac cycle. Data may be obtained from a single camera angle for first-pass studies, but when feasible the three standard cardiac views—left anterior oblique (LAO), anterior (ANT), and left lateral (LAT)—are used to give more accurate findings.

The results from the RNVG scan include the following data on heart function and structure.

FIGURE 5.13

Scintillation camera. A representative nuclear scanner, used in tests such as MUGA imaging and first-pass studies. The computer processes radioactivity counts collected by the camera into images of the heart.

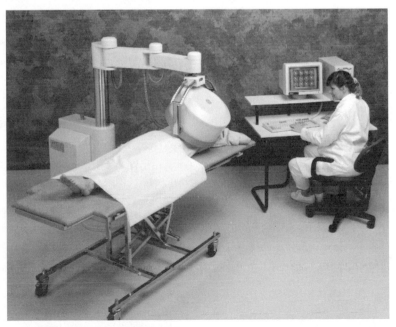

Courtesy of ADAC Laboratories.

Ejection fraction

Ejection fraction (EF) is defined as the *percentage* of blood in a heart chamber at the end of diastole (ventricular filling) that is actually pumped out of the chamber during systole (ventricular pumping). For example, if 60 mL of blood is in the left ventricle at the end of filling (diastole) and 30 mL is pumped out (during systole), then the left ventricular ejection fraction (LVEF) is said to be 50%. Normal LVEF at rest is 50% to 65%, with higher EFs found in some athletes and in patients with certain pathological conditions. The right ventricle ejection fraction (RVEF) is harder to reliably calculate because of overlying heart structures; normal RVEF is 40% to 65%.[3]

The LVEF is considered by some clinicians to be the most important single finding of the MUGA and first-pass tests because it gives an overall measure of ventricular health by looking directly at performance.[22] Others caution that LVEF must be interpreted carefully, citing the many factors that can alter a patient's ejection fraction (see below on limitations of RNVG).

Ventricular Wall Motion

In the normal heart, there is an orderly contraction of the heart muscle during each cardiac cycle; the apex and septum of the heart move less than the other ventricular walls.[3] With ischemia or infarction, the affected region of the heart muscle will not move, or will have an abnormal motion. These irregularities of wall motion are characterized as *global* (all walls similarly affected) or *regional* (some areas moving better than others). An abnormal motion may be *hypokinetic* (some motion present, but decreased), *akinetic* (no movement), or *dyskinetic* (motion in the opposite direction of normal, such as outward during systole). Both MUGA and first-pass studies show the heart in motion; the cardiologist visually assesses the film loop of the cardiac cycle and can identify abnormal movement of certain parts of the heart wall.[22]

Structural and Functional Assessment

Abnormally large or small heart chambers can be measured with MUGA and first-pass techniques. Left ventricular volumes at various stages of the heart cycle can be calculated. Heart valve function can be observed, particularly for aortic or mitral regurgitation. Areas within the heart that have low technetium 99m counts may represent clots or tumors (see text following). Structural problem areas such as aneurysms and shunts can usually be recognized on these radionuclide scans.[3,22]

Role of Exercise

As noted in the section on myocardial scans, the patient with coronary artery disease (CAD) may have adequate coronary flow at rest to permit normal heart pumping and no symptoms, and thus a normal resting radionuclide scan. A resting test may be helpful in assessing a patient with unstable angina (symptoms at rest) or known myocardial infarction (MI). But in less symptomatic patients, it may only be when the greater demands of exercise are made on the heart that ischemia may show itself. For this reason most first-pass and MUGA scans are done with exercise whenever possible.[1]

Both first-pass and MUGA studies can incorporate exercise. The usual method has been supine or upright bicycle exercise because the chest is usually more stable for imaging than when walking or running.[1,22] Some authors advocate use of treadmills because of their well-established use in other cardiac tests and the coordination/leg effort problems with bicycling.[23] In first-pass studies, separate injections of tracer may be given at various levels of exercise, with quick imaging at each dose; thus the patient need not sustain the exercise level for long periods. In MUGA, the gating process requires a relatively steady heart rate for 2 to 3 minutes at each level of exercise while images are taken. Therefore, some authors suggest that first-pass studies are superior for obtaining ejection fractions at peak exercise, while gated blood pool studies may be more sensitive for wall motion abnormalities.[24]

An increase in LVEF with exercise has been the most common criterion for a normal ventricular study; in previous studies of normal hearts, the LVEF could be expected to increase 5% or more at peak exercise. With CAD, the patient's LVEF will usually fail to rise or may even fall in response to exercise because narrowed coronary arteries cannot supply blood needed for more work; the result is less pumping ability. This ischemia may also show up as wall motion abnormalities on MUGA or first-pass tests.[23,24]

Gender differences are important when interpreting test results.[25] As with most cardiac studies in the past, the determination of "normal" LVEF response to exercise was based until recently on studies of men. However, women typically do not have a significant rise in LVEF during exercise; they create the higher cardiac output through an increase in LV end-diastolic volume, rather than in the percentage ejected. If this were not taken into account, a woman with little or no increase in LVEF on an RNVG test could be considered abnormal and thus could be diagnosed with CAD. Clearly, criteria need to be developed for women's test results, probably with a fall in LVEF or wall motion abnormalities as standards for a positive test.

First-Pass Studies

In first-pass studies, a bolus of technetium-99m pertechnetate is injected through an intravenous line, a few seconds before imaging (Figure 5.14). Scintillation cameras are then used to take separate images as little as 25 milliseconds apart. In a typical series, from 5 to 30 seconds of imaging is performed as the bolus travels through the heart. Images taken every 25 milliseconds for thirty seconds will produce some 1200 images

FIGURE 5.14

First-pass radionuclide study. A series of eight sequential images shows a bolus of technetium tracer entering the right side of the heart, separately showing the right ventricle (frame 3) and later the left ventricle (frames 6–8).

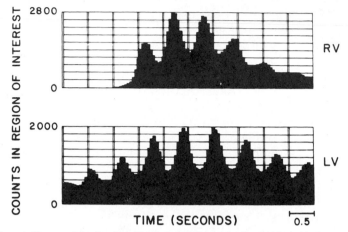

From: Gerson M. *Cardiac Nuclear Medicine.* 2nd ed. New York: McGraw-Hill; 1991:68. Used with permission.

for computer processing. A real-time film loop is produced that can be slowed down by the operator to see details of wall motion.[24]

As a rule, the more intense bolus of radioactivity delivered by the first-pass method allows better imaging of the right ventricle, which is obscured behind other heart structures in most views. Another advantage of first-pass imaging is its ability to assess the heart within a few seconds. This is an asset during exercise studies, when the heart can be studied at various levels of exercise without the patient's needing to maintain a steady effort for extended periods. For this reason, some clinicians favor first-pass studies over the gated blood pool method for studies at peak exercise.[23]

Gated Blood Pool Studies

MUGA uses the blood itself as a carrier for the radioactive technetium tracer to obtain dynamic images of the heart in motion. Once the tracer is evenly distributed in the blood, it provides a continuous source of contrast material as it moves in and out of the heart's chambers. Unlike first-pass imaging, where pictures must be taken in the few seconds after injection and repeated injections given, MUGA studies involve one injection followed by a more prolonged imaging time.[3] MUGA may use the technetium tracer already injected for a first-pass study, provided it has had a few minutes to mix with the blood.

Because technetium 99m does not adhere naturally to red blood cells (RBCs), a tin compound (stannous pyrophosphate) is first injected into the blood, where it binds with the beta-hemoglobin chain inside the RBC.[22] The technetium 99m will then bind with the stannous agent in these pretinned RBCs. Because technetium 99m has a half-life of 6 hours, it remains detectable in the blood for several hours postinjection. Thus the patient may be injected at the bedside anywhere from a few minutes to several hours before the MUGA scan.

Gating Technique

The patient is attached to an ECG machine for the MUGA. This is partly to assess the patient's performance and tolerance of exercise, but the monitor is also essential for ECG gating of the acquired images.[1,3] Gating is necessary because the low density of tracer when mixed into the entire blood pool means a low radioactivity count during any one heart cycle. By combining the images of each heartbeat into one composite image, the total counts are higher—giving a sharper, more useful picture. Triggered by the R wave on the ECG (the first upstroke of each QRS complex), a computer will activate the camera for a certain number of images in each heartbeat (usually from 16 to 64 frames per cardiac cycle). Then the image from each frame of one heartbeat is pooled by the computer with the corresponding frame of every other heartbeat during the acquisition period. Thus a heartbeat cinematic "loop" is produced that is a composite of each heartbeat imaged during the study. During an average 5- to 10-minute acquisition, data from several hundred cardiac cycles are processed to form the final images.

Problems can arise when the upright R waves on the ECG are small or if the length of the RR interval varies. Variable RR intervals occur with an irregular heart rhythm (such as atrial fibrillation, or sinus rhythm with frequent PVCs) or when the patient does not maintain a stable heart rate during exercise. As a general rule, most MUGA studies are aborted if more than 20% of the beats are premature or if the patient has runs of supraventricular or ventricular tachycardia.[22]

Indications for Radionuclide Scanning

Because it can accurately assess the pumping function of the heart, radionuclide ventriculography has been used for several purposes in cardiology. Probably its most common uses are in screening for CAD, evaluating heart function in known CAD/MI, and assessing cardiomyopathies. Other subjects for these scans include heart valve disease, cardiac transplant rejection, and monitoring the effects of cardiotoxic chemotherapy.

Screening for Coronary Artery Disease

MUGA and first-pass scans have been widely used to screen patients at high risk for CAD and those with symptoms suggestive of ischemia. The two criteria most widely used for diagnosis are (1) abnormal ventricular wall motion, and (2) a rise of less than 5% (or a fall) in left ventricular ejection fraction with exercise, bearing in mind gender differences.[23] Most RNVG screening studies are done with exercise in order to elicit any hidden ischemia.

Radionuclide ventricle studies are between 80% and 90% accurate in detecting CAD.[23] An abnormal LVEF with exercise is one of the most sensitive detectors of early CAD. In practice, the degree of abnormality of the LVEF in exercise has become a reliable predictor of the degree of heart disease and a prognostic for cardiac morbidity and mortality. An exercise LVEF of less than 30% is associated with 50% chance of MI and/or death within four years.[22,24]

After Myocardial Infarction

After an MI, the left ventricle (LV) may become dilated and show areas of decreased wall motion, even at rest. The decrease in ejection fraction is usually proportional to the size of the infarct. After several infarctions, the left ventricle may dilate even further, and this large LV may become hypokinetic. The region of the heart affected by abnormal wall motion can give clues to which coronary vessels are diseased: septal and anterior defects suggest the left anterior descending artery; posterior and lateral, the left circumflex; and the inferior wall, the right coronary artery.[23]

Evaluation of Cardiomyopathy

Abnormalities of wall motion and EF are often used to diagnose cardiomyopathy (CMP). The findings on radionuclide scans can vary, depending on the type of CMP present.[3,15] In congestive (dilated) CMP, all four cardiac chambers may be dilated, and both right and left ventricles show severe, global hypokinesis. Ischemic CMP usually shows left ventricular dilation out of proportion to that of the right ventricle, and there are generally regional wall motion abnormalities. Idiopathic CMP (that is, where the cause is unknown) may or may not have regional wall motion abnormalities. Each of these CMP types—congestive, ischemic, and idiopathic—shows a decreased LVEF.

In contrast, in hypertrophic (obstructive) cardiomyopathy the LVEF will be normal or increased, even though the cardiac output may be reduced and the patient's tissues are not being perfused well. This seeming paradox is explained by the nature of this disease and arises from the principles of LVEF calculations.[3,15] In obstructive CMP, the ventricular walls become greatly thickened, making the LV chamber much smaller. Because ejection fraction is calculated by the percentage of blood ejected during systole, the LVEF does not take into account that a much smaller volume of blood can fill the chamber in the first place. Thus a normal LVEF is not actually reassuring in the case of hypertrophic CMP.

Cardiomyopathy patients are often given RNVG studies to follow the evolution of their disease. Documentation of a low LVEF or increasing areas of abnormal wall motion can be indications for a change in therapy or reflect a more urgent need for cardiac transplantation.

Assessing Results of Therapies

Therapies for patients with congestive heart failure and cardiomyopathies might include preload- and afterload-reducing drugs (nitrates and vasodilators) and inotropics such as digitalis. Patients with CAD or AMI may be treated by angioplasty, thrombolytic agents, or bypass surgery. Once interventions to improve cardiac function have been tried, a comparison of baseline and postintervention MUGA or first-pass scans can determine whether LVEF and wall motion have improved.[22,24]

Cardiac Transplantation

The two greatest threats to patients after cardiac transplant are infection and rejection of the new heart by the recipient's body. Some degree of rejection is experienced by almost half of the patients in the first month following transplant.[26] To detect rejection early, posttransplant patients have routine invasive endomyocardial biopsy via cardiac catheterization. Finding lymphocyte infiltration in heart tissue obtained by biopsy is the usual way of diagnosing rejection. While biopsy is the "gold standard" in monitoring for rejection, it is not perfect; there are some 15% false-negatives, and a false-positive may be had by inadvertently taking a sample from a previous site of biopsy.[26]

Radionuclide ventriculography can be a useful complement to biopsy in screening for posttransplant rejection. One study found that there was little or no change in LVEF with mild rejection. However, those in moderate to severe rejection (per biopsy) showed changes in EF. Some 80% of those in moderate to severe rejection had abnormal heart wall motion seen on MUGA scan. After successful treatment of rejection, most patients' LVEF and wall motion return to normal; failure to increase LVEF with treatment suggests a poor prognosis.[26] While it will probably not completely replace biopsy, MUGA provides a noninvasive test to verify a biopsy result or quantify the functional results of rejection.

Cardiac Valve Disease

Radionuclide scans are useful in evaluating the effects of heart valve disorders on heart function. Abnormal heart valves can cause pressure and volume overloads on the ventricles. In aortic stenosis, pressure overloads on the left ventricle at first cause hypertrophy, and later, dilation of the ventricle wall. With both aortic insufficiency and mitral regurgitation, excessive volume leads to LV dilation. Ejection fractions may at first be normal, then decline as the disease progresses. Computer processing of radioactivity counts can give figures on the degree of valve regurgitation. By following the EF and other parameters, cardiologists can make better recommendations about the need for and timing of valve replacement.[3,24]

Mural Thrombi and Cardiac Tumors

Mural thrombi (blood clots inside a heart chamber) can usually be seen on MUGA as a "filling defect," with less than expected counts.[3] Only the blood on the outside of the clot or tumor is labeled with technetium, whereas the RBCs within the body of the clot give out no radioactive counts. Thus the area has a lower count density than other blood-filled regions of the ventricle. Cardiac tumors, if large enough, will change the normal outline of the chamber seen on the scans.

Other Indications

For patients receiving potentially cardiotoxic chemotherapy agents such as doxirubicin and adriamycin, radionuclide studies can evaluate for signs of adverse effects on heart muscle by measuring ejection fractions.[22] Radionuclide scans can also be used to determine cor pulmonale. This disease, an enlargement and dysfunction of the right ventricle whose primary cause is lung disease such as COPD, can be diagnosed by RNVG imaging of the right ventricle.[22]

One of the first uses of radionuclide ventricle testing was in the diagnosis of congenital heart defects in children.[24] It can highlight flow defects and altered heart chamber shapes.

Finally, MUGA imaging also detects left ventricular aneurysms with an accuracy rate of about 96% (Figure 5.15).[16]

Strengths and Limitations of Radionuclide Scans

The radionuclide ventriculogram can accurately assess the pumping function of the heart both at rest and during exercise. Given the assumption that abnormalities in ejection fraction or wall motion are a sign of myocardial ischemia or infarction, MUGA and first-pass scans can readily be used to detect and assess the consequences of CAD. They complement cardiac catheterization by detailing the effects of coronary blockages on the actual working of the heart and help establish a prognosis.[22] Scans taken over time can be used to chart improvement or decline in ventricular function with therapy or disease progression. Radionuclide tests also complement other studies for transplant rejection, valve disease, and cardiomyopathy.

FIGURE 5.15

Left ventricular aneurysm on radionuclide scan. Images of the left ventricle during diastole ("filling") and systole ("pumping") show a ventricular aneurysm at bottom right of the image, which abnormally retains some technetium 99m-labeled blood as the heart chamber empties.

DIASTOLE   SYSTOLE

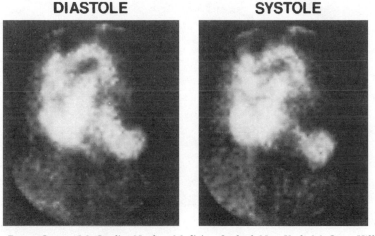

From: Gerson M. *Cardiac Nuclear Medicine*. 2nd ed. New York: McGraw-Hill; 1991: 361. Used with permission.

Compared to other cardiac testing technologies, radionuclide ventricular scanners are moderately priced and relatively portable. Many institutions have portable MUGA units that can be brought to the patient's bedside[3] (Figure 5.16).

However, while they are widely accepted as a screening and evaluation tool, radionuclide studies are not without theoretical and technical problems. Some authors object to overuse of the LVEF as a criterion, citing the factors other than CAD than can cause LVEF to be lower than expected, including dehydration, concurrent illness, drug effects, and age.[24] Others point out that the "normals" for MUGA are largely based on middle-aged male test subjects—and that an *increase* in LVEF with exercise may not be normal for women, the elderly, and some other patients.[23,25]

Technical problems can include poor R wave signal (affecting gating), arrhythmias, poor RBC labeling, camera out of position, patient motion, and errors of interpretation of wall motion.[24] False-positive findings can be due to hypertension, drugs (beta-blockers), left bundle branch block, and exercise beyond tolerance. False-negative findings can occur with anti-ischemic drugs (nitrates, calcium channel blockers), subtle abnormalities, inadequate exercise, and abnormalities out of view of camera. Interpretation of RNVG images is complex and requires adequate training and experience.

FIGURE 5.16

Portable nuclear scanner. One of the strengths of nuclear medicine tests such as MUGA is the relative portability of the equipment. Here, a portable nuclear scanner is being taken to the patient's bedside in the coronary care unit.

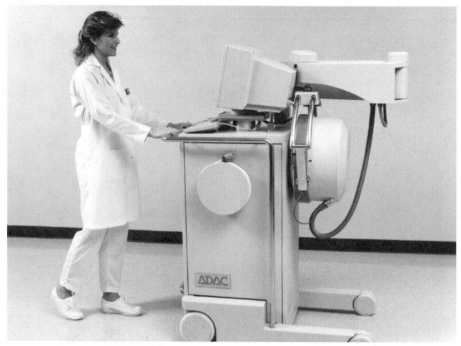

Courtesy of ADAC Laboratories.

Future of Radionuclide Ventricular Studies

Short-Acting Agents

Various substances for first-pass studies are being studied to see if intense but short-lived tracers can improve image quality while reducing overall radiation load for the patient.[24] Examples include tantalum 178 (half-life = 9.3 min), gold 195 (half-life = 30 sec), and iridium 191 (half-life = 5 sec). The challenge with some of these agents is that their half-lives are *so* short it is difficult to get them from the isotope generator to the patient quickly enough.

Myocardial perfusion testing agents such as technetium Tc 99m teburoxime and technetium Tc 99m sestamibi have been explored as doing double duty as tracers for first-pass studies.[23] These agents are being injected into the patient's IV anyway to perform perfusion studies; if the injection is made as a rapid bolus, a camera can be ready to take first-pass pictures as the bolus enters the heart. In this way the ventriculography and myocardial perfusion test can be done at the same sitting.

NURSING IMPLICATIONS OF RADIONUCLIDE TESTS

Patients undergoing radionuclide studies may range from a stable out-patient to a victim of recent myocardial infarction. The nurse must assess each patient's level of anxiety and knowledge base as well as his or her physical needs to assure the best outcome for the patient (See Patient Education Box 5.2).

Preparations will vary somewhat depending upon whether the patient is to have a resting or exercise study and on whether he or she is having first-pass studies only or also a MUGA scan. The patient's general health and inpatient/outpatient status should also be considered.

Generally, meals do not need to be withheld entirely before a radionuclide scan, but the patient should avoid eating a recent heavy meal. Medications may usually be given unless otherwise ordered. (*Note*: intravenous heparin may interfere with the marking of the red blood cells with the tracer and may be ordered held before a MUGA.[22]) The patient is encouraged to void before the procedure for the sake of comfort. An intravenous line, ECG leads, and comfortable clothing are necessary for the test. Other nuclear medicine procedures, such as bone scans, should be separated from these tests by 24 to 48 hours to prevent interference between radioactive tracers.[27,28]

The resting scan takes about 30 minutes and the patient simply lies still on the exam table with the camera close to the chest. The camera's position may be changed every few minutes. A patient having the MUGA scan will first receive an injection with nonradioactive stannous pyrophosphate (for the first-pass studies only, this step is omitted.) The technetium-99m pertechnetate injection is given 15 to 30 minutes later. Scanning usually follows a few minutes after the second injection.[27,28]

The exercise scan follows a similar procedure, except the patient is asked to pedal a stationary bicycle in either the upright or supine position. Pedaling while supine may be strange or unsettling to the patient; it helps to expect it beforehand and to know that testing personnel will provide instructions and support. The patient should give his or her best effort at exercise and try to keep the chest still during the scanning. Exercise testing extends the MUGA test to 1 to 2 hours.[27,29]

The ill patient may be anxious about his or her condition and ability to tolerate a diagnostic test. The idea of having a nuclear scan may be intimidating. It may help the patient to know that the radiation dose is low (similar to that of a GI x-ray) and that the tracer weakens over a few hours' time, leaving no lasting effects. The camera may be brought to the bedside, but it can be quite large and the patient should be fore-warned about its size.[27,28]

There is no special aftercare following a radionuclide scan. Routine universal precautions with gloves is sufficient for handling the patient's urine afterward. Visitors need not be restricted.[27]

PATIENT EDUCATION BOX 5.2

MUGA Scan

The purpose of a MUGA scan is to see how well the heart is pumping. A small amount of slightly radioactive material (which is not harmful to you) is used to make your blood visible to a special camera. The camera takes pictures of the heart as the blood moves in and out. The test takes 1 to 2 hours.

BEFORE THE TEST

It is best to not eat heavily before the test. Check with your doctor or nurse to see if any of your prescription medications should be stopped temporarily (some heart medicines might interfere with the MUGA scan). Comfortable, loose clothing is best—if you are a hospital patient, pajamas are fine. You will be asked to remove your shirt or blouse for the test and will be given a hospital gown.

DURING THE TEST

An intravenous (IV) line will be placed in your arm if one is not already in place. One or two doses of the tracer material will be given in the IV. You should not feel any side effects from the injections. The technician will attach the leads for an ECG machine to your chest and put a blood pressure cuff on your arm.

If you are having a resting MUGA scan (no exercise or extra medicines), you will go directly to the scan table, where you will lie down on your back. You may be asked to hold your arms over your head. A large camera that takes pictures of the heart will be placed next to your chest. It will be moved to take pictures from different angles.

If you are having an exercise (stress) MUGA test, you will be shown how to pedal the bicycle. This may be done either in an upright position or lying on your back. The camera will take pictures of your heart while you are pedaling. You should give your best effort, as instructed, to help the test be most accurate. The staff will check your blood pressure and pulse and will watch your heart on the monitor. *Be sure to tell them if you have any unpleasant symptoms* such as chest pain, shortness of breath, or nausea.

AFTER THE TEST

After you have finished the scan you may leave. You may go back to your usual diet and medicines. The tracer material will eliminate itself from your body in a few hours, and there are no aftereffects.

POSITRON EMISSION TOMOGRAPHY

Positron emission tomography (PET) imaging was introduced in the 1970s and has evolved into a cardiovascular imaging technique valuable in evaluating tissue viability and function. What distinguishes PET imaging from conventional imaging techniques is its ability to provide quantitative evaluation of tissue function. This means that PET imaging can identify metabolically active tissue. Identification of such tissue is especially pertinent today because more refined methods of reperfusion are becoming available to cardiologists. Reperfusion therapy via thrombolytic drugs and mechanical interventions allows preservation of myocardium and reduction of infarct size. PET imaging assists in determining which regions of the myocardium have viable but jeopardized tissue that could benefit from revascularization techniques and which areas have undergone complete infarction.[30]

Principles of PET Imaging

Imaging with PET is accomplished through the use of positron-emitting radionuclides, which are characterized by an imbalance of protons. The proton converts to a neutron to stabilize the nuclear structure and a positronium that quickly decays by annihilation, generating a pair of photons. These photons travel in opposite directions and are detected by the scanners. The major objective of PET, therefore, is to label physiologically active substrates with positron-emitting radionuclides and acquire images of the radionuclide distribution in the heart following injection of the tracer.[30]

Basic knowledge of cardiac metabolism is essential for understanding PET imaging principles. The normal heart derives most of its energy from oxidation of fatty acids. Fatty acid oxidation is sensitive to oxygen deprivation, therefore, when the heart is ischemic, glucose use is transiently increased by anaerobic breakdown of exogenous glucose and endogenous glycogen. This process continues as long as lactate is removed from the cell and depends on the level of blood flow. If blood flow is decreased, there is an increase in lactate accumulation, which stops glycolysis and results in necrosis. To determine metabolic activity, a glucose-like substance is used to measure glucose uptake in myocardial cells. The substance most frequently used is fluorodeoxyglucose 18 or [18]FDG.

Evaluation of myocardial perfusion or blood flow is accomplished through use of a second positron-emitting radionuclide. Rubidium 82 or N-13 ammonia ($^{13}NH_3$) are used to measure the degree of blood flow to the cell. These tracers are taken up by myocardial cells. By comparing the resting state to the vasodilated state, flow reserve and the functional significance of coronary lesions can be determined. Coronary vasodilation is accomplished by the use of dipyridamole, adenosine, or exercise.

Uses of PET Imaging

PET imaging may be used to evaluate the significance of coronary disease, to detect silent ischemia, to determine flow reserve during exercise, and to assess tissue viability after myocardial infarction. It can also be used to determine the degree of success after such procedures as coronary artery bypass grafting, PTCA, or other revascularization processes.

To determine the absence or presence of viable myocardium, a comparison of images obtained with ^{18}FDG and ^{13}NH$_3$ is made. If ^{13}NH$_3$ uptake is decreased or absent (indicating decreased coronary flow) and ^{18}FDG uptake is high (indicating intact metabolism), this is referred to as a *mismatch*. A mismatch predicts that there is little or no blood flow but potentially salvageable ischemic myocardium. Matched images, however, demonstrate that uptake of ^{18}FDG and ^{13}NH$_3$ is absent, which indicates no blood flow and nonviable, necrotic myocardium.

Imaging with PET allows the noninvasive evaluation of regional cardiac metabolism. The combination of tracers used for blood flow and metabolism provides the ability to identify myocardium with reduced blood flow and potentially viable tissue by determining the metabolic rate. Maintained metabolism in the presence of reduced coronary flow is indicative of myocardial tissue recovery following revascularization. This diagnostic technique is useful in identifying a myocardial infarction, distinguishing reversible from irreversible ischemic injury, and determining the extent to which revascularization techniques resulted in the salvage of myocardial tissue.[31,32]

Comparison with Conventional Imaging

The two most common types of cardiac radionuclide imaging scans are thallium 201 scintigraphy and technetium 99m ventriculography. In the first procedure, thallium, the radioactive analogue of potassium, is extracted by cardiac muscle fibers. The uptake of thallium depends on the patency of the coronary arteries. If a significant coronary artery lesion is present, the myocardium supplied by that artery will receive less blood flow; therefore, less thallium will be extracted. Coronary artery perfusion is the predominant factor affecting initial thallium uptake, which makes the thallium scan an excellent technique for evaluating perfusion.[33]

The MUGA scan or radionuclide ventriculogram is useful in determining the wall motion of the left ventricle and the ventricle's ability to eject blood. Images obtained with MUGA scanning are images representing the blood pool within the ventricular and atrial cavities. Because myocardial ischemia reduces myocardial contractility, an ischemic segment of myocardium will exhibit diminished contractility, which is detectable with a MUGA scan. Radionuclide ventriculography, therefore, is useful in evaluating function.

Imaging with PET differs from these two conventional scans by distinguishing metabolically active areas of myocardium from nonmetabolically active areas. Given that metabolic abnormalities will reflect an underlying pathologic condition, data obtained from PET imaging can indicate which tissue is viable and could benefit from revascularization techniques.

Patient Preparation

Education is the most important part of preparing a patient for a PET scan. The patient should be told that radioactive isotopes will be used to assess the function of the heart. These isotopes are not harmful to the patient and are rapidly removed from the body (half-life of $^{13}NH_3$ = 10 min; half-life of rubidium 82 = 72 sec; half-life of ^{18}FDG = 120 min). The patient will be placed inside a doughnut-shaped scanning device. Sometimes the patient's arms may be restrained at the sides to prevent movement during the scan. The $^{13}NH_3$ and ^{18}FDG are given by separate IV injections. The patient will be asked to lie still during the procedure although he or she will be able to communicate with the technologists. The technicians (and in some cases, the nurse accompanying the patient) will remain in an adjoining room to monitor the patient. The length of the scanning procedure may range from 1 to 4 hours.

Nurses should administer all medications prior to the PET scan, unless directed otherwise. Critically ill patients may need to be accompanied by a nurse or physician. Continuous ECG monitoring is available during the scan.

References

1. Alazraki N. Nuclear imaging of the cardiovascular system. In: Elliott LP. Cardiac Imaging in Infants, Children and Adults. Philadelphia: JB Lippincott; 1991.
2. Beller GA. Myocardial perfusion imaging with thallium-201. In: Marcus ML, Schulbert HR, Skorton DL, Wolf GL. Cardiac Imaging: A Companion to Braunwald's Heart Disease. Philadelphia: WB Saunders; 1990.
3. Van der Wall EE. Nuclear Cardiology and Cardiac Magnetic Resonance. Boston: Kluwer; 1992.
4. Vliegen HW, Van der Wall EE, Kuijper AF, et al. Assessment of myocardial viability with scintigraphic techniques and magnetic resonance imaging: New attainments? In: Van der Wall EE, Sochor H, Righetti A, Niemeyer MG, eds. What's New in Cardiac Imaging: SPECT, PET and MRI. Boston: Kluwer; 1992.
5. Dilsizian V, Rocco TP, Freedman NMT, et al. Enhanced detection of ischemic but viable myocardium by the reinjection of thallium after stress redistribution imaging. N Engl J Med. 1990;323:141–146.
6. Mahmarian JJ, Verani MS. Exercise thallium-201 scintigraphy in the assessment of coronary artery disease. Am J Cardiol. 1991;67:2D–11D.
7. Williams KA, Lipton MJ. Exercise thallium-201 single photon emission computed tomography for the diagnosis of coronary artery disease: What should we expect from SPECT? J Am Coll Cardiol. 1990;15:330–333.
8. Verani MS, Mahmarian JJ. Myocardial perfusion scintigraphy during maximal coronary artery vasodilation with adenosine. Am J Cardiol. 1991;67:12D–17D.

9. Coyne EP, Belvedere DA, Vande Streek PR, et. al. Thallium-201 scintigraphy after intravenous infusion of adenosine compared with exercise testing in the diagnosis of coronary artery disease. *J Am Coll Cardiol.* 1991;17: 1289–1294.

10. Beer SG, Heo J, Iskandrian AS. Dipyridamole thallium imaging. *Am J Cardiol.* 1991;67:18D–26D.

11. Ranhosky A, Kempthorne-Rawson J. The safety of intravenous dipyridamole thallium myocardial perfusion imaging. The Intravenous Dipyridamole Thallium Imaging Study Group. *Circulation.* 1990;81:1205–1209.

12. Hendel RC, Layden JJ, Leppo JA. Prognostic value of dipyridamole thallium scintigraphy for evaluation of ischemic heart disease. *J Am Coll Cardiol.* 1990;15:109–116.

13. Brown KA. Prognostic value of thallium-201 myocardial perfusion imaging in patients with unstable angina who respond to medical treatment. *J Am Coll Cardiol.* 1991;17:1053–1057.

14. Breisblatt WM, Weiland FL, Spaccavento LJ. Stress thallium-201 imaging after coronary angioplasty predicts restenosis and recurrent symptoms. *J Am Coll Cardiol.* 1988;12:1199–1204.

15. Alazraki N. Nuclear imaging of cardiomyopathies. In: Elliott LP. *Cardiac Imaging in Infants, Children and Adults.* Philadelphia: JB Lippincott; 1991.

16. Alazraki N. Nuclear imaging of coronary artery disease. In: Elliott LP. *Cardiac Imaging in Infants, Children and Adults.* Philadelphia: JB Lippincott; 1991.

17. Willerson JT, McGhie I, Parkey RW, et. al. Infarct-avid imaging. In: Marcus ML, Schulbert HR, Skorton DL, Wolf GL. *Cardiac Imaging: A Companion to Braunwald's Heart Disease.* Philadelphia: WB Saunders; 1991.

18. Berman DS, Kiat H, Leppo J, Maddahi J. Technetium-99m myocardial perfusion agents. In: Marcus ML, Schulbert HR, Skorton DL, Wolf GL. *Cardiac Imaging: A Companion to Braunwald's Heart Disease.* Philadelphia: WB Saunders; 1991.

19. Nicol PD, Khaw BA. Monoclonal antibody imaging. In: Marcus ML, Schulbert HR, Skorton DL, Wolf GL. *Cardiac Imaging: A Companion to Braunwald's Heart Disease.* Philadelphia: WB Saunders; 1991.

20. Sergi NA. When your patient needs a stress test. *RN.* 1991;54:26–31.

21. Hochrein MA, Sohl L. Heart smart: A guide to cardiac tests. *Am J Nurs.* 1992; 92:22–25.

22. Gibbons RJ. Equilibrium radionuclide angiography. In: Marcus ML, Schulbert HR, Skorton DL, Wolf GL. *Cardiac Imaging: A Companion to Braunwald's Heart Disease.* Philadelphia: WB Saunders; 1991.

23. Rozanski A. Applications of exercise radionuclide ventriculography in the clinical management of patients with coronary artery disease. *J Thorac Imaging.* 1990;5:37–46.

24. Jones RH. Radionuclide angiography. In: Marcus ML, Schulbert HR, Skorton DL, Wolf GL. *Cardiac Imaging: A Companion to Braunwald's Heart Disease.* Philadelphia: WB Saunders; 1991.

25. Taylor P, Becker RC. Noninvasive diagnosis of coronary heart disease in women. *Cardiology.* 1990;77(suppl 2):91–98.

26. Lee KL, Wallis JW, Miller TR. The clinical role of radionuclide imaging in cardiac transplantation. *J Thorac Imaging.* 1990;5:73–77.

27. Barkett, P. Cardiac MUGA scan: Taking first-rate pictures of the heart. *Nursing 88.* 1988;18:76–78.

28. Gawlinski A. New diagnostic techniques. In: Kern LS, ed. *Cardiac Critical Care Nursing.* Rockville: Aspen; 1988.

29. Brenner, Z. *Diagnostic Tests and Procedures: Applying the Nursing Process.* Norwalk, Conn: Appleton & Lange; 1987.

30. Schwaiger M, Hutchins G, Guibourg H, Kuhl D. Evaluation of myocardial blood flow and metabolism using positron emission tomography. *Am J Card Imaging*. 1989;3:266–275.
31. Schwaiger M, Brunken R, Grover-McKay M, et. al. Regional myocardial metabolism in patients with acute myocardial infarction assessed by positron emission tomography. *J Am Coll Cardiol*. 1986;8:800–808.
32. Schwaiger M, Brunken R, Krivokapich J, et. al. Beneficial effect of residual anterograde flow on tissue viability as assessed by positron emission tomography in patients with myocardial infarction. *Eur Heart J*. 1987; 8:981–988.
33. Bentley LJ. Radionuclide imaging techniques in the diagnosis and treatment of coronary heart disease. *Focus Crit Care*. 1987;14:27–36.

6

MAGNETIC RESONANCE IMAGING AND COMPUTERIZED TOMOGRAPHY

EVAN PADGITT

GLOSSARY

Adenosine (Adenocard)   A naturally occurring nucleotide with powerful vasodilating properties, used in nuclear medicine scans to induce coronary artery dilation in patients who cannot exercise. Also used to counteract supraventricular tachycardias.

Akinetic   Without movement; in cardiology, usually refers to a part of the ventricular wall that is not moving as would be expected.

Biphasic MRI   Imaging technique that focuses attention on two phases of the cardiac cycle—end-systole and end-diastole.

Bruce or Montoye protocols   Procedures for cardiac stress tests in which the patient gradually increases exercise intensity. Used with exercise portion of nuclear medicine tests.

CAT scan   Computerized axial tomography: the taking of repeated x-ray slices, with computer reconstruction of a detailed image in different planes.

Cine Mode   In ultrafast CT scanning, the method of imaging 17 frames per second at one slice level, creating a movie or "cine" film of that cross section of the heart.

Cine MRI   A technique in magnetic resonance imaging that takes from 20 to 45 "movie" frames per cardiac cycle by using gradient magnetic field methods. The movie is usually done at just one or two slice levels of the heart.

Contrast   In CT scanning, a material opaque to x-rays that is given intravenously to increase the difference on an x-ray image between vascular structures (where the contrast is more concentrated) and adjoining tissue. May have iodine (iodinated) or not (noniodinated).

Conventional CT   The first type of computed tomography, in which the x-ray source and detector rotates mechanically around the patient. Slow imaging times of 2 to 5 seconds result in blurring of moving objects such as the ventricles.

Dipyridamole (Persantine)   A potent vasodilator drug, used in nuclear medicine tests to dilate coronary arteries in patients unable to exercise. Acts by blocking reuptake of endogenous adenosine at receptor sites.

Dyskinetic   With inappropriate movement; in cardiology, refers to an area of ventricular wall that moves in the opposite direction of normal (such as outward during systole).

ECG gating   See *Gating.*

Echo planar MRI   Method for switching gradient magnetic fields very rapidly during one RF pulse, thus scanning one slice in 30 to 50 msec. The basis for fast MRI.

Ejection fraction   The percentage of blood introduced into a cardiac chamber (such as the ventricle) that is subsequently pumped out.

Fast CT   An intermediate development in computed tomography, in which the x-ray source is rotated rapidly around the patient to take images. Rotation time is about 1 second and represents the probable upper speed limit for a mechanically based CT system.

FLASH (Fast Low-Angle Shot)   MRI technique involving rapid repeated RF pulses taken at less than the usual 90° angle in relation to the magnetic field. The low angle shortens T1 times and allows for faster imaging.

Flow Mode   In ultrafast CT scanning, the method in which a bolus of contrast is injected intravenously, and several whole-heart scans are performed at 224 msec each as the bolus flows in and out of the heart.

Gantry   In CT scanning and MRI, the housing for the imaging source and detectors, into which the patient is placed.

Gating   A computerized feature of cardiac scans in which the imaging of each heartbeat is divided into a specified number of frames, or "gates," and the images from the corresponding frames of each heart cycle are combined into a composite film loop of one heartbeat.

Gradient magnetic fields   Used in MRI scanners to select the plane and slice for imaging. Allow computer to calculate coordinates in space used to construct MR image.

Gradient-refocused echo   In MRI, the use of gradient magnetic fields to focus more rapidly the echoes of radiofrequency energy coming from hydrogen nuclei. In this mode, flowing blood appears bright.

High-resolution mode   In CT scanning, the selection of closer x-ray slices (e.g. 3 mm) in order to increase resolution of the image over that of standard cardiac mode. With current technology, this results in the ability to cover a smaller area during one run.

Hypokinetic Having diminished movement; in cardiology, refers to a ventricular wall that is moving less vigorously than normal.

Magnetic resonance imaging (MRI) An imaging technique which employs a strong magnetic field and intermittent radiofrequency pulses, resulting in a natural contrast between different types of soft tissue.

Multiphasic/Multiplanar MRI Imaging technique in which multiple-slice scans can be taken by scanning different levels at varying times in the cardiac cycle, until images have been built of all levels at all time frames.

Paramagnetic contrast materials Chelated compounds of heavy metals that are used in MRI to enhance tissue contrast in some studies. Example: gadolinium-DPTA (Magnevist).

Radiofrequency (RF) Electromagnetic energy in the megaHertz (radio) band of the spectrum. Used in MRI to energize hydrogen nuclei, which reemit the RF energy, forming the MR image.

Resonance The physical property in which the nuclei of certain elements, aligned with the lines of force in an external magnetic field, will be tipped out of that alignment by an energy pulse of a specific frequency. The basis for magnetic resonance imaging (MRI).

Slice In CT and MRI scanning, the thin x-ray cut that produces a cross-sectional image; likened to slicing a cucumber and viewing it end-on.

Spin-echo MRI An imaging technique in which a radiofrequency pulse is applied to hydrogen nuclei at a 90° angle to the force lines of the magnetic field with which the nuclei are aligned. The returning RF energy and its echoes are used to form the MR image.

Standard cardiac mode In CT scanning, the usual setting for cardiac studies; generally translates as eight x-ray slices 1 cm apart, taken in flow mode.

Superconducting magnet The heart of most modern MRI machines. Made of a spool of superconducting wire immersed in supercold liquid helium, it can continue to generate an electromagnetic field even after electricity is turned off.

T1 relaxation time In MRI, the time required for the hydrogen nuclei to return to their baseline position in the magnetic field once the radiofrequency energy that has drawn them out of line has been removed. Varies with different tissues and substances. One property sensed by MRI scanners that is used to construct the image.

T2 relaxation time In MRI, the time frame in which hydrogen nuclei that have been in phase in their alignment to a radiofrequency pulse subsequently go out of phase with each other once the RF energy is removed. Varies with different tissues and substances. One property sensed by MRI scanners that is used to construct the image.

Tesla (T)   A unit for measuring the strength of a magnetic field. Modern MRI scanners generate a field up to 2.0 T.

Time of flight effects   In MRI, the effect on the MR signal of rapidly flowing blood. In spin-echo MRI, the blood shows little signal and is dark on the image; in gradient-refocused echo MRI, the blood has an enhanced signal and appears bright. These effects create a natural contrast on MRI between blood and lumen.

Ultrafast CT   The newest technology in computed tomography, in which an electron beam is magnetically steered to create x-ray scans of a patient at 50 to 100 msec per slice.

Magnetic resonance imaging (MRI) and computed tomography (CT) scans currently have a secondary place in cardiac testing. Partly due to high cost and lack of portability, MRI and CT may be used only in larger medical centers and are usually performed only when cheaper and more widely employed tests such as echocardiography and radionuclide scanning have not given satisfactory information about the patient's heart.

In spite of these limitations, MRI and CT may play a larger role in future cardiac testing if their promise is fulfilled through technical progress in the next few years. Both scans are *tomographic* or cross-sectional scans of the body and give very sharp anatomical detail of the heart and vascular structures. Researchers hope to improve the ability of CT and MRI to study the *function* of the heart as well as its structure, perhaps leading to an all-in-one cardiac examination (looking at coronary arteries, myocardial perfusion, heart structure and performance in one comprehensive scan).

Although the pictures gained from MRI and CT look somewhat similar to one another, very different principles and techniques are used to make the pictures: MRI applies strong magnetic fields and radio waves, while CT uses conventional x-rays in a unique manner. To interpret the results gained from MRI and CT cardiac tests and to best care for the patient before, during, and after the scans, it will help the nurse to understand something of the principles of each test.

MAGNETIC RESONANCE IMAGING

Magnetic resonance imaging (MRI) has become widely used in visualizing soft-tissue structures in the body, with an established role in imaging the brain, bones and joints, and other organs. MRI shows anatomy in fine detail, and can differentiate between different kinds of soft tissue.[1] It is a unique technology that uses magnetic fields to image the body. In some ways it is safer than nuclear and x-ray scans because no ionizing radiation is used, and in most cases intravenous contrast material is not needed. Like computed tomography (CT), MRI usually creates cross-sectional images, or slices, through a certain plane of the body.

Development and use of MRI for cardiovascular imaging has been slow for several reasons. Stationary organs such as the brain are easier to study than the heart, whose constant motion creates blurred images on regular MRI scans.[2] Techniques to compensate for heart motion have previously meant MRI sessions of one hour or more, longer than those of other scan techniques. MRI machines are costly, large, and require special support facilities. Some competitive technologies, such as echocardiography, are less expensive, more widely familiar and available, and can be brought to the patient's bedside.[3]

Although MRI usually has a secondary role in cardiac testing, it is important for the nurse to have basic knowledge of MRI technology and of what the test means for the patient. First, MRI is well established as a way to gain further anatomical information on structural cardiovascular problems—congenital defects, aneurysms, pericardial changes, cardiac tumors and thrombi—where the results from echocardiography are questionable.[2] Second, new technical advancements are making MRI much faster and more able to study cardiac function, not just anatomy. Proponents of MRI hope it can play a much larger role in cardiac testing in the near future, possibly as a comprehensive test that studies anatomy, ventricular function, and coronary flow all in a few seconds or minutes of scanning.[4] Third, patients undergoing MRI studies need considerable information to prepare for MRI, and the nurse must anticipate potential problems that can interfere with patient safety and the effectiveness of the test. Although MRI is generally well tolerated, the nurse's assessment, education, and support of the patient are critical for a good outcome.

Principles

The concept of nuclear magnetic resonance has been known since the 1940s.[5] Certain elements with an odd number of atomic particles in their nucleus (such as hydrogen and phosphorus) would behave in a predictable way in a strong magnetic field—the nuclei would all turn to line up along the magnetic lines of force, just like little bar magnets. Furthermore, if electromagnetic energy was beamed at the atom, the nucleus would line up with the *new* energy source while absorbing some of the beamed energy. This second source of energy had to be at a unique frequency for each element in order to match, or *resonate*, with the particular atom and magnetic field strength, thus the term *magnetic resonance*. The electromagnetic energy used was in the spectrum of radio waves, and therefore was called *radiofrequency* (RF) energy. Once the radiofrequency (RF) energy source was cut off, the atom would reemit the RF energy in a pulse that could be detected and analyzed.

Magnetic resonance became a tool for imaging the body when it was discovered that the reemitted energy from resonant atoms could be processed by a computer into an anatomical image.[1,6] This was possible because hydrogen, by far the most plentiful element in the body, is present to varying degrees in different types of tissue. So two adjacent tissues would emit different signal intensities after being placed in a magnetic field and subjected to RF energy; this difference could be measured and made into a very detailed picture of soft tissues (Figure 6.1).

FIGURE 6.1

Basic magnetic resonance images of the chest in three anatomic planes: sagittal (top left), coronal (top right), and transverse (bottom). Note how cardiac chambers and vessels, in which blood is flowing, are seen as darker than surrounding stationary tissue. These "time of flight" effects create MRI's inherent contrast between tissue and moving fluids, without the use of dye.

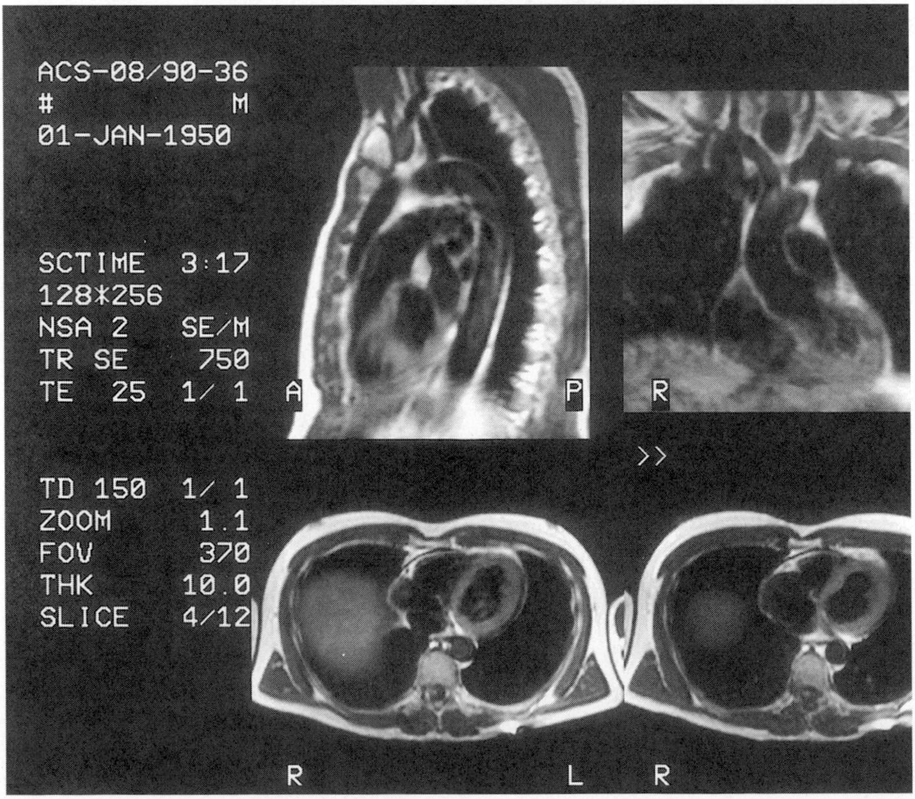

Courtesy Philips Medical Systems.

The MRI scanner has four main components:

1. A powerful *magnet* in the shape of a cylinder (the patient is placed on a sliding table in the bore of the cylinder) (Figure 6.2). Modern MRI scanners use a superconducting magnet, a spool of alloy wire immersed in liquid helium at −450°F. This device generates a static (steady) field of 0.1 to 2.0 tesla (T); one T = 10,000 gauss (G), a measurement of magnetic energy. The Earth's magnetic field is about 0.5 G. So an MRI magnet is up to 40,000 times as strong as the Earth's normal magnetic field.

2. Smaller devices produce *gradient magnetic fields* that combine with the large field to give *positional* (two- and three-dimensional) information on the area scanned; these gradient fields can be oriented at any angle to the body of the patient, and they define where cross-sectional image slices will be taken.

3. *Radiofrequency (RF) coils* inside the magnet cylinder both emit the RF pulses and receive the reemitted RF energy and send it to

FIGURE 6.2

A smaller MRI scanner, showing how patient is positioned within the bore (center) of the superconducting magnet.

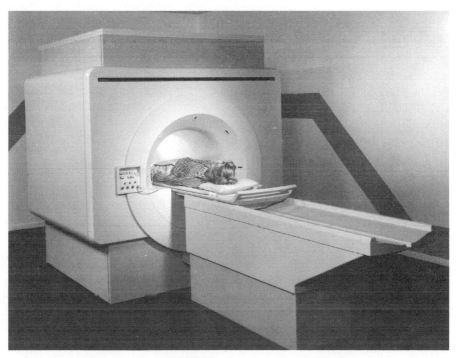

Courtesy Philips Medical Systems.

the signal processor. The angle and the frequency of the pulse can be adjusted and aimed at the body part(s) under study.
4. The *computer* not only runs the system but assembles the data into a usable image. Until sufficiently powerful small computers were available, MRI could not be performed.[1,6]

The setup is costly; in 1991 one author estimated an MRI system to cost $2 million, with operating costs at $200,000 per year.[5] This is one third higher than ultrafast CT and eight to ten times the cost of either echocardiography or radionuclide ventriculography equipment.

Scanning Techniques

The different techniques used in MRI can be complex, and an in-depth technical discussion is beyond the goals of this text. However, there are certain concepts and terms used in MRI reports that the nurse may wish to understand in interpreting results.

The *T1 relaxation time*, or *T1*, describes the time needed for the atomic nucleus to "tip back" into line with the magnetic field once the RF energy has been removed. An analogy would be a child on a swing; when no more swinging force is applied, it takes a certain time for the child to come to rest.[7] The other main measure used is *T2 relaxation time*, or *T2*, which describes the different rates at which the different atoms go out of sync with each other as they tip back into line with the magnetic field. To continue the analogy, if three children are swinging in line and the swinging force is stopped, they will begin to swing out of phase with each other as they slow down. Various substances and tissues inherently have different T1s and T2s, and these differences are used by the MRI computer in constructing images.[6] Furthermore, the scanner can be adjusted for frequencies and angle of the RF pulse so that T1 or T2 can be given more importance; these T1- or T2-weighted images can better show the differences between tissues.

As with other cardiac imaging methods, the images obtained with MRI have much poorer quality if the motion of the heart is not compensated for.[2] Also, although some new MRI techniques are rapid, other procedures require up to 45 minutes of imaging time; thus the images are gathered over many heartbeats, and the timing must be precise in order to pool the data into images. MRI generally uses *ECG gating*, in which the R wave of each QRS complex (or every other one), triggers RF pulses and imaging.

Certain MRI studies *do* employ a kind of contrast material. Such substances are primarily made from heavy metals, and have their own magnetic qualities when subjected to an external magnetic field.[6] When injected intravenously and distributed into body tissues, *paramagnetic contrast agents* can increase the contrast between tissues by decreasing T1 and T2 relaxation times. An example is gadolinium-DTPA, which can increase MRI contrast between ischemic and healthy myocardium.

MRI has great flexibility in the *imaging planes* selected for viewing. In other imaging systems, the patient's body must be positioned to align with the machine to achieve proper orientation of the heart for viewing. MRI allows unrestricted image plane selection through the use of gradient magnetic fields to select the angle and area of interest[5] (Figures 6.3–6.8). MRI studies can be set up in standard planes (sagittal, coronal, and transverse), but because of the oblique placement of the heart itself, these views can distort dimensions or miss areas of interest. In the same way as echocardiography, MRI can produce views which are oriented to the axis of the heart, rather than the axis of the body as a whole. Image orientation can also be customized to any structure, such as lengthwise slices of the thoracic aorta.[5]

Spin-echo MRI is probably the most widely used technique.[3,5] Spin-echo begins with an RF pulse aimed at a 90° angle to the magnetic field, followed by several RF pulses oriented at 180° to the field that create

FIGURE 6.3

"Scout" views, which resemble a conventional A-P and lateral chest x-ray, are often taken of the patient before the full scan. The lines represent the imaging slices the operator has selected. With most modern MRI scanners, slices can be made at almost any angle or view desired.

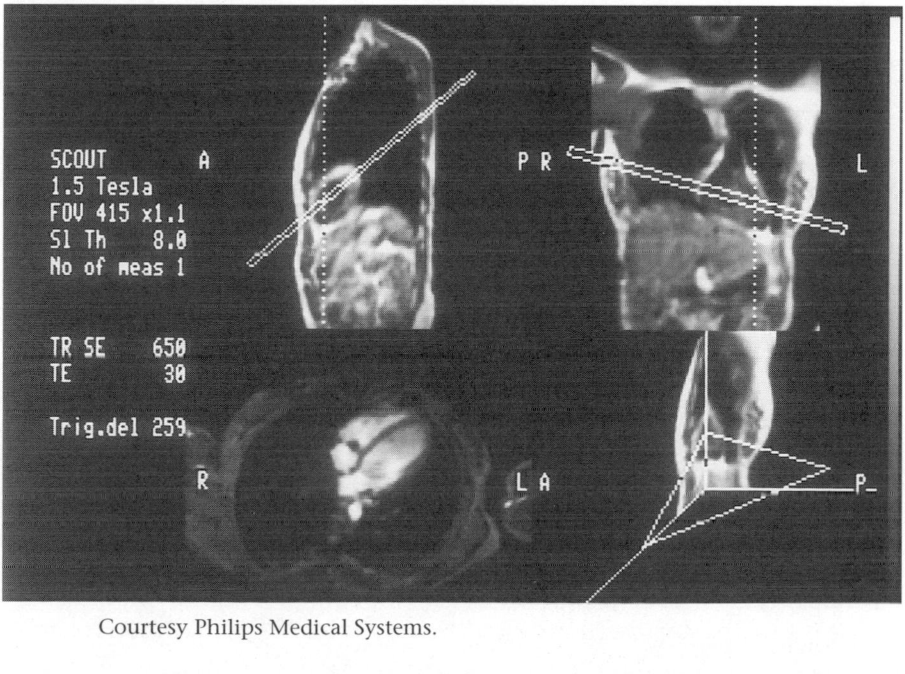

Courtesy Philips Medical Systems.

FIGURE 6.4

In this coronal slice approximately midway through the heart, clearly seen are the right atrium and ventricle (RA, RV), aorta (AO), left ventricle (LV), and pulmonary artery (PA). Note the diaphragm, on which the heart rests, and the liver at lower left.

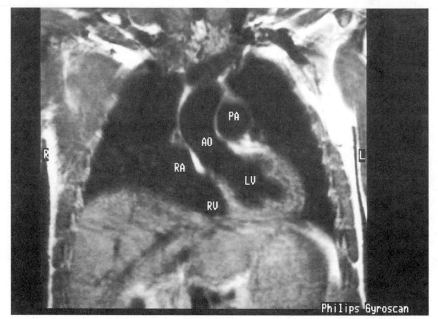

Courtesy Philips Medical Systems.

echoes with the initial 90° pulse. Highly detailed still images of the heart can be generated through analysis of the complex signal return of the pulses and their echoes. Spin-echo MRI is unsuitable for functional studies, but does deliver excellent anatomical information. Blood or other fluids that are flowing rapidly appear dark in spin-echo images, while stationary fluids and structures are lighter. A common scan sequence produces eight slices of the heart, about 1 cm apart, in 7 to 10 minutes of scanning.

Multiphasic/multiplanar MRI takes spin-echo techniques a step further by using multiple sequences of several slices.[6,8] Multiphasic imaging constructs a composite view of several slices by varying the sequence in which the slices are imaged within each cardiac cycle. Slice views of the entire heart at several points in the cardiac cycle are produced; total imaging time is long, however, at some 30 to 40 minutes.

Gradient-refocused echo (GRE) uses more rapid RF pulsing and interprets the echoes of the pulses for faster imaging. Whereas spin-echo sequences usually start with an RF pulse at 90° to the field direction, GRE

FIGURE 6.5

A sagittal view (along the length of the body) also shows the left atrium (LA) and, faintly, the mitral valve (MV) separating the left atrium and ventricle. Note the detail of vertebrae, sternum, and descending aorta.

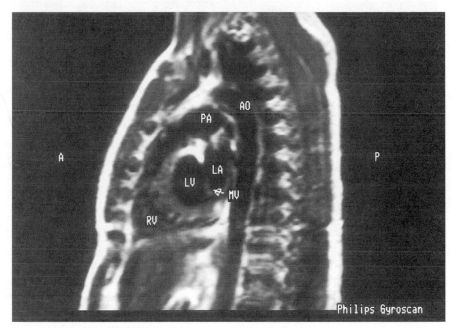

Courtesy Philips Medical Systems.

uses a pulse at less than 90°—commonly, a 30° angle.[2,6] This technique gives a shorter T1 (faster return to equilibrium) and so the RF pulses can be done faster. Unlike spin-echo images where the flowing blood is dark, in GRE images the fast-traveling blood is actually brighter than surrounding slow or stationary objects, and turbulent, slower blood is darker. Thus GRE is ideal for evaluating flow phenomena and valvular regurgitation. Image resolution and tissue contrast are less for GRE than for spin-echo, so GRE is better for evaluating function than for anatomical details.

Cine MRI produces a "film loop" of one cardiac cycle.[7,8] Fast GRE techniques are used, with each slice acquired as rapidly as every 5 miliseconds. A single-slice 30-frame sequence of one heartbeat requires 3 to 5 minutes scanning time; the entire heart can be scanned in about 30 minutes. The resultant "movie" is a truly dynamic study of the heart during one cardiac cycle. While image resolution is less than in spin-echo MRI, it is still adequate for reliable studies of heart function, including ejection fraction, segmental wall dynamics, flow abnormalities, and valvular regurgitation.[3,9]

FIGURE 6.6

A transverse slice midway through the heart, with a clear view of all four chambers and the descending aorta (DA). Cardiac fat is represented as the brighter tissue.

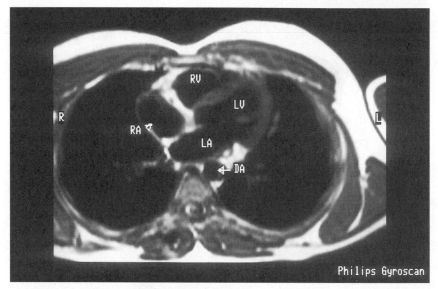

Courtesy Philips Medical Systems.

Flow-encoded (velocity-mapping) MRI shows turblent blood flow (such as around a regurgitant heart valve) by computerized color coding of the different RF signal intensities created by the flowing blood.[4,8] The result is much like color Doppler echocardiography, but with a longer imaging time.

High-speed MRI has been a goal for at least the last decade, and several approaches have been tried. In *echo-planar imaging*, the gradient magnetic fields are changed very rapidly, making it possible to gather all the data needed for an image in the space of one RF pulse.[6,8] The imaging time is described as only 30 to 50 milliseconds, essentially real-time imaging. Thus an entire scan of the heart can be accomplished in a few seconds, with the patient holding his breath to reduce motion artifact. Disadvantages include a lower-resolution image, restricted imaging orientations, and possible adverse biological effects such as muscle stimulation.[2]

Indications for Cardiac MRI

With its inherent contrast between kinds of soft tissue, magnetic resonance imaging is particularly well suited to studying cardiac anatomy, although the relatively slow speed of conventional MRI makes studies of heart function more challenging. Furthermore, due to its cost

FIGURE 6.7

Another transverse slice, this time at the base (top) of the heart, shows cross sections of the great vessels. In addition to the aorta (AO), descending aorta (DA), and pulmonary artery (PA), the right and left pulmonary veins (RPV, LPV) are visible, as is the right atrial appendage (RAA).

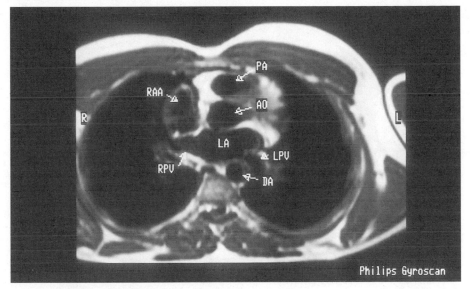

Courtesy Philips Medical Systems.

and unwieldiness, MRI is rarely the test of first choice in cardiac diagnosis. However, with its high-resolution imaging (showing details of 1 mm or less), MRI can add useful information if more commonly used tests such as echocardiography give inconclusive results. If technical problems can be overcome and the cost of scanners is not prohibitive, MRI may someday be used as an all-in-one test of cardiac anatomy and function. For now, these are the current indications for cardiac MRI.

Pericardial disease is well evaluated by MRI; the high resolution helps define the healthy pericardium (2–4 mm in thickness) and its thickening in disease. MRI may be the procedure of choice for diagnosing the constrictive pericarditis that can follow cardiac surgery.[3,4] Echocardiography is used to diagnose most pericardial effusions, but MRI has equal accuracy and can better characterize the kind of effusion (hemorrhage, inflammatory, uremic).[3,5] Pericardial tumors and their degree of infiltration into tissue can be well imaged by MRI.

Cardiac masses, tumors, and thrombi are often first recognized by echocardiography, with further information then gathered using MRI. Tumors can be precisely sized and localized, and the point of attachment of masses within the cardiac chambers described for the benefit of the sur-

FIGURE 6.8

Upper left scout view shows setup for three slices along the long axis of the heart, a diagonal plane that compensates for the normally oblique position of the heart in the chest. (Because this is a gradient-echo study, the blood-filled chambers and aorta are light-colored, rather than dark as in more conventional spin-echo MRI.)

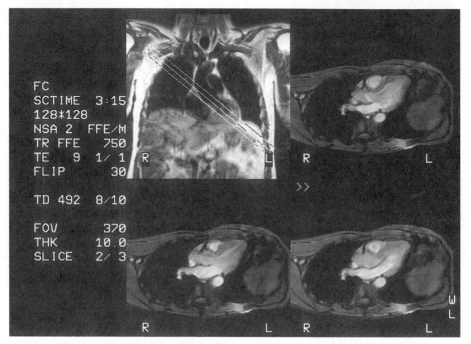

Courtesy Philips Medical Systems.

geon[4] (Figure 6.9). The motion pictures of cine MRI show the effect of the tumor or clot on cardiac function, and other MRI techniques can give limited definition of the type of mass (cyst, lipoma, solid tumor).[3,5]

Congenital heart defects can be explored with MRI for both anatomic and functional problems (Figures 6.10 and 6.11). Echocardiography is usually employed first, as it is equally noninvasive and cheaper and is better tolerated by patients, usually children under 6 years old (who require sedation to endure the long MRI study).[5] Therefore, echocardiography remains the primary means for congenital anomaly assessment, with MRI reserved for use when echo is technically inadequate. MRI can accurately image many congenital abnormalities, such as great vessel defects, chamber variations, and septal defects.[3] Flow characteristics and heart function can be assessed accurately with cine and flow-encoded MRI. The high resolution of MRI is sometimes used to check the effectiveness of surgical repairs.[8,9]

Valvular heart disease is usually imaged by echocardiography or color Doppler to evaluate the anatomy and degree of abnormal blood

FIGURE 6.9

In this transverse section, a myxoma (tumor) can be seen within the left atrium (bottommost of the four chambers, just above the spine). Compare to the normal anatomy shown in Figure 6.6.

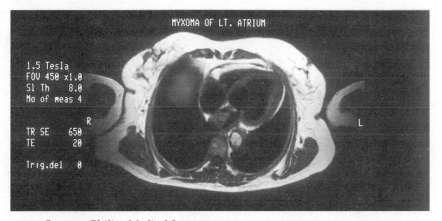

MYXOMA OF LT. ATRIUM

1.5 Tesla
FOV 450 x1.0
Sl Th   8.0
No of meas 4

R

TR SE   650
TE   20

Trig.del 0

L

Courtesy Philips Medical Systems.

flow through the tight (stenotic) or incompetent (regurgitant) valve.[5] MRI has a similar accuracy rate, however, in assessing mitral and aortic regurgitation.[3] The disordered flow from a stenotic valve has been technically more difficult for MRI to analyze, but the newer flow-encoded MRI techniques can focus on the fine differences in flow velocity and enable a study similar to that by color Doppler.[4,8] The morphology of natural and artificial valves can be studied with MRI, but the older metallic artificial heart valves cause signal interference and artifact, and cannot be evaluated with MRI.[5]

Aortic disease is easily assessed with MRI due to its ability to produce cross-section views in any plane—in this case, both widthwise (transaxial) and lengthwise (paraxial) through the aorta.[5] In aortic dissection, MRI easily defines intimal flaps, detects the slower blood flow in false lumens, and can assess for hemorrhage outside the vessel. Only transesophageal echo (TEE) appears to approach MRI in accuracy, and since that technique is faster than MRI, it may be the first choice in acute, life-threatening dissection. Patients with abdominal aortic aneurysm (AAA) and thoracic aneurysms may require repeated studies over time to determine if the aneurysm is large enough to warrant surgical repair.[5] Strictly on technical quality and noninvasiveness, MRI is probably the test of choice. But because of cost, TEE is often used instead of MRI for serial testing. After surgical repair of aneurysms, MRI is valuable in checking patency and stability of surgical repairs and grafts[9] (Figure 6.12).

Coronary arteries and bypass grafts have been viewed in cross section by MRI, allowing a crude assessment of their patency.[6] At present, however, only the larger coronary arteries can be studied, and cardiac

FIGURE 6.10

Although practical matters make MRI in infants difficult, the technical detail can be impressive. Here a congenital hypoplasia (underdevelopment) of the aorta can be seen in sagittal section. Compare to Figure 6.5.

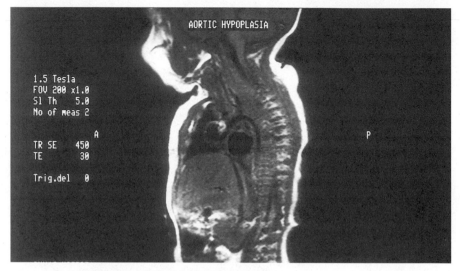

Courtesy Philips Medical Systems.

cathetherization remains superior in defining the patency of vessels. In spite of problems with MRI signal artifact from metal sternal clips, MRI studies of coronary bypass grafts have been 90% to 95% accurate in diagnosing graft stenosis.[6] A technique called *magnetic resonance angiography*, which has already produced images of the coronary arteries, is being investigated[10] (Figures 6.13 and 6.14). More widespread use of MRI studies of these vessels awaits further technical developments.

Ventricular mass, volume, and performance are well measured with MRI, using three-dimensional data gathered from multislice scans, perhaps more accurately than in two-dimensional methods such as MUGA scans.[3,8] These measurements, taken at different times in the cardiac cycle, enable reliable descriptions of ventricular ejection fraction and cardiac output.[4]

Cardiomyopathies are evaluated with MRI by physical measurements of ventricle mass, wall thickness, and chamber volume, as well as with cine MRI assessment of the ventricle's function. Some cardiomyopathies result from sarcoidosis, myocarditis, and systemic lupus erythematosus, which cause myocardial tissue changes that can be detected by MRI as altered T1 and T2 times.[4,5]

Cardiac transplant rejection can be assessed with MRI. Preliminary studies suggest a measurable rise in T2 relaxation times in the myocardium of patients with moderate to severe rejection. These changes

FIGURE 6.11

Spin-echo MRI. In this sagittal view, a coarctation (narrowing) of the descending thoracic aorta can be seen clearly.

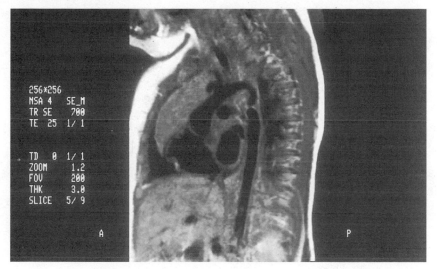

Courtesy Philips Medical Systems.

are probably due to edema. Up to three weeks postoperatively, however, patients may have *expected* edema due to surgery—so MRI would not be able to detect early rejection. MRI may have some utility as a non-invasive test for rejection, but more study is needed.[5,11]

Myocardial ischemia is traditionally diagnosed with nuclear medicine scans such as thallium scans. Like echocardiography, MRI can currently only detect ischemia by finding the abnormalities of heart wall motion caused by ischemic myocardium, as seen on cine MRI.[6] The lack of practical exercise testing has limited the use of MRI in detecting ischemic heart disease; the patient is inside the bore of the magnet, and not able to move freely. Some studies have been made using pharmacologic stress tests, where a drug such as dobutamine is given intravenously, causing vasodilation and tachycardia that simulate an exercise response.[4,8] As long as stress thallium and stress echocardiography are more practical, development of stress MRI is unlikely; however, ultrafast MRI machines of the future may make such studies possible.

Myocardial infarction (MI) causes tissue changes that can be detected by MRI. Probably because of edema, infarcted tissue has a strong MRI signal on scans adjusted to highlight T2 relaxation times.[6] These changes begin 3 to 6 hours after coronary occlusion and last about 20 days. Some studies have questioned whether these changes are specific to infarcted tissue or may also happen in ischemia. The use of a paramag-

FIGURE 6.12

A massively dilated thoracic-abdominal aortic aneurysm is vividly seen on MRI without the use of contrast dye.

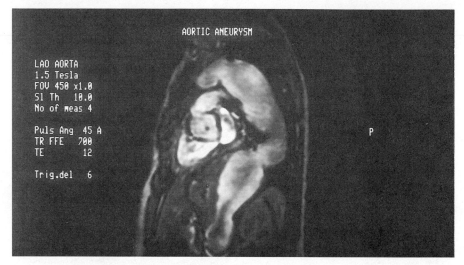

Courtesy Philips Medical Systems.

netic contrast agent, gadolinium-DPTA (Gd-DPTA; Magnevist), increases signal intensity of infarcted tissue on T1-weighted MRI, and may improve the test's accuracy for MI.[12] Gd-DPTA is able to enhance an MI beginning a few minutes after occlusion, and this effect lasts for several days postinfarct. The other use of MRI in detecting MI is by analysis of abnormal wall thinning and motion. Cine MRI will show the abnormal movements of a part of the myocardium that has been infarcted.[6] Also, whereas normal myocardium thickens during each systolic cycle, infarcted regions stay abnormally thin walled; this also can be seen on MRI[4] (Figure 6.15).

In spite of these abilities to detect myocardial infarction, MRI in its present stage of development will probably not gain wide use in MI diagnosis. The test is more expensive than echocardiography and nuclear scans, cannot be made truly portable, and has practical problems in doing stress studies and evaluating acutely ill patients.[6]

Summary of Indications for MRI

One author has summarized the indications for MRI scanning:[5]

Test of first choice for:
    Stable aortic dissection or coarctation
    Thoracic aortic aneurysm
    Aortic arch abnormalities and surgery follow-up

FIGURE 6.13

Two MRI slices along the long axis of the heart using the MR angiography technique. This very rapid scan is obtained in 14 seconds, well within the breath-holding capability of most patients. Arrows indicate a cross section of the right coronary artery, showing excellent anatomical detail.

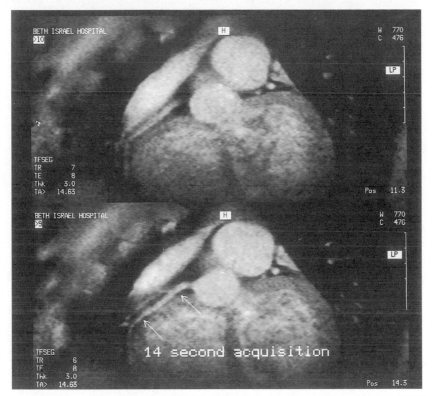

Courtesy Robert Edelman, MD, Beth Israel Hospital, Boston, and Siemens Medical Systems.

Constrictive pericarditis
Anomalous pulmonary venous connection
Systemic/pulmonary artery shunts
Imaging superior/inferior vena cava or central pulmonary
   artery

Use if echocardiography/nuclear scans give inadequate information:
Abdominal aortic aneurysm
Pericardial effusion/tumor
Intracardiac mass
Complex congenital abnormality and its postoperative
   evaluation
Ventricular function analysis

FIGURE 6.14
Another MR angiography image, this time showing the loss of signal (darker area) at the point of stenosis in the right coronary artery.

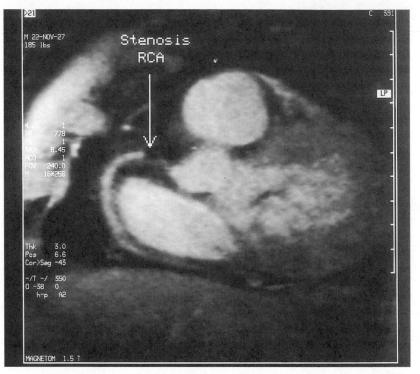

Courtesy Robert Edelman, MD, Beth Israel Hospital, Boston, and Siemens Medical Systems.

Further study needed for MRI use in:
 Myocardial infarction/ischemia
 Cardiac transplant rejection
 Myocarditis
 Coronary artery and CABG vessel stenosis

Future of MRI

Whether MRI increases in acceptance as a cardiac diagnostic test depends on both economic and technical factors. Increasing speed of MRI scans may make them more practical and useful in functional studies of the heart. But MRI facilities are still the most expensive diagnostic technology to establish and will be compared with the expanding and less expensive techniques in echocardiography.

Comprehensive cardiac testing through MRI may one day be accomplished through high-speed scanners and the use of pharmacologic

FIGURE 6.15

Short-axis images are taken at (left) end-diastole (ED) and (right) end-systole (ES); the computer analyzes ventricular wall thickness during these phases of the heartbeat. Cardiac ischemia or infarction may be detected by seeing ventricular wall tissue that is too thin or that does not thicken normally by the end of systole.

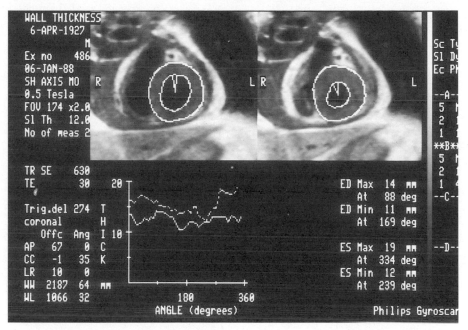

Courtesy Philips Medical Systems.

stress agents such as dobutamine to study the heart in exercise mode.[3] Greater image resolution and ability to study blood flow at the coronary artery level are awaited developments that may help MRI compete with cardiac catheterization in diagnosing coronary artery disease.

Magnetic resonance spectroscopy (MRS) has been studied for some years as a means of analyzing the metabolic state of the myocardium and other body tissues. In the same way MRI studies the resonance of hydrogen atoms to form an image of tissue, MRS focuses on phosphorus, another resonant atom in body tissues.[6] Phosphorus is not plentiful enough to send back enough MR signal for an image to be made, but a spectroscopic graph of the various signals is possible. The important phosphorus compounds—such as adenosine triphosphate (ATP) and creatinine phosphatase—have a characteristic appearance on the graph. ATP and the other phosphorus compounds in the myocardium change in response to ischemia or infarction. Therefore, magnetic resonance spectroscopy can be used to test the metabolic health of the myocardium, as does positron emission tomography (PET). This technology is still in the research phase.

Real-time MRI is a goal of some MRI researchers.[10] This near-instantaneous imaging would look like x-ray fluoroscopy, enabling clinicians to use it for guidance in surgical and diagnostic procedures. *Three-dimensional (3-D) MRI* awaits the combination of very fast imaging and high-capacity computers to create an essentially lifelike reconstruction of the heart on-screen that can be rotated to any view and opened up at any portion to examine anatomy and function.[4]

Nursing Implications of Cardiac MRI

The nurse caring for the patient undergoing MRI has an important role in promoting a good outcome of the test and assuring safety for the patient and staff. Careful preparation and assessment of the patient, preparation of equipment, and education of the patient are especially important in cardiac MRI (Figure 6.16).

FIGURE 6.16

As the patient is placed completely into a large MRI scanner, the difficulties can be seen in monitoring and accessing the patient during a scan lasting up to an hour. In the future, faster MRI machines are expected to lessen some of the problems in scanning patients who are claustrophobic or physiologically unstable.

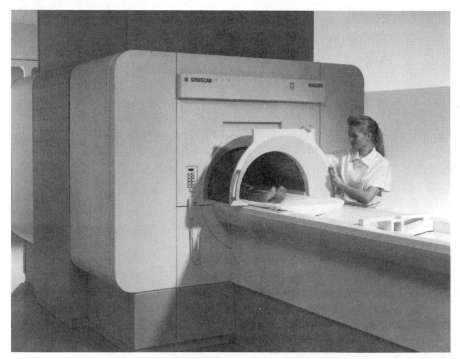

Courtesy Philips Medical Systems.

Patient Preparation and Assessment

The fundamental concept to remember in preparing a patient for MRI is the *presence of an extremely strong magnetic field*, not only within the scanner but anywhere in the MRI room itself. Promoters of MRI suggest the biological effects of the magnetic field are minimal, certainly having fewer damaging aspects than the ionizing radiation used in x-rays and CT scans.[13] The patient should be reassured that no nuclear radiation is involved. Early concerns about the potential of fluctuating magnetic fields to cause epileptic seizures or heart fibrillation have not been borne out in practice; animal studies indicate much stronger field changes than those seen in a typical MRI scan are needed to induce ventricular fibrillation.[6] However, the shifting fields of certain imaging techniques can cause retinal neuron discharges; these perceived flashes of light, called "visual phosphenes," don't seem to be associated with any damage to the eye.[1] Because biological effects on the fetus are inadequately studied, MRI in pregnancy is generally contraindicated.

Any object made of metal, either inside or outside the patient's body, may cause injury or interfere with the accuracy of the scan.[13] Items made of ferrous metals (containing iron) are particularly hazardous since they may move within the body during the scan. Even nonferrous metals should be removed if possible because they can create artifact in the scan, reducing its accuracy.[14]

Patients should be actively questioned about the presence of *any* metal implants or foreign objects in or on their bodies. The radiology department may provide a checklist of items to ask about; if in doubt, consult the radiologist or MRI staff. Generally, *all* metal objects should be kept out of the MRI room.[1,15]

Patients with these items should be excluded from MRI:
- Implanted cardiac pacemakers and automatic cardiac defibrillators (MRI may cause shutdown of pacing, rapid firing, or dislodgment of pacer wires)
- Certain implanted devices such as chemotherapy or insulin pumps
- Cochlear (inner ear) implants
- Metal vascular or aneurysm clips, especially cerebral
- Metal shrapnel and certain types of bullets (includes occupational exposure to metal fragments in eyes, etc.)
- Metal artificial heart valves
- Metal shank anchoring artificial eye

MRI may be allowed, but patient should be assessed by the radiologist:
- Artificial joint replacements
- Dental braces and bridges
- Surgical wires and clips from well-healed surgeries

- Metal meshes and plates that are firmly anchored
- Any other foreign objects in the body

Have not been shown to be a problem in MRI:
- Dental fillings
- Intrauterine devices (IUDs)

The patient's personal items should be reviewed and any metal left outside the MRI room. Specifically, the patient should remove all jewelry, eyeglasses, removable dental bridges, hairpins and barrettes, watches, and hearing aids. Eye cosmetics may contain metal flakes and should be removed. Clothing going into the scanner should be free of metal snaps, hooks and zippers. The patient should not bring in any items such as coins, keys, or cigarette lighters. Electronic devices and magnetic items such as credit cards, computer disks, and tapes may be damaged by the magnetic field. (*Note*: these precautions also pertain to visitors and staff entering the MRI room.)[13,15]

Before going to MRI, the patient should be asked to void. Only if IV contrast is being used does the patient need to be NPO (four hours before the scan), but it may be wise to restrict fluids about two hours beforehand to promote patient comfort.[13]

The patient should be assessed to determine his or her ability to tolerate the MRI procedure and to cooperate for a good result. He or she should be able to lie still for the expected 60 to 90 minutes some scans require and to follow directions. Certain characteristics may make an MRI scan difficult for the patient:

- A medically unstable patient cannot be easily monitored and accessed inside the MRI magnet chamber.
- A very large patient (typically, over 300 lb or 52 in. in girth) may not fit inside the scanner.
- Compromised renal function may inhibit use of contrast dye, which is excreted by the kidneys; check serum BUN/creatinine before procedure.
- Inability to lie still due to muscle spasms, frequent cough, seizures, or restlessness will cause blurred imaging.
- Claustrophobia (estimated 2–5% of patients) may induce high anxiety and make the scan impossible to tolerate; distraction and/or sedation may help.
- Children may also be unable to lie still; sedation may be needed.
- If the patient is unable to comprehend or follow instructions (i.e. "hold breath," "lie still"), the test may be less useful.[13,15]

Preparation of Equipment

Medical equipment made of metal can endanger patient and staff if it is drawn into the powerful magnetic field of the MRI scanner. *Remem-*

ber, the magnetic field of a modern MRI machine is ALWAYS "on"! Oxygen tanks, IV poles, wheelchairs, and tools have actually become airborne in MRI rooms, causing damage and serious injury as they fly toward the magnet. Nurses should consult with MRI staff about special equipment such as nonferrous infusion pumps and IV poles. Specifically do the following:

- Change IVs to heparin locks when possible.
- If IV is required, add extra extension tubing to reach inside scanner; notify the MRI staff of special needs. Flow rate may need to be monitored manually.
- Leave *all* wheelchairs, stretchers, oxygen tanks, and metal IV poles outside the MRI room.
- Check with the MRI staff if patient needs cardiac monitoring.[14,15]

Special procedures and equipment for resuscitation are needed. The patient is usually taken outside the MRI room for treatment. *Under no circumstances should the standard metal crash cart be wheeled next to an MRI scanner.*

Patient Education

Patient education for MRI should include safety matters as well as anticipatory information on what to expect and how to cooperate for the test (see Patient Education Box 6.1). The patient's MRI experience should not involve any pain, but may be bewildering and a bit overwhelming. The MRI scanner is quite large; the patient lies on a padded table that is moved into the center of the scanner. Vision is restricted and the wall of the scanner is close to the face. Most scanners incorporate a ventilation system, intercom, call button, and sometimes earphones with music to make the patient more comfortable and secure. There is a loud, pulsating sound during the scan, like a drumbeat. The technician will ask the patient to lie as still as possible and sometimes to hold a breath for a few seconds. The patient should not experience any special sensations during the scan, but sometimes parts of the body become warmer. If IV dye is used, the patient may feel transient flushing, nausea, or headache for a few moments after injection. The technician can hear and speak with the patient, who should report any discomfort. Depending on the kind of scan, the MRI may take from 30 to 90 minutes.[1,14,15]

Aftercare

Aftercare is minimal for MRI. On emerging from the scanner, the patient should sit a few moments to recover from any postural dizziness. Medications, diet, and activity may be resumed immediately following an MRI. If contrast dye was used, the patient should receive extra fluids over the next few hours to aid in elimination of the dye. If the patient was sedated, he or she should be monitored for recovery from its effects; an outpatient should be driven home by another person.

Magnetic Resonance Imaging

The purpose of the magnetic resonance imaging (MRI) scan is to take very detailed pictures of the heart, using a strong magnetic field and radio waves. The pictures are taken *across* the body, in thin "slices," giving the doctor a picture of the heart in cross section at several different levels and angles. The test usually takes 60 to 90 minutes.

BEFORE THE TEST

It is important that you tell the staff before the test if you have any metal objects in your body (such as surgical clips, wires, artificial joints, or shrapnel). Most people with heart pacemakers, heart defibrillators, or ear implants should not have an MRI because of the magnet. Do not bring any metal objects into the MRI room (jewelry, watches, keys, etc.). If you have any questions about any of the above, do not hesitate to ask the MRI staff.

Women who are (or might be) pregnant should discuss this with their doctor or the MRI staff before having an MRI scan.

Normally, it is permitted to eat and drink lightly before an MRI test. If your test is to include contrast dye, however, you must not eat or drink for 4 hours before your test time.

If you have had a reaction before to intravenous (IV) dye, or contrast, tell the staff before the test is started.

DURING THE TEST

You will lie on a flat, padded table that will be rolled inside the MRI machine. The machine is quite large and will surround you completely. You will be asked to lie still during the scan. You may be asked to hold your breath at times. There is a microphone and speaker so that you may talk to the technician while inside the MRI machine. If you have a fear of close places (claustrophobia), have trouble lying still, or feel short of breath, tell the staff before the test.

If you are having a test using contrast (IV dye), a needle will be placed in an arm vein temporarily. You may feel nauseated or have a warm, flushed feeling when the dye is injected into your IV. This is normal and usually passes in a few seconds. *If you are having discomfort, tell the staff.*

AFTER THE TEST

If you had a regular MRI scan, there is nothing special to do after the test. If you had a scan using contrast dye, the dye will leave the body in a few hours in your urine. You should drink several glasses of water or other fluids over the next 3 to 4 hours, to help this happen. Should you develop a rash or feel short of breath later, tell your nurse or doctor.

COMPUTED TOMOGRAPHY

Since its introduction in the mid-1970s, computed tomography (CT) has revolutionized x-ray technology. CT has become the method of choice for x-rays of most soft-tissue structures, especially in the thorax, abdomen, and brain. It has proved invaluable in the diagnosis of tumors, soft-tissue injury, and effusions. However, for one very important area of soft-tissue—the heart—CT has not yet found wide usage, despite its improving ability to perform cardiac studies.

Early CT machines required exposure times of several seconds, and so the movement of the heart produced blurred images. But even after the introduction of faster CT scanners that can freeze the image of a beating heart, other tests such as echocardiography and radionuclide scans continue to have greater acceptance among most clinicians. Although CT is used most commonly to image cardiovascular anatomy, it has shown promise in studying certain heart functions as well. In the near future, more capable CT scanners may give more cardiac information than any other single test, and CT may be used more widely than it is now.

Principles

Conventional CT

Standard x-ray pictures are taken by exposing a photographic plate to a beam of x-ray energy, with the patient located between the x-ray source and the film. As the x-rays penetrate the patient, they pass through less dense tissue with little change, but are scattered or weakened by denser structures such as metal or bone. The energy reaching the photographic film will therefore form an image of the materials it has passed through, with dense materials seen as darker than adjoining soft tissue. Although it provides much useful information, conventional x-ray does not define soft tissue well and has trouble with structures that overlie one another.

A different method of x-ray imaging is to take cross-sectional pictures, rather like slicing a cucumber and looking at the inside. A very thin x-ray beam must be generated—either a pinpoint beam that sweeps across the body or a fan-shaped beam.[16] However, taking such pictures from just one angle gives limited information. The solution is to have the x-ray source rotate around the patient in one plane, taking multiple views of that "slice" of the body from all different angles. Rather than striking a photographic plate, the x-rays are picked up by detectors on the other side of the patient. Data from the detectors are organized in digital form and correlated by a computer, then formed into a two-dimensional "map" of the cross section.[16]

The CT technique gained its name from this computerization and from *tomography*, a generic term for imaging through a certain body plane. It is also called computerized axial tomography (CAT), referring to the rotation of the imaging system around an axis. The first CTs required 5 minutes to acquire one total slice, with 2 to 5 seconds needed for each image.[16] The patient was required to lie quite still to avoid motion artifact. In spite of the slow scanning speed, the early CT was recognized as a revolution in imaging. It provided sharp detail and a new cross-sectional view of organs. It was found that iodine-based contrast dyes given intravenously improved the contrast between certain tissues and highlighted vascular structures. Because of its much better definition of soft tissues than regular x-ray, CT soon became the new standard for imaging the brain and was useful for imaging the thorax and abdomen as well.

Conventional CT has not been widely useful in cardiothoracic studies because its slow image acquisition causes the image of the moving heart and lungs to blur. Studies have been limited to structures that have relatively less movement, such as the pericardium, aorta, and vena cava.[17,18] Attempts were made to use ECG gating (as in nuclear medicine studies) to improve the image quality, but results were still not satisfactory.[19] Since 1980, coronary bypass grafts have been studied with conventional CT. A bolus of contrast dye, coordinated with the scan, is used to illuminate the lumen of grafts—seen usually end-on, as small circles in the cross-section view.[20] Note that this procedure is technically difficult.

In an effort to make CT more useful, various hardware changes in the second generation of CT scanners led to fast CT[19] (Figure 6.17). A stationary ring of detectors also incorporated a rapidly rotatable x-ray source; the x-ray emitter could rotate completely around the patient in about one second, completing the slice in that period of time. Although this improved the speed of the CT scan, the need to physically rotate the x-ray source around the patient put a "speed limit" on imaging that made studies of the moving heart difficult.

Ultrafast CT

The next generation of CT scanners was designed to bypass the speed constraints imposed by mechanical movements of the x-ray source and detectors around the patient. In what has come to be known as ultrafast CT, magnetic fields are used to direct the x-ray beams in a very rapid scan of the patient's body. For the first time, the time needed to image one slice can be measured in milliseconds (one thousandth of a second), and the CT is capable of freezing the motion of the human heart.

Ultrafast CT (UFCT) depends on both high-precision x-ray technology and a sophisticated computer connected to an array of x-ray detectors.[16,19] The business end of a UFCT consists of a cylindrical set of magnetic coils through which a high energy electron beam is fired (Figure 6.18). The magnetic field generated by the coils is adjusted to focus

FIGURE 6.17

A fast CT scanner performing a transverse (long-axis) cardiac scan. Using slip ring technology, this machine performs each slice in 1 to 2 seconds—the upper speed limit of conventional CT, in which the x-ray source is physically rotated around the patient. While some blurring of cardiac motion is present, fast CT is adequate for many structural studies of the heart.

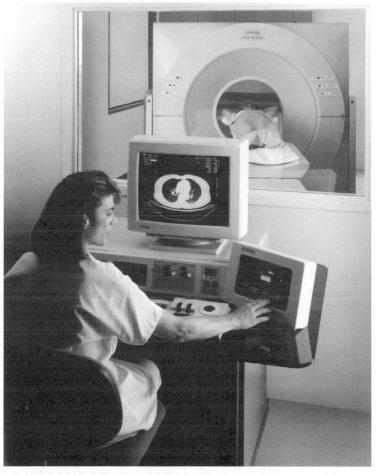

Courtesy Picker International, Inc.

the electron beam onto a large ring set perpendicular to the floor. The bottom part of the ring, constituting about 210° of arc, is made up of four rows of tungsten deflectors. The electron beam is steered onto these deflectors, and the impact generates x-rays that are directed toward the upper part of the ring. The top section of the ring is a double set of x-ray detectors, making up the remaining 150° of arc. The patient lies on a couch positioned lengthwise through the center of the ring[16,19] (Figure 6.19).

FIGURE 6.18

Ultrafast CT scanner for cardiac studies. The electron beam is deflected by magnetic coils onto the target rings surrounding the patient, creating a highly focused x-ray scan of the heart. Because there are no moving parts in the ring, scans can be performed in a few milliseconds—thus freezing cardiac motion.

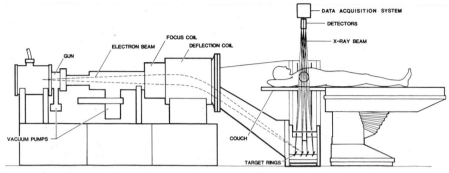

Courtesy Imatron Corporation.

Each pass produces two 1-cm-wide slices as the beam strikes the two detector rings set side by side. Therefore, in four passes, eight 1-cm-wide slices are generated. The beam takes 50 milliseconds (one twentieth of a second) to sweep over each tungsten ring and 8 milliseconds to reset to the next ring.[16,19]

The couch of a UFCT can be moved back and forth to position the patient very precisely for imaging. Usually the 8-cm scan area is enough to cover the part of the heart that is of most interest; if not, the table can be repositioned and additional scans made. Most UFCT imaging is performed along the long axis of the heart (base to apex—as in that sliced cucumber). But the heart axis is off by several degrees from the axis of the body; therefore the UFCT couch can be skewed diagonally up to 30° to align the heart correctly for the scanner. The couch can also be moved at a diagonal sufficient to scan along the short axis of the heart ("slicing" the heart lengthwise).[21]

The x-ray input collected by the detectors is gathered in a built-in computer system that stores the results as digital data. Once in the computer, the imaging data on the patient can be manipulated in many different ways. Using the digitized "maps" of various densities within the heart, images at many levels and at many points in the cardiac cycle may be selected by an operator at a computer workstation. With enough computer power, three-dimensional images of the heart may be constructed on the computer screen.[19,22]

Scanning Methods

The UFCT hardware and software can be configured in different ways to provide different kinds of data. The eight 1-cm slices generated

FIGURE 6.19

Ultrafast cardiac CT scanner showing adjustable patient couch.

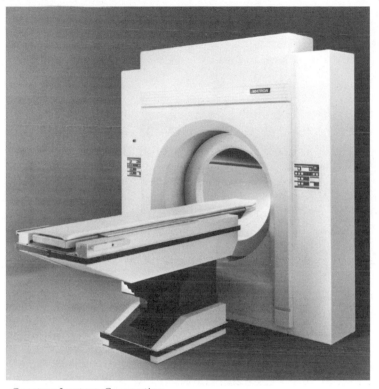

Courtesy Imatron Corporation.

in the arrangement described above are considered *standard cardiac mode*. Objects down to 1.5 mm in size can be resolved on the image, and this is usually adequate for most cardiac studies.[17] The UFCT can also be set for a different, *high-resolution mode* that provides finer detail—resolving objects as small as 0.5 mm. In high-resolution mode, the slices are only 3 mm apart. Because of the restrictions on computer storage and manipulation, the number of slices is limited, so high-resolution mode covers a smaller area.

There are two main methods of using UFCT, depending on the type of images and data desired. These are *flow mode* and *cine mode*. Application of UFCT to exercise or stress tests is still being developed.

Flow Mode

Flow mode involves using the UFCT to follow the flow of a bolus of intravenous contrast material as it makes its first pass through the chambers of the heart.[23] A 40-ml dose of contrast material is injected IV at a rate of 5 to 10 ml per second. The operator sets the UFCT to begin scanning as the bolus enters the heart. The scanning is repeated, usually for a total of ten heartbeats. The bolus is seen changing through the frames as it enters first the right side of the heart, then the left, then washes out. The cardiac structures are sequentially "lit up" by the dye going through the heart in the successive beats. The computer is able to calculate flow rates, cardiac output, and other parameters of interest.[19]

Cine Mode

Cine mode, also called "movie mode," creates moving pictures of the heart at various levels.[19,23] Contrast is injected at a slower rate—60 to 80 ml of contrast is delivered at 1.5 to 2.0 ml per second, usually by an automated power injector. The computer constructs a film loop of 10 to 20 images taken at each cross-section level of the heart. A skilled operator can view the cine sequences and spot abnormal ventricular wall motions that correlate with ischemia or infarct. Computer analysis can estimate ejection fraction, cardiac output, and ventricular wall mass. Sophisticated software can process cine UFCT data to construct three-dimensional models of the heart's chambers in action.[19,22]

Exercise and Stress CTs

Some studies have been performed on the use of ultrafast CT during exercise.[24] Because the heart at rest may not show symptoms or signs of coronary artery disease, exercise may highlight areas of ischemia. UFCT can image the heart during exercise, detecting ischemia through changes in wall motion and thickness. Future methods for CT may allow testing for myocardial perfusion as well.

However, practical problems in exercise CT have yet to be overcome. The sheer bulk and physical arrangement of the CT scanner makes supine bicycle exercise the only practical stress method. During exertion patients may easily move out of position for the scan, so the chest must be kept as still as possible. Because the cardiac cycle is shorter with the faster heart rates during exercise, cine UFCT can take only 8 to 10 frames per cycle, versus the usual 10 to 20 frames per cycle at rest.[24] This produces less useful detail than do the images from a resting study. The same problem with poorer images during faster heart rates has limited development of pharmacologic stress CT scans, such as with dobutamine or dipyridamole (Figure 6.20).

Indications for CT Scanning

Computed tomography has the ability to contribute valuable information to the clinician about the structure, function, and pathology of a patient's heart. Like MRI, CT is rarely the test of first choice for eval-

FIGURE 6.20

Supine bicycle ergometer being used for exercise ultrafast CT. After a resting study, the patient is exercised to evaluate ejection fractions, wall motion, and other ventricular performance measurements under stress.

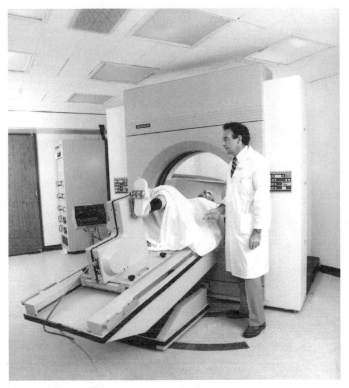

Courtesy Imatron Corporation.

uating cardiac patients. Certain technical problems, cost, and size of the equipment may be reasons for these preferences. (See "Strengths and Limitations" on p. 257.) However, with continuing improvements CT may stand out from other kinds of tests not by studying one aspect of the heart best, but by encompassing many different kinds of findings all in one procedure.

Coronary Artery Disease

UFCT in flow mode may be used to view the patency of coronary arteries as contrast flows through them.[19] Correct anatomic placement of the slices is critical, and usually high-resolution mode must be used. As with other flow studies, the computer "sees" the progress of contrast through the arteries and uses this data to calculate flow and diameter of the vessels.

Another method of viewing coronary arteries takes advantage of the presence of calcium in most atherosclerotic plaques.[17,19] The calcium lining coronary arteries shows up well on CT, even without contrast. Computer programs are able to quantify the calcium present, giving a rough estimate of the degree of coronary plaque buildup. This can be followed over time, and evaluated after interventions for any signs of improvement (Figures 6.21 and 6.22).

Conventional CT scans have been used to detect myocardial infarction (MI) by comparing myocardial uptake of tracer in different regions of the heart.[25] As with thallium and other nuclear tests, the iodine-based dye is taken up less readily by damaged heart muscle cells. Ultrafast CT may add extra details and localization to diagnosing MI. More research is needed to support this application of CT, however, and it has not been adopted widely by clinicians.

Ventricular wall motion can be assessed quite well in cine-mode UFCT, with regions of abnormal wall motion correlating highly with ischemic or infarcted myocardium.[24] Ventricular wall thinning occurs after

FIGURE 6.21

Multilevel ultrafast CT study of 27-year-old man with family history of CAD shows several small calcifications in the coronary arteries.

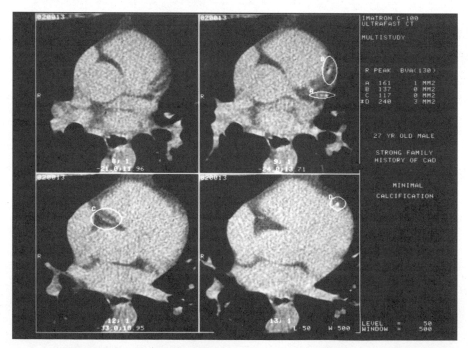

Courtesy Imatron Corporation.

FIGURE 6.22

Photograph of a three-dimensional image of the heart reconstructed from twenty to thirty 3-mm slice images. Calcified coronary artery plaques are visible, and the computer has estimated the volume of plaque based on 3-D volume calculations.

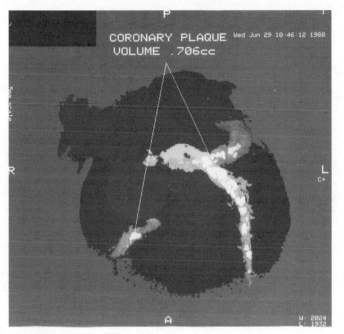

Courtesy Imatron Corporation.

myocardial infarction, and the high resolution of CT is ideal for measuring heart wall thickness.[25]

Coronary Artery Bypass Grafts

One of the earliest uses of CT in cardiac studies was the evaluation for patency of coronary artery bypass grafts (CABG).[20] Because the upper region of the heart where grafts are located moves less than, say, the ventricles, even conventional and fast CT could often get clear images of grafts illuminated with contrast material. Scanning at the level of the aortic root, the grafts are usually seen end-on as small white circles. Blockage by thrombus or plaque will prevent all or part of the contrast from flowing through, and a dark spot where a graft should be indicates some obstruction (Figure 6.23).

Ventricular Volume, Mass, and Performance

With its rapid imaging of cardiac chamber dimensions at different levels, ultrafast CT (UFCT) provides computer data for precise mea-

FIGURE 6.23

Flow study on ultrafast CT using contrast dye to determine patency of coronary artery bypass grafts. Shown is one of 13 transverse images taken during injection. The computer counts the density of contrast in each graft vessel during each image and places the data on a time-density graph (at bottom). The bell-shaped curve for the aorta (A) and the right coronary graft (R) show they are patent, while the flat lines of the circumflex (C) and left coronary (L) grafts indicate those vessels are occluded.

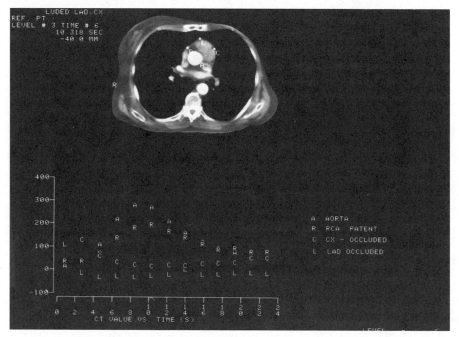

Courtesy Imatron Corporation.

surement of cardiac volumes, ejection fraction, and cardiac output.[26] UFCT precisely outlines the inner and outer walls of the heart, allowing accurate estimates of ventricle mass and wall thickness—important factors in diagnosing cardiomyopathies and ventricular hypertrophy[17] (Figure 6.24).

Pericardial Disease

The pericardium is well visualized on CT because it has less intrinsic movement than the heart itself.[17] Echocardiography is the most practical method for imaging the pericardium, but CT is helpful when technical problems make the echocardiogram unreliable or if more detail is needed on pericardial thickness and type of effusion.[27] Calcified pericardium "lights up" on CT even without contrast dye. Ultrafast CT shows the motion of the heart and pericardium in relation to each other, which

FIGURE 6.24

Transverse ultrafast CT images of (left) end-diastole and (right) end-systole are made at multiple levels during one cardiac cycle. The data are analyzed with wall-motion software to yield end-diastolic and stroke volumes, ejection fraction, and myocardial mass.

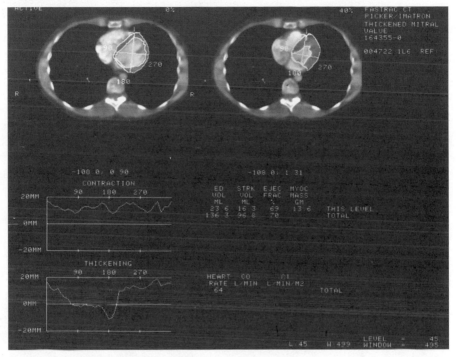

Courtesy Imatron Corporation.

helps to differentiate constrictive pericarditis (where the thickened pericardium restricts the heart's filling and pumping).

Cardiac Valve Disease

Two-dimensional and Doppler echocardiography are the most frequently used tests for studying cardiac valves. Ultrafast CT can be used to image all four cardiac valves, but the patient and scanner must be aligned very precisely in order to slice along the valve surface. In spite of these challenges, UFCT has been used to diagnose disorders of the mitral valve (prolapse, regurgitation, stenosis) and the aortic valve (stenosis, regurgitation).[17]

Aortic and Ventricular Aneurysms

Although angiography and echocardiography are the usual methods for detecting aortic aneurysms, CT has shown promise as an alternative with a lower radiation load and a unique cross-sectional view.[17] Peripheral injection of contrast is sufficient to give excellent CT images of the aortic lumen. Flow-mode studies can diagnose dissections and leaks, and define any obstruction of branch vessels. Cine-mode images will show movement of the aneurysm structures.

UFCT can also diagnose ventricular aneurysms effectively. They appear on flow images as a structural outpouching of the ventricular wall. The wall-motion studies in cine mode can detect the paradoxic outward movement of the aneurysm during systole.[17] (Figure 6.25)

Thrombi and Tumors

Echocardiography is frequently used to diagnose clots in the heart. CT can, however, provide a minimally invasive alternative and add information where echo results are equivocal.[27] Thrombi within the heart, seen as contrast-poor filling defects within the chamber, are often associated with areas of abnormal wall motion or wall thinning—all vis-

FIGURE 6.25

A transverse ultrafast CT image using contrast dye, which shows as bright areas on the scan. The central bright area represents the dye normally seen in the ventricles, but the outpouching of an aneurysm into the pericardial space is readily seen (arrow) as the dye fills it.

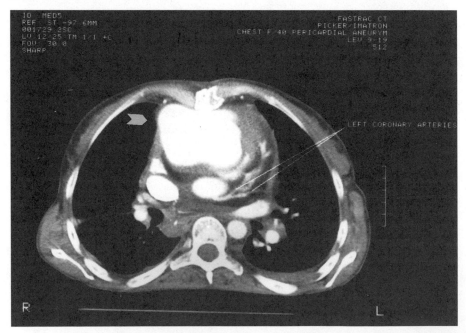

Courtesy Imatron Corporation.

ible on CT. When attached to a wall (mural thrombus), the clot may be verified by its movements as seen on cine-mode CT. The left atrial appendage is a common site for thrombi; UFCT shows it in cross section, providing better information than does echocardiography.[27]

CT also may be used to diagnose and define tumors of the heart, pericardium, and mediastinum. Primary cardiac tumors, such as myxomas, often lie within the heart chambers and may be either firmly attached to the wall or on a peduncle (stalk). Like thrombi, tumors in the heart chambers appear as filling defects. Initially best seen in flow-mode CT, the tumors can be further characterized by observing their movements in cine-mode imaging. Tumors that grow in the pericardium and mediastinum (including metastases from distant tumors) can also be detected with CT.[27]

Congenital Heart Defects

CT has largely been superseded by magnetic resonance imaging (MRI) and echocardiography in the diagnosis of congenital heart defects. However, CT is capable of detecting great vessel transposition, coarctation of the aorta, and other structural abnormalities.[28] An advantage over current MRI systems is the very fast imaging of UFCT, especially useful for high-resolution pictures in children who may be restless.

Strengths And Limitations Of CT

Strengths

For cardiac studies, most of the advantages of computed tomography are specific to ultrafast, rather than conventional, CT. The cross-sectional format gives information on structure not available with some of the planar imaging techniques, such as radionuclide scans and 2-D echocardiography. UFCT gives substantial information about cardiac structure, and is improving its ability to assess function. Computer storage of the data allows extensive manipulation and reformatting of the images; CT-linked computers can construct three-dimensional images of the heart, and this ability is expected to improve.[29] While UFCT is an expensive technology, it can also be performed quickly (in about 30 minutes), allowing a quicker turnover of patients, which may offset the cost somewhat.

UFCT has shown high accuracy in delineating the inner and outer surfaces of cardiac walls, thus making possible more exact calculations of chamber volumes, ventricular mass, wall thickness, and cardiac output.[17] Cine CT shows wall motion abnormalities, perhaps better than does radionuclide ventriculography. Good detail is available for most masses, tumors, and thrombi.[27] Resolution of structures as small as 0.5 to 1 mm makes CT competitive with magnetic resonance imaging, which is generally more expensive.[18,22]

CT falls in the medium range of invasiveness. While contrast is used, the amount is usually less than in cardiac catheterization. The radiation load is modest, and with UFCT is even less than conventional CT. Easier-to-establish peripheral IV contrast injection is used, rather than injection via central line as in catheterization. More information on wall motion and myocardium can be gained with UFCT than with catheterization.[18,22]

In summary, ultrafast CT is a modestly invasive technology for evaluating cardiac structures. Although other tests are often considered to be superior in measuring cardiac function, few offer as many measurements in one quick procedure. Technical improvements are predicted that may realize UFCTs potential for heart studies.

Limitations

Ultrafast CT is a relatively expensive technology that is yet to find a strong place in cardiac testing. More experience and studies are needed to know its true utility. Current CT machines are large and stationary, unable to travel to the bedside as can echocardiographic machines and even some nuclear scanners.

Technical limitations make evaluation of heart structure difficult. UFCT is inferior to both echo and MRI in the evaluation of valves. Studies of myocardial perfusion, exercise performance, and CABG vessels are difficult and not widely used. Patient placement must be exact in order to scan the correct area. Although resolution is high, the interslice areas are not imaged at all. High-capacity computers will be needed for projected increases in speed and resolution.[17,19,20]

Although it is considered a noninvasive test, CT may result in a contrast reaction. Contrast often causes temporary flushing and nausea in the patient and can precipitate allergic reactions, including anaphylaxis. Contrast can also cause acute renal failure, and therefore, is contraindicated in patients with renal insufficiency.[17] The patient is exposed to ionizing radiation in the form of x-rays (about the same as in a standard abdominal CT or skull x-ray series).[30]

Conventional CT machines may be quite large and confining, and patients with claustrophobia may become acutely anxious—likely changing their cardiac output as well. The patient must be able to lie still for long periods for conventional CT and may be asked to hold his or her breath for up to 45 seconds.[18,22] (UFCT is done much more quickly, and breath holding is not as essential.) UFCT machines are less likely to induce claustrophobia as they are more open, and the procedure much shorter.

The Future and CT

Optimists project improvements in UFCT that will allow testing of coronary arteries, cardiac function, and myocardial perfusion in the near future. In fact, the stated goal of those working to develop ultrafast CT for cardiac studies is to make CT "the only exam needed for cardiac diagnosis."[19] To do so will require further improvements in scanning speed, resolution, computer memory, and computer processing time. The equally impressive cost of UFCT systems will no doubt be debated in the future and will be a factor in the acceptance and use of cardiac CT.

Further developments in three-dimensional (3-D) CT imaging are expected, including cine 3-D and color imaging of various densities. Faster image processing may allow real-time imaging, essentially CT fluoroscopy, in the future. Promoters of CT project the use of UFCT as the primary whole-body screening tool, in which 300 to 1000 1.5-mm cuts could be taken during one held breath, with complete 3-D reconstruction of the patient's body on-screen.[31,32]

NURSING IMPLICATIONS OF CT SCANS

CT scans are usually well tolerated by the patient. There are, however, certain contraindications and precautions of which the nurse must be aware in assessing, preparing, and providing aftercare for the patient undergoing cardiac CT. Explanations will help educate patients about the procedure and elicit their cooperation for more useful test results.

Patient Assessment

Certain patients should probably not have a CT scan. Pregnant women are usually not given x-ray tests such as CT due to possible negative effects on the fetus. Most patients with iodine allergy or previous reactions to IV contrast dye may be excluded from CT testing. If the test is considered essential, those with previous mild (nonanaphylactic) reactions to contrast may be pretreated with IV methylprednisolone (Solu-Medrol) and an IV antihistamine such as diphenhydramine (Benadryl). Renal failure and renal insufficiency will inhibit kidney excretion of the contrast dye, predisposing the patient to toxicity and further renal compromise. The nurse should check recent lab results before the CT scan for an elevated serum BUN or creatinine.[29,30]

Physical abilities as well as mental and behavioral factors should be assessed in the patient having a CT scan. The patient will need to lie very still for prolonged periods with conventional CT scan, and with all types of CT may be asked to hold his or her breath or otherwise cooperate with the procedure. The patient must be stable enough to be alone in the scan room for 30 to 60 minutes (a technician monitors the patient from the next room). The usual position is flat and supine, with arms over the head. The patient may be anxious about radiation exposure; it may help to reassure him or her that the radiation dose is no more than that in a series of normal x-rays. The large, enclosing nature of the conventional CT scanner may induce anxiety in a patient with claustrophobia, so the nurse should ask about any fears of confined places. (This is not as much an issue with the more open design of the ultrafast CT scanner.)[29,30]

Patient Preparation

The patient should take nothing by mouth for 4 hours before the procedure. (Some institutions allow clear liquids to be taken.) An intravenous line is necessary for the injection of contrast dye. Medications may typically be given as usual before the CT scan. The patient should wear a hospital gown top and should expect the chest to be exposed. ECG leads may be attached for certain studies.

For conventional CT, the patient should expect to lie on the table between 30 and 90 minutes, depending on the type of study (see Patient Education Boxes 6.2 and 6.3). The technician is usually in the next room and speaks to the patient through an intercom. The technician will tell the patient when to lie still; the patient should not talk during this time. Breath holding may be requested, perhaps up to 30 to 45 seconds at a time. The scanner may emit clicking or whirring sounds as the mechanism repositions itself.[29,30]

In ultrafast CT, the procedure is usually much shorter, and breath holding and lying still are for much briefer periods. The entire scanning sequence may take just a few seconds; including setup, the patient may be on the table less than 30 minutes.

Contrast administration is a similar experience in all types of CT scans. Depending on the type of study, contrast may be given by rapid IV bolus or by a slower IV infusion. Many patients experience flushing, tingling, headache, or nausea during injection and for a few moments after. The patient should be told to expect this and informed that the effect should pass in a few minutes or seconds. The patient should report any chest pain, severe itching, shortness of breath, or other symptoms to the test personnel.[29,30]

Aftercare

After the CT scan, diet and medications may be resumed. The patient should be closely assessed for any signs of contrast reaction for the next few hours: respiratory distress, palpitations, hypotension, itching, urticaria (hives), or diaphoresis. (There should be emergency equipment close at hand to treat allergic or cardiorespiratory reactions both during and after the scan.) Oral or IV fluids should be increased to aid renal excretion of the contrast, and an adequate urine output documented. A drop in urine output may signal renal problems from the dye.[29,30]

PATIENT EDUCATION BOX 6.2

Conventional CT Scan

The purpose of the CT scan is to take detailed x-ray pictures of the heart. The pictures are taken *across* the body, in "slices," giving the doctor a picture of the heart at different levels. The test takes 1 to 1½ hours.

BEFORE THE TEST

Take nothing by mouth for at least 4 hours before your test. Otherwise there is no special preparation. If you are a woman who might be pregnant, however, you should tell the doctor before the test.

If you have an allergy to iodine (which is in the dye), *or have had a reaction to IV dye, or contrast, tell the staff before the test is started.*

If you have a fear of close places (claustrophobia), have trouble lying still, or cannot hold your breath, tell the staff before the test.

Comfortable, loose clothing is best—if you are a hospital patient, pajamas are fine. You will be asked to remove your shirt or blouse for the test, and will be given a hospital gown.

An intravenous (IV) line will be inserted in your arm if one is not already in place.

DURING THE TEST

You will lie on an x-ray table that will be rolled inside the CT machine. The machine is quite large and will surround you completely. The technician will speak to you by intercom. You will be asked to lie still during the scan, which takes 30 to 60 minutes. You may be asked to hold your breath at times.

After the first scan, you may be given a second scan in which IV dye (contrast) is used. This can make for much clearer pictures of your heart. When the dye is injected into your IV, you may feel nauseated or have a warm, flushed feeling. This is normal and passes in a few seconds. *If you are having discomfort, tell the staff.*

AFTER THE TEST

After you have finished the scan you may go back to your usual diet and medicines. Make sure you drink extra glasses of water or other fluids for the next few hours. This will help eliminate the dye from your body.

A small number of people may have a reaction to the dye used in the CT scan. Report at once to your doctor or nurse if you develop itching, swelling, rash, shortness of breath, or dizziness, or if you make a lot less urine in spite of drinking fluids.

PATIENT EDUCATION BOX 6.3

Ultrafast CT Scan

The purpose of the CT scan is to take detailed x-ray pictures of the heart. The pictures are taken across the body in thin "slices," presenting a picture of the heart in cross section. The test takes 30 to 45 minutes.

BEFORE THE TEST

Take nothing by mouth for at least 4 hours before your test. Otherwise there is no special preparation. If you are a woman who might be pregnant, you should tell the doctor before the test.

If you have an allergy to iodine (the dye), or have had a reaction to IV dye, or contrast, tell the staff before the test is started.

If you have a fear of close places (claustrophobia), have trouble lying still, or cannot hold your breath, tell the staff before the test.

Comfortable, loose clothing is best—if you are a hospital patient, pajamas are fine. You will be asked to remove your shirt or blouse for the test, and will be given a hospital gown.

An intravenous (IV) line will be inserted in your arm if one is not already in place.

DURING THE TEST

You will lie on an x-ray table inside a ring next to a large machine. The technician will speak to you by intercom. The table may be moved during the test to position you for different pictures.

The scans themselves take only a few seconds. You may be asked to hold your breath at times, and to lie still during the scans.

You may be given IV dye (contrast) during the study. This can make for much clearer pictures of your heart. When the dye is injected into your IV, you may feel nauseated or have a warm, flushed feeling. This is normal and usually passes in a few seconds. *If you are having discomfort, tell the staff.*

AFTER THE TEST

After you have finished the scan you may go back to your usual diet and medicines, making sure you drink extra glasses of water or other fluids for the next few hours.

A small number of people may have an allergic reaction to the dye used. Report at once to your doctor or nurse if you develop itching, swelling, rash, shortness of breath, or dizziness, or if you make a lot less urine in spite of drinking fluids.

References

1. Rudy EB. Magnetic resonance imaging: New horizon in diagnostic techniques. *J Neurosurg Nurs.* 1985;17:331–337.
2. White RD, Van Rossum AC. Introduction to the use of magnetic resonance imaging. In: Elliott, LP. *Cardiac Imaging in Infants, Children and Adults.* Philadelphia: JB Lippincott; 1990.
3. Higgins CB, Caputo GR. Role of MR imaging in acquired and congenital cardiovascular disease. *Am J Roentgenol.* 1993;161:13–22.
4. Pettigrew RI. Magnetic resonance imaging in cardiology: Attractive for clinical cardiologists? In: Reiber JHC, van der Wall EE, eds. *Cardiovascular Nuclear Medicine and MRI: Quantitation and Clinical Applications.* Boston: Kluwer; 1992.
5. Rehr RB. Cardiovascular nuclear magnetic resonance imaging and spectroscopy. *Curr Prob Cardiol.* 1991;16:127–215.
6. Van der Wall EE. *Nuclear Cardiology and Cardiac Magnetic Resonance.* Boston: Kluwer; 1992.
7. Peshock RM, Moore DM. Magnetic resonance imaging: Technical aspects. In: Brundage BH, ed. *Comparative Cardiac Imaging.* Rockville, Md: Aspen; 1990.
8. Sechtem U, Theissen P, Baer FM, Schicha H. Evaluation of cardiac function using MRI. In: Reiber JHC, van der Wall EE, eds. *Cardiovascular Nuclear Medicine and MRI: Quantitation and Clinical Applications.* Boston: Kluwer; 1992.
9. Underwood R. Magnetic resonance imaging of the cardiovascular system. In: Reiber JHC, van der Wall EE, eds. *Cardiovascular Nuclear Medicine and MRI: Quantitation and Clinical Applications.* Boston: Kluwer; 1992.
10. D'Agincourt L. Advances push imaging past recognizable limits. *Diagn Imaging.* 1991;13(January: suppl A):A23–A55.
11. Doornbos J, Verwey H, Essed CE, et al. MR imaging in assessment of cardiac transplant rejection in humans. *J Comput Assist Tomogr.* 1990;14:77–81.
12. Wolfe CL. Application of contrast agents in magnetic resonance imaging: Additional value for detection of myocardial ischemia? In: Van der Wall EE, Sochor H, Righetti A, Niemeyer MG, eds. *What's New in Cardiac Imaging?* Boston: Kluwer; 1992.
13. Schoenbeck SB. Your role in caring for patients undergoing MRI. *J Pract Nurs.* 1991;41:33–35.
14. Rauscher N. Understanding magnetic resonance imaging (MRI). *J Orthop Nurs.* 1990;9:60.
15. Plankey ED, Knauf J. What patients need to know about magnetic resonance imaging. *Am J Nurs.* 1990;90:27–28.
16. Gould RG. Principles of ultrafast computed tomography: Historical aspects, mechanism of action and scanner characteristics. In: Stanford W, Rumberger JA, eds. *Ultrafast Computed Tomography in Cardiac Imaging: Principles and Practice.* Mount Kisco, NY: Futura; 1992.
17. Marcus RL, Weiss RM. Evaluation of cardiac structure and function with ultrafast computed tomography. In: Marcus ML, Schulbert HR, Skorton DL, Wolf GL. *Cardiac Imaging: A Companion to Braunwald's "Heart Disease."* Philadelphia: WB Saunders; 1991.
18. Stanford W. Computed tomography and ultrafast computed tomography in ischemic heart disease. In: Elliott LP. *Cardiac Imaging in Infants, Children and Adults.* Philadelphia: JB Lippincott; 1991.
19. Boyd DP. Cardiac computed tomography: Technical aspects. In: Brundage BH, ed. *Comparative Cardiac Imaging.* Rockville, Md: Aspen; 1990.

20. Stanford W. Introduction to the use of computed tomography and ultrafast computed tomography. In: Elliott LP. *Cardiac Imaging in Infants, Children and Adults*. Philadelphia: JB Lippincott; 1991.
21. Stanford W. Normal cardiac anatomy as seen with ultrafast computed tomography. In: Stanford W, Rumberger JA, eds. *Ultrafast Computed Tomography in Cardiac Imaging: Principles and Practice*. Mount Kisco, NY: Futura; 1992.
22. Omvik P. Magnetic resonance imaging and cine computed tomography as future tools for cardiac output measurement. *Eur Heart J*. 1990;11(suppl 1):141–143.
23. Rumberger JA. Ultrafast computed tomography scanning modes, scanning planes and practical aspects of contrast administration. In: Stanford W, Rumberger JA, eds. *Ultrafast Computed Tomography in Cardiac Imaging: Principles and Practice*. Mount Kisco, NY: Futura; 1992.
24. Roig E, Chomka EV, Castaner A, et al. Exercise ultrafast computed tomography for the detection of coronary artery disease. *J Am Coll Cardiol*. 1989; 13:1073.
25. Brundage BH. Myocardial imaging with ultrafast computed tomography. In: Zaret BL, Kaufman L, Berson AS, Dunn RA, eds. *Frontiers in Cardiovascular Imaging*. New York: Raven Press; 1993.
26. McIntyre WJ. Potential application of new imaging modalities in the measurement of cardiac volumes and characteristics. *Eur Heart J*. 1990;11 (suppl 1):133–140.
27. Stanford W, Rooholamini SA, Galvin JR. Assessment of intracardiac masses and extracardiac abnormalities by ultrafast computed tomography. In: Marcus ML, Schulbert HR, Skorton DL, Wolf GL. *Cardiac Imaging: A Companion to Braunwald's Heart Disease*. Philadelphia: WB Saunders; 1991.
28. Husayni TS. Ultrafast computed tomographic imaging in congenital heart disease. In: Stanford W, Rumberger JA, eds. *Ultrafast Computed Tomography in Cardiac Imaging: Principles and Practice*. Mount Kisco, NY: Futura; 1992.
29. Pagana KD, Pagana TJ. *Diagnostic Testing and Nursing Implications: A Case Study Approach*. St. Louis: CV Mosby; 1990.
30. Gawlinski A. New diagnostic techniques. In: Kern LS, ed. *Cardiac Critical Care Nursing*. Rockville, Md: Aspen; 1988.
31. Boyd DP. New applications speed ultrafast CT into the spotlight. *Diagn Imaging*. 1991;13(January: suppl A): A72–A73.
32. Rumberger JA, Stanford W. The future of ultrafast computed tomography. In: Stanford W, Rumberger JA, eds. *Ultrafast Computed Tomography in Cardiac Imaging: Principles and Practice*. Mount Kisco, NY: Futura: 1992.

7

CARDIAC CATHETERIZATION

CATHERINE GAGE RICCIUTI

GLOSSARY

Bioptome   A special instrument used to obtain a biopsy of cardiac tissue.
Ectopic   Referring to an electrical impulse that originates from an unexpected area.
Fluoroscopy   A radiographic technique used to examine a part of the body that allows for immediate serial images.
Intima   Innermost lining of the artery.
Orifice   An entrance or opening.
Ostia   An entrance or outlet of a vessel.
Percutaneous   Referring to a procedure performed through the skin via a puncture wound.
Shunt   A pathway through which blood flows in an unusual or abnormal direction.
Stenosis   Narrowing or closure of a blood vessel due to the buildup of plaque on the intimal surface.
Transseptal   Across the septum.
Vasovagal reaction   Stimulation of the vagus nerve resulting in a decreased heart rate and decreased blood pressure.

Cardiac catheterization is a relatively new procedure in the history of cardiology. In the short time that it has been available, cardiac catheterization has changed from a purely diagnostic procedure to one with significant therapeutic implications. Many procedures may be performed in the cardiac catheterization laboratory, including right and left heart catheterization, evaluation of stenotic valves, valvuloplasty, shunt detection, coronary angiography, ventriculography, percutaneous transluminal coronary angioplasty, coronary artery stent deployment, coronary atherectomy, and cardiac biopsy. The purpose of this chapter is to provide the clinician with a general picture of what occurs in the cardiac catheterization laboratory and to assist in the integration of this knowledge into clinical practice.

HISTORY OF CARDIAC CATHETERIZATION

The concept of cardiac catheterization has evolved over the past 150 years. The first cardiac catheterization was performed in 1844 by Claude Bernard, with a horse as the patient, using the carotid artery and the internal jugular vein.[1] However, it was not until 1929 that the first human catheterization was performed. Werner Forssmann inserted a catheter via his antecubital vein into his right atrium and then walked up two flights of stairs to the x-ray department in order to document his accomplishment. Since that historic feat, investigators have been developing and improving mechanisms of cardiac catheterization in humans. Some of the accomplishments include catheter passage into the right ventricle with cardiac output calculation (Klein, 1930); passage of a catheter into the pulmonary artery (Dexter, 1947); development of a percutaneous insertion technique (Seldinger, 1953); transseptal catheterization (Ross and Cope, 1953); and passage of a balloon-tipped, flow-guided catheter into the heart (Swan and Ganz, 1970).

In 1977, Andreas Gruentzig performed the first successful percutaneous transluminal coronary angioplasty (PTCA).[2] Anderson and others described the use of streptokinase to salvage myocardial tissue during an acute myocardial infarction in 1983.[3] The following year, studies were begun to determine the efficacy of several thrombolytic agents in limiting infarct size. As a result, a number of thrombolytic agents are now used in the catheterization laboratory, often in conjunction with PTCA, to minimize cardiac damage during an acute myocardial infarction. In the late 1980s, implantation of coronary artery stents and pulverization or the removal of plaque using an atherectomy catheter began to have a place in combating the effects of coronary artery disease. The continuing refinement of both equipment and technique has resulted in sophisticated and highly effective management of patients with cardiac disease.

Approaches

Most authors agree on the general definition of cardiac catheterization. It is a combined hemodynamic and angiographic invasive procedure undertaken to confirm the presence of a clinically suspected heart condition, define its anatomy and physiology, and perhaps provide a mechanism to treat the condition.

Just as there are several different procedures that may be done in the cardiac catheterization laboratory, there are also several different techniques to carry out those procedures. The most common approaches are described below.

The Direct Approach

The direct approach (developed by Sones) involves a cutdown under local anesthesia in the antecubital area, which provides access to the brachial artery and vein. Once isolated, catheters will be placed in each vessel. First, right heart catheterization is done via the vein, and then the left heart catheterization is done via the brachial artery. When the procedure is completed, the catheters are removed and the artery is repaired with suture. The direct approach may be used on patients with peripheral vascular disease, obesity, hypertension, aortic regurgitation, and wide pulse pressure. This approach may also be used on patients who have tortuous femoral vessels or vascular grafts in the femoral area. The advantages of this technique are increased catheter control and increased catheter choice. The major disadvantages of this approach are: (1) the artery must be repaired and consequently is at risk for incomplete repair, resulting in hemorrhage or embolic formation due to arterial damage, and (2) the small size of the vessels limits the types of catheters that may be used for this approach.

The Seldinger Approach

This approach, also known as the *percutaneous femoral approach*, is more popular because it does not involve arterial cutdown or repair. Using a guide wire, catheters are inserted via an introducer into the femoral artery and vein after local anesthesia is injected into the groin area. Blood pressure monitoring is done via a stopcock system that allows for heparin flush, injection of contrast material, and transducer access to the artery. After the procedure, the catheters are removed and manual pressure is held over the site for 20 to 30 minutes to promote arterial clotting at the insertion site. One advantage of this approach is that the catheters may be left in place so that there is easy access to the coronary arteries for interventional purposes. Another advantage is that the artery does not need to be repaired. The Seldinger approach is quicker and easier to perform because the larger blood vessels of the groin are less likely to be damaged by the catheter and are easier to locate. The major disadvantages of this approach include decreased catheter control and the necessity for bed rest after the procedure to promote hemostasis and arterial wall healing.

Contrast Material

The most commonly used contrast material in the United States is meglumine sodium diatrizoate, a solution containing sodium and iodine.[1] When contrast material is injected into the coronary arteries, it opacifies the vessels so that they can be seen clearly on the fluoroscope.

Because of the high osmolality of the contrast material, transient electrocardiographic and hemodynamic changes are produced during injections into the coronary vessels. Injection into the right coronary artery produces T wave inversion in the inferior leads and T wave peaking in the anterior leads. Injection into the left coronary artery produces T wave peaking in the inferior leads and T wave inversion in the anterior leads. With each injection, heart rate and blood pressure usually decrease. If these conditions persist or if the patient develops ventricular extrasystoles, the patient will be asked to cough, which increases intrathoracic pressure and helps to clear the contrast from the coronary vasculature. The sodium content of the contrast helps to discourage ventricular dysrhythmias.

Although reactions are relatively rare (approximately 5%), the majority seem to occur in certain high-risk patients in whom contrast with high osmolality is used.[4] Renal failure may occur after contrast injection in patients who have mild to moderate renal insufficiency due to chronic hypertension or diabetes mellitus. Elderly or dehydrated patients are also at risk, as are those who have congestive heart failure or undergo several contrast exposures in a short period of time. Note also that high osmolality contrast, such as meglumine sodium diatrizoate, is sluggishly filtered through the renal tubules and may result in acute renal failure secondary to acute tubular necrosis. This sequelae may be prevented if the patient is well hydrated postcatheterization.

Other adverse reactions may also occur following the injection of contrast. Rash, anaphylaxis, and hypotensive reactions can be prevented if it is noted that the patient has had a previous reaction to contrast or has a history of allergic reactions to food containing iodine, such as shellfish. In this case, prednisone or another steroid is given 12 to 18 hours precatheterization and an antihistamine is given just prior to the procedure.

A special contrast such as iohexol, may be used in high-risk patients or in those who are likely to have an adverse reaction due to contrast material injection. Because it is lower in osmolality than meglumine sodium diatrizoate, iohexol produces a lesser degree of hemodynamic and electrocardiographic changes in the patient. Iohexol is more expensive than meglumine sodium diatrizoate and consequently is used only when indicated.

PROCEDURES

Many procedures or combinations of procedures may be done to confirm or rule out the patient's tentative medical diagnosis. During the catheterization, a series of films, called cineangiograms or cineventriculograms depending upon which part of the heart is recorded, are taken. These "cines" document the findings of the cardiac catheterization. Once the procedure is completed, the information is used to plan the patient's treatment. Valvuloplasty, PTCA, stent deployment, and atherectomy are interventions that may be done immediately after the medical diagnosis is made, thereby alleviating symptoms and preventing further cardiac damage. Cardiac catheterization provides a roadmap of the heart's anatomy and furnishes the information needed to alter the roadmap for the best possible outcome.

Diagnostic Procedures

Right and Left Heart Catheterization

The purpose of right and left heart catheterization is to measure hemodynamic pressures in the right atrium, right ventricle, pulmonary artery (both intraluminal and wedge), left atrium, and left ventricle. Two different methods may be used: (1) transseptal left heart catheterization, or (2) right and left heart catheterization.

Transseptal left heart catheterization is rarely done because of the potential complications and degree of difficulty associated with the procedure. A catheter is introduced via the brachial vein. It is guided under fluoroscopy into the superior vena cava and then into the right atrium. The right atrium pressure is noted and then a guide wire is passed into the fossa ovalis, across the atrial septum, and into the left atrium. After the pressure is noted in the left atrium, the wire and catheter are advanced into the left ventricle, where a pressure reading is also taken. The right ventricular pressure is usually not noted during this procedure. The patient must not be anticoagulated prior to the procedure because perforation of the aorta or pericardium, resulting in hemorrhage, is possible. This procedure is difficult to do in patients with mitral stenosis because the stenotic valve inhibits catheter passage into the left ventricle. Transseptal left heart catheterization is done more frequently in patients with cyanotic congenital heart disease or chest deformities or in patients who cannot lay flat.[1]

Right and left heart catheterization is the preferred method for evaluating cardiac chamber pressures. A brachial or femoral approach may be used. After guide wires are inserted into the artery and vein, right heart catheterization is done via the vein. Either a balloon-tipped, flow-guided (Swan-Ganz) catheter or a simple catheter is guided under fluoroscopy from the vein, through the inferior or superior vena cava, and into the right atrium, where the pressure is recorded. It is then passed through the tricuspid valve into the right ventricle for pressure measurement. The catheter is next passed into the pulmonary artery via the pulmonic valve and eventually into the pulmonary capillary wedge pressure

(PCWP) position. When the PCWP is measured during diastole, it is considered to be an indirect measure of the left ventricular pressure during diastole (except in patients with pulmonary hypertension or chronic obstructive pulmonary disease). The catheter is then withdrawn. At this point, direct left heart catheterization may be done. A new catheter is guided under fluoroscopy from the access artery up through the aorta. The catheter is then guided through the aortic valve into the left ventricle, where a pressure reading is done and recorded. The left atrium is then entered by moving the catheter across the mitral valve.

Normal pressure readings for all of the chambers are found in Table 7.1. In general, elevation of pressures on the right side of the heart indicate right-sided heart failure and elevation of pressures on the left side of the heart indicate left-sided heart failure. Other causes of elevated right heart pressures include pulmonary hypertension, obstructive pulmonary disease, and tricuspid and pulmonic valve impairments. Mitral and aortic valve impairments may be the cause of elevated left heart pressures. Complications of right and left heart catheterization include ventricular irritability resulting in ectopic beats. Other complications are discussed at the end of this chapter.

Coronary Angiography

Coronary angiography is done to determine the degree of coronary artery disease in patients with angina pectoris, to confirm the presence of variant angina, to assess the complications of myocardial infarction, or to evaluate positive stress tests. Since angiography can cause ischemia, this procedure should be done immediately after the right and left heart catheterization so that hemodynamic pressures will be as close to the patient's baseline as possible.[1] A special catheter is guided under fluoroscopy through the aorta into the left and right coronary arteries, and several injections using contrast (diluted with normal saline) are given so that the anatomy and patency of the coronary arteries may be noted. Individual coronary arteries and their branches are injected sepa-

TABLE 7.1

Normal Cardiac Pressure Readings

Cardiac Chamber	Pressure (mm Hg)
Right Atrium	2–10
Right Ventricle*	15–30/0–8
Pulmonary Capillary Wedge	3–15
Left Atrium	3–15
Left Ventricle*	100–140/3–15

* Ventricular pressures are stated in terms of systolic pressure over diastolic pressure.

rately and viewed from different angles so that the entire coronary artery circulation may be visualized (Figure 7.1). A stenosis is considered significant if it is 50% or greater in the left main coronary artery and 75% or greater in the major branches, such as the left anterior descending, the circumflex, or the right coronary artery.

The American Heart Association and the American College of Cardiology have agreed on a three-tiered classification system for coronary lesions, based on the characteristics of the lesion, including size, contour, presence of calcification, and location.[5] The purpose of this classification system is to describe the lesion in terms of its applicability to successful angioplasty. Thus, a type A lesion is small (< 10 mm in length), noncalcific, not totally occluded, nonostial, and concentric, and has a smooth contour. Type A lesions are associated with very high success rates following angioplasty. A type B lesion is moderate in size (10–20 mm in length), has moderate calcification, is irregular in contour and somewhat tortuous, is ostial in location, may occur at a bifurcation, and may have some thrombus present in the artery. A type C lesion is diffuse (greater than 2 cm), very tortuous, and often totally occluded. Successful treatment of each of these lesion types is possible with angioplasty; however, the success rate decreases and the morbidity increases with type C lesions[5] (Table 7.2).

Once the anatomy has been carefully analyzed, an appropriate intervention is decided upon. Often an angioplasty will be attempted first unless the disease is diffuse or there is a very risky left main coronary lesion. If there is a clot detected in the artery, a thrombolytic agent (such as urokinase or tissue plasminogen activator) may be injected directly into it. In some cases, medical management will be recommended.

Coronary artery spasm, a temporary closure of the coronary artery, may be documented during routine angiography. If it is suspected, all nitrates and calcium antagonists must be discontinued 48 hours prior to the procedure (chest pain episodes are treated with sublingual or intravenous nitroglycerin). After a catheter is placed in the left ventricle to monitor hemodynamic pressure, ergonovine (a vasoconstrictor) is injected intravenously or directly into the coronary artery. The patient is observed for 2 minutes for electrocardiographic, hemodynamic, or symptomatic changes. If spasm is produced, it is treated with intracoronary nitroglycerin until the artery returns to normal.

Coronary angiography serves as a guide for medical and/or surgical management of cardiac patients. If angioplasty or another medical intervention is indicated it will be attempted first because of the potential risks and longer recovery associated with coronary artery bypass grafting. When nonsurgical intervention is unsuccessful or not possible, coronary artery bypass grafting may be done. However if there are several coronary artery lesions or if the disease is quite diffuse, it is possible that the patient will not be a candidate for surgical management and one of the sev-

FIGURE 7.1

(A) Normal right cine angiograms viewed in the LAO (left anterior oblique) position. (B) Normal left cine angiogram viewed in the RAO (right anterior oblique) position.

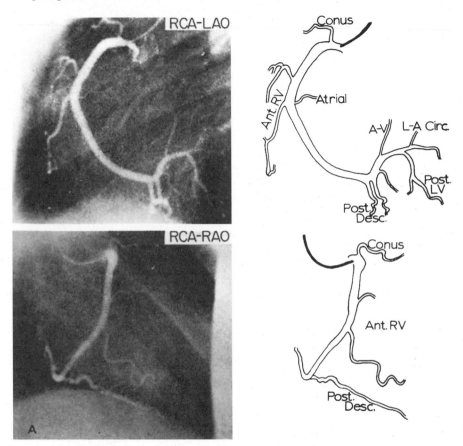

From: Friesinger GC, Ross RS. Coronary angiography: Review of technique and a report of experience with selective angiography. In: Cooley R, Schreiber M, eds. *Radiology of the Heart and Great Vessels*. 2nd ed. Baltimore: Williams & Wilkins; 1967: 4.408, 4.414.

eral interventional techniques, such as intracoronary stent implantation or atherectomy, will be attempted. If these interventions fail, the patient's medication regimen is optimized for the best possible control of angina.

Ventriculography

Left ventriculography is used along with hemodynamic data to evaluate ventricular function, aortic and mitral valve competence, and presence and location of ventricular aneurysms and septal defects.[1] Right ventriculography is usually only done in patients with congenital heart

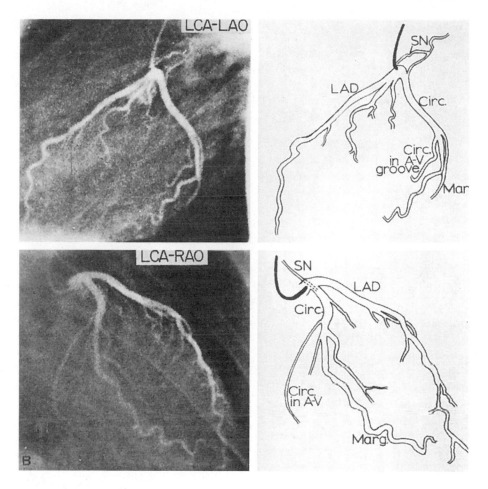

disease.[1] It provides information about the tricuspid valve and right ventricular function. The following discussion will be confined to the left ventricle, with the understanding that similar techniques can be used to evaluate the right ventricle.

Contrast is injected directly into the left ventricle. As the ventricle contracts and then relaxes, the contrast helps to outline ventricular wall motion and to highlight areas of decreased, abnormal, or absent movement. A simple method for determining left ventricular ejection fraction (EF) is described in the following formula:

$$FF (\%) = \frac{EDV - ESV}{EDV} \times 100$$

where

        EDV = end-diastolic volume
        ESV = end-systolic volume

TABLE 7.2

Descriptions of Coronary Lesion Characteristics

ECCENTRIC	Lesion that is located on one side of the artery wall only
CONCENTRIC	Lesion that is evenly spread around the lumen of the artery
DISCRETE	Small lesion
DIFFUSE	Disease that is widely disseminated
ANGULATED	Taking a sharp turn
TORTUOUS	Twisted, not straight
FRIABLE	Easily breakable
OSTIAL	At the opening of an artery
BIFURCATED	At the junction of two vessels

Simply stated, ejection fraction is the percentage of blood ejected from the left ventricle during each contraction. It is normally 50% or greater in a patient at rest. Ejection fraction is a valuable predictor for survival in patients with heart disease.[6] Postmyocardial infarction patients with an ejection fraction of less than 20% have a 50% mortality rate during the first year after the event.[7] Consequently, ejection fraction is an important measurement to obtain in postmyocardial infarction patients (Figure 7.2).

Evaluation of Valve Disease

Orifice area of stenotic valves is evaluated during right and left heart catheterization. A valve that is stenotic is less pliable and does not open as easily as a normal valve. Calculation of the valve orifice involves noting the pressure difference on both sides of the valve during ventricular filling and emptying and then applying appropriate mathematical formulas to the results obtained. If the orifice is too small, blood flow will be restricted and the chamber proximal to the valve will enlarge to accommodate the increased pressure generated by the increased blood volume. In the case of the mitral valve, not only will the left atrium enlarge but blood will back up into the lungs, resulting in pulmonary edema. In some patients, pulmonary edema will not occur until the heart is stressed (e.g. during exercise); in other patients, pulmonary edema occurs at rest. When the valvular stenosis results in pulmonary edema with minimal or no stress, the valve is considered to be critical. The critical mitral valve orifice is less than 1 cm² in area (5 cm²/m² BSA is normal), while the critical aortic valve orifice is less than 0.5 cm² in area (3 cm² is normal). Surgical valve replacement or valvuloplasty is usually necessary for these pa-

FIGURE 7.2

Calculated ejection fraction of 33% during ventriculography. Outline of systole and diastole; the systolic/diastolic volume difference is represented by a percentage. Normal ejection fraction is 50% to 60% at rest.

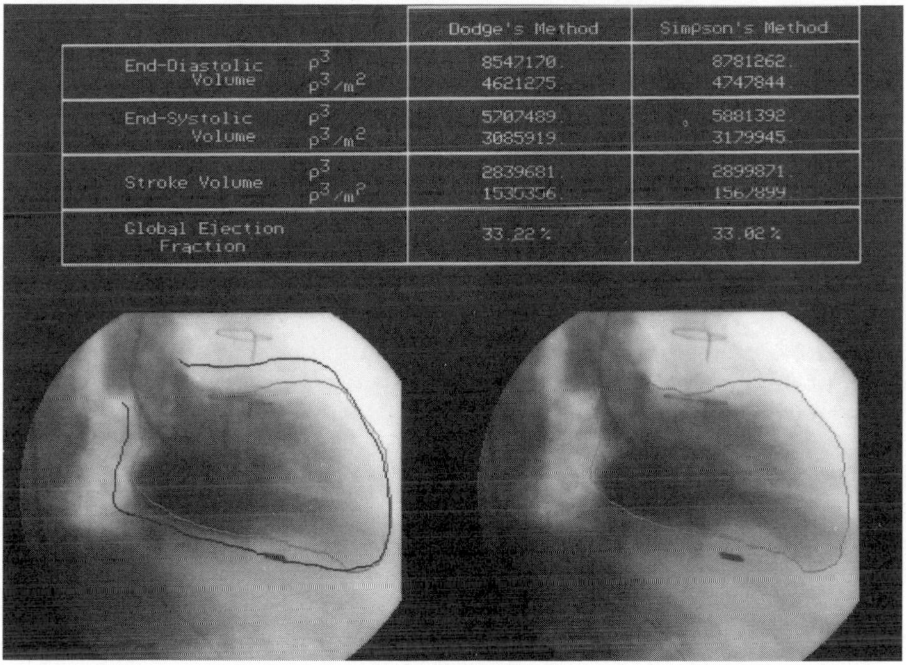

		Dodge's Method	Simpson's Method
End-Diastolic Volume	p^3 p^3/m^2	8547170 4621275	8781262 4747844
End-Systolic Volume	p^3 p^3/m^2	5707489 3085919	5881392 3179945
Stroke Volume	p^3 p^3/m^2	2839681 1530356	2899871 1567899
Global Ejection Fraction		33.22 %	33.02 %

Courtesy Dr. Steven Werns, University of Michigan Hospitals, Ann Arbor, Mich.

tients. In patients with valvular regurgitation, a grading system is used to distinguish between minimal regurgitation and severe regurgitation. The degree of regurgitation is measured from grade 1 to grade 4, with grade 4 being the most severe,[8] Regardless of the regurgitation grade, the symptomatic patient may require valve replacement.

Shunt Detection

Shunt detection is done in conjunction with right and left heart catheterization. It is done in patients with known or suspected cyanotic congenital heart disease or in patients who are suspected of having an acquired ventricular septal defect secondary to myocardial infarction. The procedure involves withdrawing blood via the catheter from each chamber in the heart so that it may be analyzed to determine its oxygen saturation. The right atrium and ventricle normally have a low oxygen saturation (75%) because they contain primarily unoxygenated blood from the systemic venous circulation.[9] The left atrium and ventricle have a high oxygen saturation (96%).[9] If the right heart oxygen saturation is abnormally high and the left heart oxygen saturation is abnormally low, a left-to-right shunt is diagnosed.

Cardiac Biopsy

Cardiac biopsy is a means to diagnose and evaluate primary myocardial disease, myocarditis, or heart transplant rejection. While the biopsy may be taken from either the right or left ventricle, it is more commonly done on the right. If the right ventricle is biopsied, the right femoral vein or, more often, the right internal jugular vein is the insertion site. If the left ventricle must be biopsied, the right femoral artery is used as the insertion site. Once the insertion site is selected, a bioptome is threaded through a catheter into the selected ventricle. The bioptome has a scissor-like handle controlling a collection device at the other end. This allows the operator to scrape a small amount of tissue from the interior of the right ventricle (Figure 7.3). The bioptome is then withdrawn and the tissue is microscopically examined.

Biopsy of cardiac tissue yields important information necessary to guide medical treatment, especially in patients who have heart failure for unknown reasons. In most cases, types of cardiomyopathy may be distinguished from myocarditis based on the types of cells found.[10] Once the cause of heart failure is known, the proper intervention can be started.

Cardiac biopsy is the preferred method to monitor for heart transplant rejection. Heart transplant rejection is evidenced by the presence of inflammatory cells and myocardial degeneration and is the most common indication for cardiac biopsy.[10] Heart transplant patients routinely have a cardiac biopsy at regular intervals for the first year posttransplant and whenever symptoms of rejection are manifested.

Therapeutic Procedures

Percutaneous Transluminal Coronary Angioplasty

Percutaneous transluminal coronary angioplasty (PTCA) has become the treatment of choice in patients with one or two significant coronary artery stenoses. After coronary angiography has proven that a significant stenosis is present, a small catheter with a balloon near the tip is passed through the stenosed coronary artery. The balloon is then inflated several times for progressively longer periods of time in the stenosed area in an attempt to reduce the stenosis (Figure 7.4).

Scientists are uncertain as to the mechanism of action in PTCA. Several theories have been proposed: compression and redistribution of plaque which enlarges the lumen of the artery; stretching of plaque-free segment of wall in an eccentric lesion; localized stretching of arterial wall; splitting or tearing of the plaque and the intima at its weakest point.[2]

FIGURE 7.3

Bioptome used for endocardial biopsy. (**A**) Bioptome in open position, illustrating "jaws." (**B**) Bioptome in closed position next to a pencil. (**C**) Squeeze handle used to open and close the tip of the catheter to harvest a tissue sample from the right ventricle. The catheter can be reshaped so that a different area of heart is used for each subsequent biopsy.

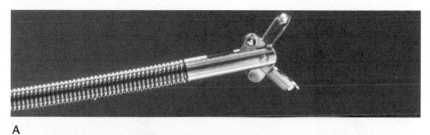

A

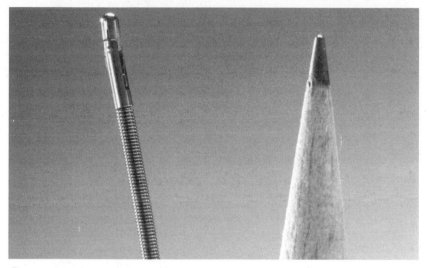

B

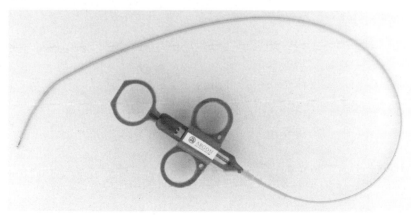

C

Courtesy Argon Medical, Inc.

FIGURE 7.4

(**A**) Tubular lesion of the left anterior descending artery. (**B**) After several sequential balloon inflations, a smooth lumen contour was obtained with a < 20% residual stenosis.

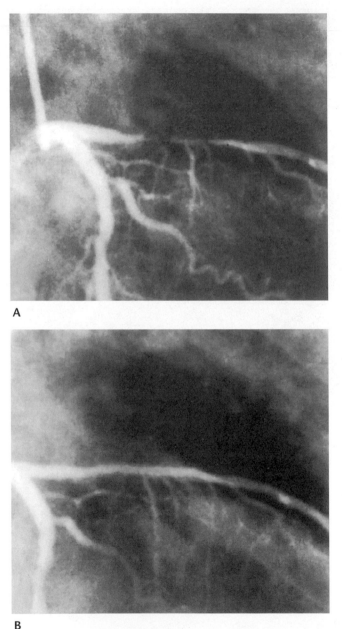

A

B

From: Popma JJ, Leon MB, Topol EJ et al. *Atlas of Interventional Cardiology*. Philadelphia: WB Saunders; 1994: 158. Used with permission.

Regardless of the mechanism of action, scientists do know that PTCA works. Success rates have been up to 99% in certain patients with type A lesions. Even the most complex lesions (type C), are associated with about a 65% to 70% success rate.[11] Success is defined as a decrease in stenosis to less than 50% of the lumen diameter or by an increase in flow through the artery.[11] Flow can be measured by using the TIMI scale, which evolved from the *Thrombolysis In Myocardial Infarction* trials in the 1980s. The TIMI perfusion scale is in Table 7.3.[11]

The mortality rate for angioplasty is about 0.7%, compared to 1.0% for coronary artery bypass grafting. Morbidity following angioplasty includes a 1% to 3% need for emergent bypass surgery, a 2% to 3% incidence of myocardial infarction, and a 25% to 35% restenosis rate that will require a second revascularization procedure.[12]

Despite improvement in techniques and types of balloons available, restenosis continues to be a problem. During angioplasty the intima of the coronary artery is traumatized and an inflammatory response is initiated, resulting in vascular smooth muscle cell buildup and tissue hyperplasia. Thrombus forms on the jagged edges of the angioplasty site and partially or completely reoccludes the artery. Heparin is administered continuously up to 24 hours postangioplasty and aspirin is prescribed indefinitely to prevent thrombus formation. However, in 25% to 35% of patients, this treatment is insufficient and restenosis occurs within 3 months.[13] Scientists are investigating other possible interventions to inhibit the inflammatory response and therefore decrease the rate of restenosis.

Califf et al[13] noted that risk factors for restenosis fall under three categories: Patient-related factors, lesion-related factors, and procedure-related factors. Patient-related factors include male sex, smoking postangioplasty, diabetes mellitus, and the presence of unstable angina. Lesion-related factors include angioplasty of left anterior descending and sapheneous graft lesions as well as proximal, multivessel, and multilesion angioplasty. Procedure-related factors include using a large number of balloon inflations and obtaining a widely patent vessel, which may indicate a large amount of damage to the intimal wall. This results in an exaggerated healing response with proliferation of smooth muscle cells and

TABLE 7.3

TIMI Coronary Flow Scale

TIMI-0	No flow through the artery
TIMI-1	Very sluggish flow through the artery
TIMI-2	Slightly slower than normal flow through the artery
TIMI-3	Normal, brisk flow through the artery

intimal hyperplasia. Thus, the greater the enlargement of the lumen after the angioplasty, the greater the injury to the wall and the higher the risk for restenosis.[14]

Atherectomy

Atherectomy is a relatively new procedure that takes place in the cardiac catheterization laboratory. It shows great potential in the treatment of coronary artery disease. The procedure involves removal of the atherosclerotic plaque using one of several types of devices (Figure 7.5). The first device, the transluminal extraction catheter (TEC), is a motorized stainless steel tube with a conical cutting head that is placed in the vessel with a guide wire. The plaque is shaved by the cutting head, and a vacuum on the end of the device extracts the excised material. A second method, directional coronary atherectomy, using the Simpson Directional AtheroCath uses a balloon-tipped catheter with a special cutting blade on one side. The balloon is inflated against the opposite wall of the artery and the blade is passed through the plaque. The directional atherectomy catheter works best on noncalcified lesions. Remnants are caught by the blade housing and extracted when the catheter is removed. The third device is the Rotablator, which has a diamond-studded burr that rotates at over 200,000 rpm. This device is particularly effective on heavily calcified lesions. The plaque is pulverized, and the debris then travels distally down the artery. Measurements taken of this debris show an average size of < 5 μm, which is smaller than blood cells and too small to clog capillaries.[15]

The primary advantage of atherectomy is that the intima of the coronary artery is left smooth and the plaque is removed from the artery (Figure 7.6). Since an erratic intimal surface and residual plaque seem to be the impetus for restenosis after PTCA, it was hoped that restenosis after atherectomy would be less common. Two recent studies compared the results of atherectomy vs. PTCA. Although atherectomy resulted in greater lumen size, the restenosis rate and outcome for patients was the same in both groups. In addition, atherectomy resulted in a greater number of complications such as abrupt closure and acute myocardial infarction. There was also an increase in cost associated with the atherectomy procedure.[16] Investigators conclude that atherectomy in selected patients could be used to debulk atheromas and enhance the benefits of PTCA.

As with PTCA, the postatherectomy patient is placed on intravenous heparin for up to 24 hours postcatheterization, and a follow-up catheterization may be done after the procedure to assess vessel patency.

Coronary Artery Stent

The coronary artery stent is a coiled metal apparatus that is permanently imbedded in the plaque-filled coronary artery after the lesion has been reduced by PTCA. Stents can be deployed on an angioplasty bal-

FIGURE 7.5

Atherectomy devices. (**A**) The transluminal extraction catheter. (**B**) The Rotablator with its abrasive burr. (**C**) The directional coronary atherectomy device (Simpson Coronary AtheroCath).

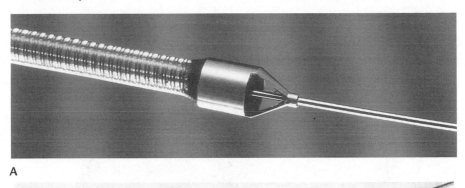

A

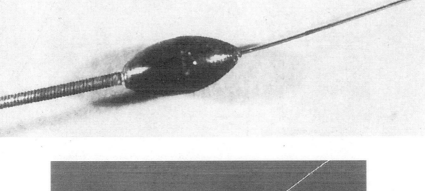

B

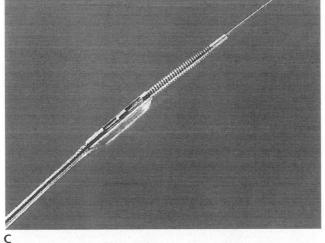

C

A. Courtesy International Technologies, Inc., San Diego, CA. B. From: Bertrand ME, Bauters C, LaBlanche JM. Percutaneous coronary rotational angioplasty with the Rotoblator. In: Topol EJ, ed. *Textbook of Interventional Cardiology*. 2nd ed. Philadelphia: WB Saunders; 1994, p. 660. C. From: Hinohara T, Robertson GC, Simpson JB. Directional coronary atherectomy. In: Topol EJ, ed. *Textbook of Interventional Cardiology*. 2nd ed. Philadelphia: WB Saunders; 1994, p. 643. Used with permission.

FIGURE 7.6

(A) A stenosis of the proximal left anterior descending artery was treated with directional atherectomy. (B) After retrieval of an abundant amount of tissue, no residual stenosis was seen at the site of atherectomy.

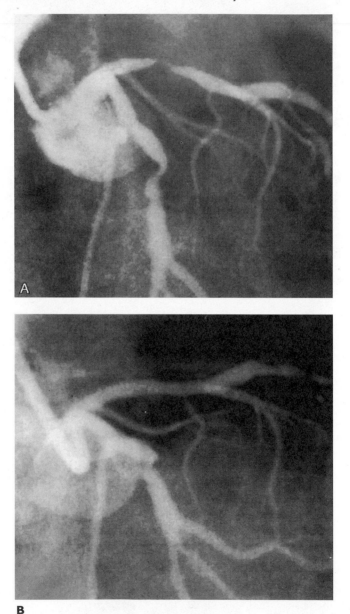

From: Popma JJ, Leon MB, Topol EJ. *Atlas of Interventional Cardiology*. Philadelphia: WB Saunders; 1994: 205. Used with permission.

loon or can be self-expanding. For balloon deployment, the stent is guided under fluoroscopy to the stenosed area of the coronary artery and then imbedded into the coronary vessel as the balloon is inflated (Figure 7.7). The balloon is then deflated and withdrawn from the vessel. The stent stays in place for the duration of the patient's life and helps keep the artery open. Most patients can be managed with aspirin and other antiplatelet agents such as dipyridamole and ticlodipine. Occasionally short-term post-procedural anticoagulation with warfarin is done for about 6 weeks to minimize the risk of thrombosis in patients whose lumen diameter remains somewhat compromised after the stent.

Since stents have shown tremendous promise in decreasing the incidence of restenosis following angioplasty, research is ongoing to develop improved stent materials. Biodegradable stents and stents coated with biologically active materials that prevent thrombosis and cellular hyperplasia (both of which contribute to restenosis) await further development.

Valvuloplasty

In the early 1980s, studies were begun on the use of balloon valvuloplasty in patients with valvular stenosis. The aortic valve was the primary focus because patients with aortic stenosis are usually elderly and debilitated and consequently poor surgical candidates.[17] Typically the patient has symptoms of congestive heart failure as a result of a stenotic valve that prevents complete emptying of the ventricle during systole. The blood backs up into the pulmonary vasculature, resulting in pulmonary edema.

The valvuloplasty procedure takes place in the catheterization laboratory. The balloon involved is 18 to 25 mm when inflated and is used to make the orifice larger. A large insertion catheter is necessary to accommodate the valvuloplasty balloon size, thus increasing the potential risk of bleeding from the femoral artery. Following the procedure, most patients have relief of symptoms for approximately 6 months before restenosis of the orifice occurs. Patients with higher baseline left ventricular ejection fractions seem to do better.[18] Possible complications from valvuloplasty include hemorrhage, cerebral vascular accident, atrial fibrillation, ventricular tachycardia, pulmonary edema, and, most frequently, damage to the femoral artery. Although valvuloplasty is not done with great frequency, it may provide a window of short-term relief of symptoms to an elderly patient who is a poor surgical risk, and who would otherwise spend considerable time in the hospital for symptom management.

PATIENT PREPARATION FOR CARDIAC CATHETERIZATION

Preparation protocols for cardiac catheterization vary from institution to institution. Both physicians and nurses have a responsibility to ensure that the patient has the safest procedure possible. This collaborative care

FIGURE 7.7

A 35-year-old heart transplant recipient with accelerated atherosclerosis of the right coronary artery was angioplastied (**A**) and then given a 3.5-mm Johnson & Johnson Palmez-Schatz stent (**B**). The result was excellent (**C**).

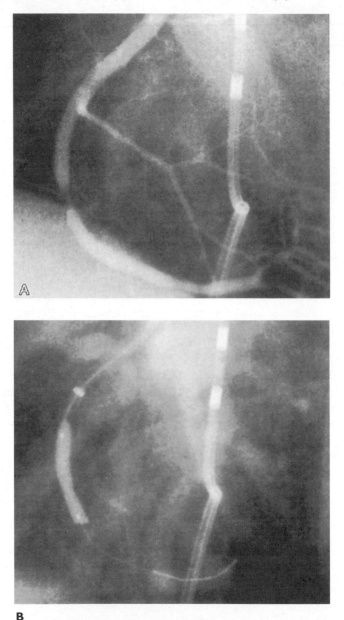

B

From: Popma JJ, Leon MB, Topol EJ. *Atlas of Interventional Cardiology*. Philadelphia: WB Saunders; 1994: 266. Used with permission.

FIGURE 7.7

(continued)

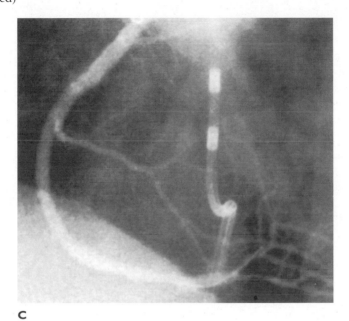

C

effort is illustrated in Fig 7.8, which shows sample care path for cardiac catheterization. Ideally, patient preparation for the catheterization should begin as soon as it is known that the patient will be undergoing the procedure.

Physician orders should include the following: no food or drink for 6 to 8 hours prior to the procedure, baseline coagulation and electrolyte studies, discontinuation or decrease of heparin 4 to 6 hours before the procedure or of warfarin 1 to 2 days before (if necessary), and premedication orders. Possible premedication orders include diphenhydramine or diazepam for sedation and sublingual nitroglycerin just prior to the catheterization to prevent coronary artery spasm. For those patients who are allergic to contrast, a steroid may be given along with diphenhydramine.

Patient Education

When the catheterization is imminent, information about the purpose of the catheterization and the physician's expectations of the patient are most likely to reduce the patient's anxiety. It is important to review the sensations the patient will experience during the catheterization. Anxiety about the procedure is normal; it might be helpful to request a sedative if the patient's anxiety seems to be impairing coping.

FIGURE 7.8

A sample critical pathway for the care of the patient undergoing PTCA. Pathways can be modified to include specific care following atherectomy or stent deployment.

Collaborative Problems	Nursing Diagnoses	Expected LOS
• Chest pain	• Anxiety	
• Coronary artery disease	• Knowledge deficit	**Admission Date**
• Increased right heart pressures	• Pain related to cardiac ischemia	**Discharge Date**
• Left ventricular dysfunction		

Night/Morning Before	Day of Procedure	Postprocedure
MEDICAL		
Assessment	**Assessment**	**Assessment**
• Include allergies, health history	• Assess change from baseline	• Assure WNL
• Physical exam, labs, EKG		• Assess groin and peripheral pulses
Medical Orders	**Medical Orders**	**Medical Orders**
• Diet: low chol, NAS	• Resume diet, 2 L fluid po or IV	
• NPO after MN except meds		• D/C IV
• Order/evaluate electrolytes, CBC, PT, PTT, and EKG	• Assess change from baseline	• Write prescriptions and F/U appts
• IV access	→	• Review risk factors, advise patient to stop smoking if appropriate, advise to follow low cholesterol diet
• Order patient's routine meds	• Resume or change previous medication orders	• Consider cardiac rehab program
• ASA, Cardizem	• Resume Coumadin (if indicated)	• Provide patient direction on returning to work, hobbies, usual activities.
• D/C or decrease Heparin	• Resume Heparin (if indicated)	• D/C monitor
• Premedication orders: (if indicated) Predinose Benedryl Valium		
• Telemetry monitoring if indicated	• Monitor prn	

BOTH
Patient and Family Education
• Pre, intra, and post procedure expectations. Use audiovisual material

Planning
• Assess for rehab dietary, home care

NURSING

Assessment
• Health hx: chest pain, syncope, SOB
• Vital signs, heart sounds, lung sounds, pulses, labs, presence of chest pain, syncope or SOB, coping skills, anxiety, knowledge level

Nursing Orders
• IV access
• Assure NPO after MN
• I&O

• Administer meds
• Telemetry
• Prep groin site prn

• Up ad lib

Patient and Family Education
• Activity (arm use) limitations or bedrest duration →
• Review results of tests
• Make further treatment plans
Discharge Planning →

Assessment
• q 8 hr and prn
• Vital signs, pedal pulses and circ., and groin site q 15'' × 4, q 30'' × 4, q1hr × 4, q4hr × 4, then q 8 hr. Maintain q1hr checks if sheaths still in place.

Nursing Orders
• Maintain patient IV (change to HL after 2L intake)
• Resume diet, assure intake 2L of fluid (if patient unable to drink, notify M.D.)
• Administer meds for back discomfort as needed
• Monitor urine output closely for first 4–6 hours

• 10# sandbag to groin site x2-3 hrs after sheaths out

• Complete BR until sheaths out and 8–10 hrs after, then up

Patient and Family Education
• Reinforce importance of attending F/U appts, and importance of notifying MD if chest pain reoccurs
• Instruct on insertion site care
• Explain further treatment plans**Discharge Planning**
• Make final arrangements for F/U care

Assessment
• Assure WNL before D/C

Nursing Orders
• D/C IV →

Teach patient to take meds as ordered →

• Remove dressing, assess site for hematoma, ecchymosis, erythema and/or drainage: if site bleeds cover w/pressure drsg; notify M.D.
• Up ad lib, resume usual ADL's

The patient should expect to see a room filled with large diagnostic equipment. He or she will be asked to lay very still on a hard table during the procedure. At this point, a nurse or technician will drape the patient and prepare the insertion site(s). The physician numbs the area with a local anesthetic and then places the introducers. Catheters are then advanced into the heart, and the patient may feel some chest discomfort or shortness of breath. These symptoms may continue throughout the duration of the procedure. The patient should be instructed to report these symptoms to the staff as they occur.

It is very important to instruct the patient about coughing when he or she is asked to do so during the catheterization. *The importance of coughing cannot be overemphasized when one considers that coughing can often eliminate potentially life-threatening dysrhythmias.* The patient will also be asked to hold his or her breath while cines are taken of the coronary arteries: The cessation of movement helps to ensure that high-quality cines will be obtained.

In teaching the patient what to expect postcatheterization, the caregiver should emphasize the need to lay flat for 6 to 12 hours (and possibly overnight if the catheters are left in the groin). The patient should also be told that frequent measurement of vital signs and checking of the dressing and distal pulses are necessary postcatheterization to assess for potential complications. The patient will be asked to drink 1 to 2 liters of fluids after the catheterization to facilitate contrast material elimination. Patient education materials including videotapes and pamphlets (see Patient Education Box 7.1) are helpful in reinforcing what has been taught.

Diagnostic cardiac catheterization is usually performed on an outpatient basis. When this occurs, the nurse and physician must assess the patient while he or she is in the catheterization laboratory. A family member or friend should accompany the patient to the hospital to drive the patient home afterward. However, the patient should be prepared to stay at the hospital overnight in case of complications or if an intervention (such as PTCA) is necessary.

Just prior to the procedure, the patient may be given diazepam or morphine sulfate intravenously. These drugs enable the patient to rest comfortably during the catheterization yet allow the patient to be alert enough so that he or she may cough or hold a breath when necessary. During the procedure, the patient is closely monitored for hypotension, arrhythmias, and angina. Should any of these alterations in cardiac output occur, the patient must be treated promptly so that serious complications do not develop. Consequently, emergency medications and a defibrillator need to be immediately available in the catheterization laboratory.

Patient Care After Catheterization

After the catheterization, the catheters are removed. Pressure is manually held on the artery for 20 to 30 minutes; then a pressure dress-

PATIENT EDUCATION BOX 7.1

Cardiac Catheterization

The purpose of a cardiac catheterization is to evaluate the function and blood flow to your heart and see if there has been any damage. The test takes 1 to 2 hours.

BEFORE THE PROCEDURE

You should not eat or drink anything beginning about 6 hours prior to the test.

If you take a medicine called Coumadin, you should not take this medicine the day before the test. Also, if you are allergic to any medications or dyes you must inform your doctor prior to the procedure.

DURING THE PROCEDURE

You will be placed on a small hard table and probably will be asked to keep your arms above your head. Let your doctor or nurse know if you have any discomfort at any time during the procedure.

Next, one side of your groin (your arm may be used if the doctor decides that it is necessary) will be shaved and sterile drapes will be placed to keep the area as clean as possible. Do not touch these drapes.

A doctor will then place a catheter (similar to an IV) into the groin after giving you some local numbing medicine.

It will be very important for you to cough and hold your breath when you are asked to do so. Tell the staff if you have chest pain or any other discomfort.

A large camera will rotate around you and take pictures of your heart as the doctor injects dye into your coronary arteries and into the heart. The dye will make you feel very hot for a few seconds and you may have some chest pain.

AFTERCARE

Your doctor will be able to tell you the results of your test shortly after the catheterization. Together, you will both be able to plan what to do about your heart disease.

After the procedure, the catheter(s) will be removed from your groin and pressure will be held on your groin for about 30 minutes to prevent bleeding. You then must lay flat for 4 to 8 hours as directed.

During the recovery period your vital signs, the groin dressing, and the pulses in your feet will be checked frequently. It is very important to maintain bedrest as you are instructed.

After the catheterization, you will be encouraged to drink as many fluids as possible to flush the dye out of your body.

ing is applied to promote hemostasis. For brachial approaches, the artery must be repaired with sutures. The patient must not bend the affected extremity for six to eight hours after catheter removal to promote complete arterial repair. Oral and intravenous fluids (at least 2000 cc) are given to encourage elimination of the contrast material through the kidneys and to prevent renal damage.

Shortly after the procedure is completed, the important findings and/or treatments done during the procedure are explained to the patient. Changes in medications and future interventions may also be discussed.

Vital signs, circulation checks, and dressing checks must be done frequently during the postcatheterization period to ensure that circulation to the affected extremity has not been impaired. This routine is crucial for all postcatheterization patients. Diminished or absent pulses, increased heart rate, increased blood pressure, or bleeding at the insertion site may indicate incomplete arterial repair, retroperitoneal bleeding, pseudoaneurysm, or femoral artery dissection and warrant further investigation by a physician.

Overall, postprocedure complications are relatively rare.[1] Potential complications include arterial thrombosis, hemorrhage or (pseudo-) aneurysm, perforation of the heart or great vessels, coronary artery spasm, vasovagal reaction, dysrhythmia, cerebral vascular accident, phlebitis, and infection. The overall mortality rate is less than 0.14%.[19] In general, the more catheterizations a laboratory does, the less likely it is for a patient to experience a complication.

Complications

Complications are always possible when an invasive procedure is performed on a patient. However, during cardiac catheterization the likelihood of complications is relatively rare, with the highest incidence associated with patients who have left main coronary artery disease. This is because injection of contrast may result in a lack of blood supply to a large portion of the heart. Other patients who are more likely to have complications are those with severe left ventricular dysfunction, acute MI, critical aortic stenosis, overt insulin-dependent diabetes mellitus, or unstable angina with a crescendo pattern. It is often preferred that these high-risk patients not undergo catheterization unless surgeons and an operating room are immediately available.[1]

If these high-risk patients are identified prior to the catheterization, the intra-aortic balloon pump (IABP) may be used prophylactically. The IABP is a device that decreases the workload of the heart while maintaining myocardial oxygen supply. As a result, the heart receives maximum blood flow during the catheterization and is less likely to suffer infarction during the procedure.

However, since any patient is potentially a high-risk patient, certain preventive measures are taken in all patients. Laboratories are equipped with the necessary staff and equipment for full cardiopulmonary resuscitation. In many hospitals, back-up cardiac surgery is available. For those that do not have cardiac surgery, patients are often triaged and transferred if they have any indications of high-risk lesions or other comorbidities.

Patients with acute myocardial infarction and unstable angina may receive a combination of thrombolytics, anticoagulants, antithrombins, and/or antiplatelet agents to reduce the risk of thrombosis during or after the procedure. Heparin is used for the patient with unrelieved chest pain because greater than 85% of myocardial infarctions are secondary to coronary artery thrombosis.[20] Heparin is also given during the procedure to reduce the risk of thrombis formation and embolization around the catheters while they are in the heart. Recently, new drugs, such as the glycoprotein IIb/IIIa antagonists, Reopro and Integrelin, have been shown to be potent platelet inhibitors and may play a vital role in reducing the platelet aggregation and ischemic complications that are seen after angioplasty.[11] Much research is underway to investigate possible agents to reduce thrombosis following angioplasty.

THE FUTURE OF CARDIAC CATHETERIZATION

It is likely that cardiac catheterization will remain an important diagnostic and therapeutic medical intervention for patients with cardiac disease. Researchers are continuously developing new techniques, instruments, and medications that can be used in the catheterization laboratory.

There are several technologies currently under investigation that may allow significant improvements in diagnosing coronary anatomy and the effectiveness of therapeutic interventions. These include intravascular ultrasound, intracoronary Doppler studies, coronary angioscopy, and qualitative and quantitative angiography. *Intravascular ultrasound* (IVUS) allows the researcher to assess the complete thickness of the plaque beneath the luminal surface[21] (Figure 7.9). This device may be used to guide directional atherectomy catheters or other types of therapeutic interventions. *Intracoronary Doppler* measures flow through the coronary arteries. Although Doppler technology within coronary arteries is very complex and limited in its applications, its use is helping researchers better understand the physiology of coronary blood flow[22] (Figure 7.10). Coronary angioscopy permits direct visualization of the coronary arteries through a fiberoptic percutaneous coronary angioscope. It is hoped that this emerging technology will provide assistance in diagnosing coronary pathology and in selecting and evaluating treatments such as stenting or atherectomy.[23] *Qualitative and quantitative angiography* uses computer-assisted arterial edge-detection al-

FIGURE 7.9

Intravascular ultrasound. (A) An ultrasound catheter within the coronary is used to assess the characteristics of the plaque. Calcifications are seen as bright white areas within the wall of the artery. (B) A discrete atherosclerotic lesion within the coronary artery is treated with a stent.

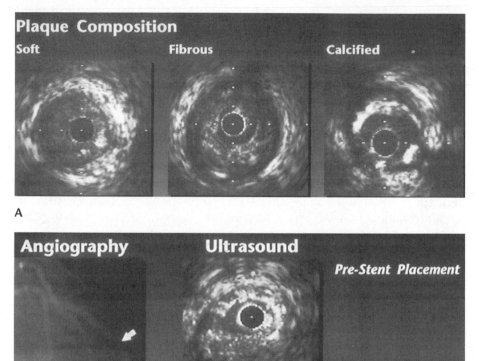

Courtesy of Mansfield, a division of Boston Scientific Corp. Used with permission.

FIGURE 7.10

Intracoronary Doppler. (**A**) Resting coronary artery flow velocity in the left anterior descending artery of a patient with atypical chest pain and angiographically intermediate coronary artery stenosis. The average peak velocity (APV) was 29 cm/s. (**B**) After intracoronary injection of adenosine (18 µg), the APV was increased to 71 cm/s. Therefore the calculated coronary reserve was 2.6. A coronary reserve between 2 and 3 is considered normal, thus no further intervention was needed at this time.

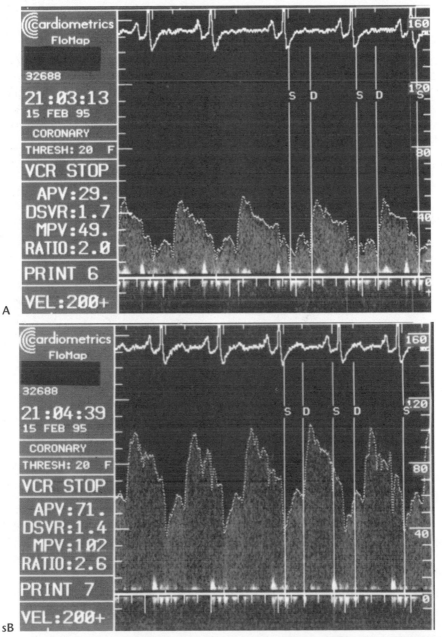

Courtesy Dr. Steven Werns, University of Michigan Hospitals, Ann Arbor, Mich.

gorithms to evaluate coronary dimensions and thus promote more accurate evaluations of therapy.[24]

In addition to technologies for improving diagnostic capabilities, there is much research ongoing relative to improving treatment options using catheterization. These include various additions to angioplasty such as improved stents or atherectomy devices and laser-assisted angioplasty. In addition, direct delivery of drugs into the coronaries and exciting work in gene therapy lie just on the horizon.

Several devices to reduce risks and maximize blood flow during angioplasty are also currently in clinical trials. The usefulness of the *cardiopulmonary bypass machine* during PTCA in patients with severe coronary artery disease is being investigated. The bypass machine is inserted via a cutdown procedure into the femoral artery and vein. Damage to the heart is prevented because blood is shunted through the bypass machine to the periphery while angioplasty of the vessel is done.

Lasers have been the subject of much research on their use in debulking lesions, assisting in PTCA, or directly removing plaque from vessel walls. Current laser technology is very expensive, requires special construction and safety designs in the catheterization laboratory, and has not yet shown results that improve on current PTCA therapy. Nonetheless, researchers believe that laser angioplasty, when perfected, will produce a smoother intima and therefore will prevent platelet aggregation and consequential restenosis.[25]

Synchronized retroperfusion during PTCA is another future option for patients with coronary artery disease. A separate balloon is inserted into the great cardiac vein via the coronary sinus and inflated during diastole while the PTCA balloon is inflated in the coronary artery. Occluding the coronary sinus during diastole results in retrograde blood flow back into the artery that is temporarily occluded by the angioplasty catheter. Consequently, the angioplasty balloon can be inflated for longer periods of time at reduced pressures, thus decreasing the likelihood of intimal tearing or dissection.[26]

Other devices that provide antegrade perfusion into the occluded coronary artery during PTCA are being developed.[26] The *autoperfusion catheter* is an angioplasty catheter that allows antegrade blood flow during PTCA into the distal part of the coronary artery once the guide wire is pulled back. Another possibility is the infusion through the central lumen of the angioplasty catheter of oxygenated fluorocarbon (Flurosol) emulsions, which provide high oxygen levels and seem to reduce the effects of prolonged balloon inflation.

Endoluminal polymer paving, still mostly a theoretical concept, holds to the idea that the coronary arteries could actually be coated with a substance to smooth the intima and prevent ongoing atherosclerosis.[27] Gene therapy, another hope for the future, holds potential for direct manipulation of the process of atherosclerosis.[28]

Modern-day researchers are charged with the formidable task of finding less expensive and more effective ways of treating coronary artery disease. Prevention and plaque regression therapies are making headway in an environment that previously had been focused on illness treatment and damage control. As we approach the next century, we can expect further research on nonsurgical revascularization interventions and pharmacologic therapies. While we have little hope of eradicating coronary heart disease in our society, we can be optimistic that our future strategies to both decrease its incidence and treat it effectively and cost efficiently will enjoy success.

REFERENCES

1. Grossman W. *Cardiac Catheterization and Angiography*. 2nd ed. Philadelphia: Lea and Febiger; 1980.
2. Vliestra RE, Holmes DR. *Percutaneous Transluminal Coronary Angioplasty*. Philadelphia: FA Davis; 1987.
3. Kennedy JW. Thrombolytic therapy for acute myocardial infarction. *Heart Lung*. 1987;16:740–745.
4. Hill JA, Lambert CR, Pepine CJ. Radiographic contrast agents. In: Pepine CJ, Hill JA, Lambert CR, eds. *Diagnostic and Therapeutic Cardiac Catheterization*. Baltimore: Williams and Wilkins; 1989.
5. Ryan TJ, Faxon DP, Gunnar RP, et al. and ACC/AHA Task Force. Guidelines for percutaneous transluminal coronary angioplasty. *J Am Coll Cardiol*. 1988;12:529.
6. Yang SS, Bentivolglio LG, Maranhao V, Goldberg H. *From Cardiac Catheterization Data to Hemodynamic Parameters*. 3rd ed. Philadelphia: FA Davis; 1988.
7. The Multicenter Postinfarction Research Group. Risk stratification and survival after myocardial infarction. *N Engl J Med*. 1982;306:1065–1070.
8. Mendel D, Oldershaw P, eds. *The Practice of Cardiac Catherization*. 3rd ed. Oxford: Blackwell Scientific Publications; 1986.
9. Sanderson RG, Kurth CL. *The Cardiac Patient: A Comprehensive Approach*. 2nd ed. Philadelphia: WB Saunders; 1983.
10. Billingham ME. Histopathological diagnosis of acute myocarditis and dilated cardiomyopathy. In: Bawaldi G, Camerini F, Goodwin JF, eds. *Advances in Cardiomyopathies*. Berlin: Springer-Verlag; 1990.
11. Topol EJ, Serrays PW. *Current Review of Interventional Cardiology*. 2nd ed. Philadelphia: Current Medicine; 1995.
12. Ellis SG. Elective coronary angioplasty: Technique and complications. In: Topol E, ed. *Textbook of Interventional Cardiology*. 2nd ed. Philadelphia: WB Saunders; 1994.
13. Hillegass WB, Ohman M, Califf RM, Frid DJ, et al. Restenosis: The clinical issues. In: Topol E, ed. *Textbook of Interventional Cardiology*. Philadelphia: WB Saunders; 1990.
14. Califf RM, Fortin DF, Frid DJ. Restenosis after coronary angioplasty: An overview. *J Am Coll Cardiol*. 1991;17:2B.
15. Ahn SS, Auth DC, Marcus DR, et al. Removal of focal atheromatous lesions by angioscopically guided high speed rotary atherectomy: Preliminary experimental observations. *J Vasc Surg*. 1988;7:292–300.

16. Umans VA, Beatt KJ, Rensing BJ, et al. Comparative quantative angiographic analysis of directional atherectomy and balloon coronary angioplasty. *Am J Cardiol.* 1991;68:1556–1563.

17. McKay RG, Safron RD, Lock JE, et al. Balloon dilatation of calcific aortic stenosis in elderly patients: Postmortem, intraoperative and percutaneous valvuloplasty studies. *Circulation.* 1986;74:119–125.

18. Davidshore CJ, Bashore TM. Late clinical and hemodynamic follow-up after balloon aortic valvuloplasty. In: Bashore TM, Davidshore CJ, ed. *Percutaneous Balloon Valvuloplasty and Related Techniques.* Williams & Wilkins: Baltimore; 1991.

19. Kennedy JW, Baxley WA, Bunnel IL, et al. Mortality related to cardiac catheterization and angiography. *Cathet Cardiovas Diagn.* 1982;8:323–340.

20. DeWood MA, Spores J, Notske RN, et al. Prevalence of total coronary occlusion during the early hours of acute transmural infarction. *New Engl J Med.* 1980;(303):897–903.

21. Yock PG, Fitzgerald PJ, Sudhir K. Intravascular ultrasound. In: Topol EJ, ed. *Textbook of Interventional Cardiology.* 2nd ed. Philadelphia: WB Saunders; 1994.

22. Serruys PW, Di Mario C, Kern MJ. Intracoronary Doppler. In: Topol EJ, ed. *Textbook of Interventional Cardiology.* 2nd ed. Philadelphia: WB Saunders; 1994.

23. Ramee SR, White CJ. Percutaneous coronary angioscopy. In: Topol EJ, ed. *Textbook of Interventional Cardiology.* 2nd ed. Philadelphia: WB Saunders; 1994.

24. Popma JJ, Bashore TM. Qualitative and quantitative angiography. In: Topol EJ, ed. *Textbook of Interventional Cardiology.* 2nd ed. Philadelphia: WB Saunders; 1994.

25. Sanborn TA. Laser angioplasty: What has been learned from experimental studies and clinical trials? *Circulation.* 1988;78:769–774.

26. Jacobs AK, Faxon DP. Retroperfusion and PTCA. In: Topol EJ, ed. *Textbook of Interventional Cardiology.* Philadelphia: WB Saunders; 1990.

27. Sigwart U. An overview of intravascular stents: Old and new. In: Topol EJ, ed. *Textbook of Interventional Cardiology.* 2nd ed. Philadelphia: WB Saunders; 1994.

28. Forrester JS. Laser angioplasty: Current and future prospects. In: Topol EJ, ed. *Textbook of Interventional Cardiology.* 2nd ed. Philadelphia: WB Saunders; 1994.

8

ELECTROPHYSIOLOGY TESTING

MARGARET RICKLEMANN
SHARON VANRIPER

GLOSSARY

A Wave   Represents atrial activation on an intracardiac electrocardiogram.

Accessory Pathway   A pathway that connects atrial muscle to ventricular muscle or to the lower part of the conduction system and allows either antegrade or retrograde impulse conduction.

AH Interval   Represents AV nodal conduction time and is measured from the A wave to the initial deflection seen on the His bundle electrogram.

Automaticity   The capability of a cell to depolarize spontaneously, reach threshold potential, and initiate an action potential.

Cardiac Action Potential   The rapidly progressive series of changes in electrical potential that occur across the cell membrane.

Cycle Length   The distance between depolarizations (the RR interval), generally expressed in milliseconds (ms).

Delta Wave   Slurring of the initial part of the QRS due to early depolarization of ventricular muscle. Seen in preexcitation syndromes, particularly Wolff-Parkinson-White (WPW) syndrome.

Excitability   The property by which a cardiac cell can give rise to an action potential when driven by an adequate stimulus.

H Wave   Represents His bundle activation on the His bundle electrogram.

His Bundle Electrogram (HBE)   A direct recording of the electrical activity in the bundle of His.

HV Interval   The conduction time through the His-Purkinje system, measured from the beginning of His bundle activation to the onset of ventricular activation.

Infranodal   Originating beneath the AV node or nodal junction.

Intracardiac Recording/His Bundle Electrocardiogram   A visual representation of the electrical events taking place within the heart. These events are obtained through the use of intracardiac electrode catheters and are displayed on a strip chart recorder.

Overdrive Suppression   The inhibitory effect of a faster pacemaker on a slower one.

PA Interval   A measurement of intra-atrial conduction time. Represented by the time interval between the initial deflection in the high right atrium and the A wave on the HBE.

Preexcitation   Activation of part of the ventricular myocardium earlier than would be expected if the activating impulses traveled only along the normal pathways.

Proarrhythmia   The effect of an antiarrhythmic drug that causes an increase in tachyarrhythmias, usually ventricular tachyarrhythmias.

Programmed Electrical Stimulation   The use of electrical pacing to produce a tachyarrhythmia.

Reentry   Tachycardia mechanism in which the electrical impulse travels in a circular pattern, resulting in self-perpetuation of the tachycardia. Reentry frequently occurs within the AV node and results in narrow complex tachycardia.

Refractoriness   The inability of a cell to respond to a second stimulus after a depolarization.

Refractory Period   The period during the repolarization process in which the cell resists stimuli that would normally initiate a depolarization. There are three main divisions: the absolute refractory period, during which the cell will not respond to any stimulus; the relative refractory period occurring during phase three, when the cell will respond to very strong stimuli; and the supernormal period at the end of phase three, during which the cell will respond to a weaker stimulus than is usually required to produce depolarization.

Resting Membrane Potential   The voltage that exists across the cell membrane when the heart muscle is at rest.

SA Electrogram (SAE)   A direct recording of the electrical activity in the SA node.

Syncope   A transient loss of consciousness followed by spontaneous recovery.

Threshold Potential   The transmembrane potential that must be achieved before an action potential can be initiated.

V Deflection   Represents ventricular depolarization.

Effective treatment of complex tachyarrhythmias has historically been difficult, primarily because of the many mechanisms of arrhythmia generation, the limitations of the ECG in diagnosing the rhythms, and the unpredictable effects of antiarrhythmic agents in controlling rhythms.

Over the past few years, significant progress has been made in the diagnosis and treatment of complex tachyarrhythmias. Electrophysiologists have discovered arrhythmogenic mechanisms and have researched a number of pharmaceutical agents to identify more effective antiarrhythmic drugs. With the development of the electrophysiology (EP) study, there is a safe, effective method to study the conduction system and electrical activity of the heart from within the chambers. Accurate diagnosis of tachyarrhythmias and efficient drug testing using EP have become widely accepted.[1]

Much valuable information can be gained from an EP test. For example, the EP test helps to differentiate ventricular from supraventricular tachyarrhythmias, determine which antiarrhythmic drug or therapeutic intervention is most effective, and assess abnormalities of the conduction system. By determining the type of tachyarrhythmia or conduction abnormality, the EP test provides information the physician can use to efficiently direct and evaluate the therapeutic course of the patient. Often a shorter hospital stay may be an added benefit. Many medical centers have incorporated the EP test into the standard cardiac diagnostic workup for patients who present with syncope or malignant tachyarrhythmias because of its cost effectiveness and reliability in providing an accurate diagnosis. Figure 8.1 gives an example of a care path for an electrophysiology study.

CARDIAC ELECTROPHYSIOLOGY

The Action Potential

There are four phases in the cardiac cell action potential. A myocardial cell has a polarized membrane separating the negatively charged interior of the cell from the positively charged ions outside the cell. At rest, the membrane potential is usually −90 millivolts (mV).

When a stimulus is applied to the cell, electrical forces alter the cell membrane, resulting in less negativity in the membrane potential. This is *depolarization*. The stimulus must be strong enough to depolarize the cell to a certain level, usually around −60 mV, before the threshold potential is met. The *threshold potential* is the point at which the cell will progress automatically through the process of depolarization. If the stimulus is not strong enough to excite the cell to this level, the stimulus is ignored and the cell returns to its resting state. The strength of the stimulus needed for the cell to reach threshold determines the excitability of the cell. Very excitable cells require relatively small stimuli. Once threshold potential is reached, a rapid depolarization ensues. This is *phase 0* of the action potential. Physiologically, a rapid influx of Na^+ ions causes this to occur.

FIGURE 8.1

A sample critical pathway for the care of the patient following an electrophysiology study.

Collaborative Problems	Expected LOS
• Arrhythmias	
• Syncope	
Nursing Diagnoses	**Admission Date**
• Anxiety	
• Potential for Injury	**Discharge Date**

Night/morning Before	After EPS

MEDICAL

Assessment	**Assessment**
• Include allergies, health hx	
• Labs, physical exam, ECG	• Assess change from baseline

Medical Orders
- Diet: Regular; NPO after MN
- IV access
- D/C antiarrhythmics
- Order routine medications
- Obtain baseline ECG and ECG for change in rhythm

Medical Orders
- Resume diet
- ——————→
- Order antiarrhythmics if indicated
- ——————→
- ——————→

- BR until _____ time (3–6 hours)
- Order diagnostic tests if indicated

BOTH

Patient and Family Education
- About procedure; purpose, protocol, activity after
- Obtain consent
- Give written material

Patient and Family Education
- About results of EPS; plan of action including new medications or devices

- ——————→

Discharge Planning
- Assess need for social work, dietary, or home care referrals

Discharge Planning
- ——————→

- Discharge when recovered unless pt requires further invasive intervention

NURSING

Assessment
- Health hx
- Vital signs, telemetry, heart sounds, lung sounds, pedal pulses, labs, coping

- Chest pain, SOB, palpitations, light-headedness, syncope, discomfort

Assessment
- Vital signs, pedal pulses, groin dressing every 15 minutes × 4, every 30 minutes × 4, every hour × 4, then remove pressure dressing and assess site for erythema, ecchymosis, hematoma, or drainage; cover site with adhesive strip
- Document and report to physician

Nursing Orders
- Ensure NPO after MN
- Administer meds; hold antiarrhythmics
- Ensure IV access
- Up ad lib

Nursing Orders
- Resume diet
- Resume medications
- Maintain IV access until stable
- BR for 3–6 hours→then up ad lib→recheck groin

Phase 0 is immediately followed by the repolarization process, which returns the cell to its resting membrane potential. The first rapid repolarization phase is *phase 1*. This initial phase corrects the overshoot of phase 0, turning the transmembrane potential back toward zero. This phase may be due to the inactivation of the fast Na^+ channel and/or the repolarizing effects of K^+ and Cl^- ion influx. This phase is most prominent in the Purkinje fibers. Phase 1 leads into *phase 2*, or the *plateau phase*. In this phase the slow channel is opened, allowing the gradual influx of Na^+ and Ca^{2+} ions. As calcium enters the cell, myocardial contraction occurs. The slow influx of these ions into the cell maintains phase 2 in a steady state for a short time. As the influx of Na^+/Ca^{2+} ions decreases, outward K^+ current activation is increasing. This leads into *phase 3*, the more rapid phase of repolarization.[2]

During phase 3 repolarization, the sodium-potassium pump removes extra Na^+ and Ca^{2+} ions from the cell and allows K^+ ions to enter. This brings the cell back to *phase 4*, the resting state. The entire sequence, from phase 0 through phase 4 (depolarization through repolarization), forms the cardiac cell action potential[3] (Figure 8.2).

Once the cell has been depolarized, it will resist any further stimulus until it has had a chance to recover and reestablish the resting mem-

FIGURE 8.2

An illustration of the major ionic movements during a Purkinje cell action potential. Arrows indicate approximate times when the ion movement influences membrane potential.

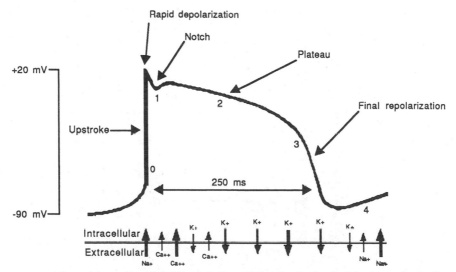

Adapted from: Ten Eick RE, et al. Ventricular dysrhythmia: Membrane basis. *Prog Cardiovasc Dis.* 1981;24:159 and Fozzard HA, Gibbons WR. Action potential and contraction of heart muscle. *Am J Cardiol.* 1973;31:183. Used with permission.

brane potential. However, this ability to resist depolarization weakens as the process of repolarization continues. Early on in the process there is a period known as the *absolute refractory period* during which no stimulus, no matter how strong, will cause the cell to depolarize. This period corresponds to the interval between the onset of the QRS complex and the beginning of the T wave on the ECG. During the period known as the *relative refractory period*, the cell may be depolarized but only with a very strong stimulus. There is one brief period at the end of phase 3 and the beginning of phase 4, called the *supernormal period of excitability*, during which certain cells (usually Purkinje cells) will respond to a weaker stimulus and undergo depolarization. This may occur because the cell has repolarized near threshold potential, but has not yet reached membrane potential. A stimulus at that critical time can push the cell back toward threshold, and depolarization then occurs[2] (Figure 8.3).

The duration and shape of the action potential varies among fiber types and may be altered by various physiological and pharmacological

FIGURE 8.3

Excitability during the cardiac action potential. Different parts of repolarization are illustrated. During the effective refractory period (ERP), a stimulus of any size is unable to initiate an impulse. The ERP is followed by the relative refractory period (RRP), during which only a stimulus of greater intensity than normal can result in an action potential. The RRP is followed by the supernormal period (SNP), during which stimuli slightly less than those that normally reach threshold can cause a propagated action potential. The action potentials generated during the RRP and SNP usually propagate slowly. The cardiac cycle is the entire period from depolarization, after which the threshold returns to normal and stimulation produces a normally propagated action potential.

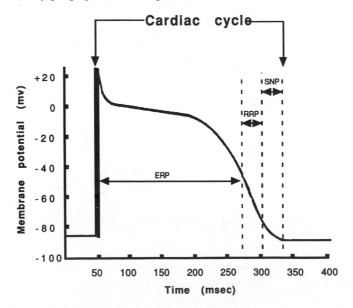

factors. Usually, conduction is slower as it travels from atrial fibers through the AV node and His bundle to the Purkinje fibers in the ventricle. Chemical or neurologic stimuli can also affect cycle length. An example is the slower heart rate produced by vagal stimulation and the associated increase in action potential duration. In short, the slower the heart rate, the longer it takes for the process of repolarization to occur and vice versa. Any changes in the cell's excitability, automaticity, or refractoriness may play a role in the generation of cardiac arrhythmias.

Certain cardiac cells are unique in that they have the ability for spontaneous membrane depolarization and the formation of individual impulses. This is called *automaticity*, and is usually found only in the fibers of the specialized conducting system consisting of the sinus node, intra-atrial conduction pathways, junctional tissue around the AV node, His bundle, bundle branches, and peripheral Purkinje network.

The characteristic feature of automaticity is the speed with which cells can restore themselves to their resting membrane potential, thereby enabling them to initiate another impulse. The SA node is the usual pacemaker of the heart: Because the fibers of the SA node have the shortest action potential duration, the SA node repolarizes more quickly than the other fibers and assumes control of the conduction sequence in the heart. When the SA node fails or its excitability is changed due to mechanical, chemical, or electrical factors, other cells with properties of automaticity, such as AV junctional tissue, take over this pacemaking function.

The Conduction System

Since abnormalities of the conduction system may cause a variety of symptoms, ranging from lightheadedness to palpitations to syncope, an assessment of the electrical pathways is essential. Normal conduction begins with an electrical impulse, which originates in the sinus node, located in the high right atrium. The impulse then travels through the atrium to the AV node, located in the lower right atrium. The rate of conduction is normally slowed as the stimulus passes through the slower conducting fibers of the AV node and bundle of His. The AV bundle is the pathway that connects the atria to the ventricles. As the stimulus passes through the His bundle it begins to excite the ventricles by traveling down the bundle branches, where speed of conduction is greatly increased. The impulse races through the bundle branches into the fine Purkinje fiber network, finally exciting ventricular myocardial cells and initiating contraction of the ventricles (Figure 8.4).

The measurement of intervals and of the conduction times between various points along the stimulus pathway is done on selected patients during the electrophysiology study. The information obtained is recorded on a special graph and represents the electrical activity taking place inside the heart. Intracardiac electrophysiology recordings provide information pertaining to sinus node function, conduction intervals and

FIGURE 8.4

(A) Schematic diagram of the PQRST complex illustrating the sequence of activation of the atria and specialized conduction system. SN = sinatrial node, HIS = bundle of His, BB = bundle branches, P = Purkinje fibers. (B) Illustration of a single cardiac cycle showing the intervals measured during an electrophysiologic study. HRA = high right atria, HBE = His bundle electrogram [which records low atrial (A) activity], H = His bundle, V = ventricular septal activity. Retrograde conduction from the His bundle to the atria is 45 ms (HA interval) Adapted from: El-Sherif N, Samet P. *Cardiac Pacing and Electrophysiology*. 3rd ed. Philadelphia: WB Saunders; 1991:141. Used with permission.

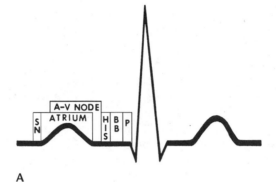

A

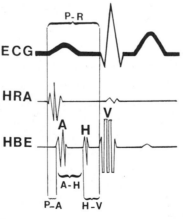

B

From: Damato AN, Lau SH. Clinical value of the electrogram of the conduction system. *Prog Cardiovasc Dis*. 1970;13:119. Used with permission of Grune and Stratton.

cycle lengths of the AV node, intrabundle (His) conduction times, and refractory period analysis.[4] Through analysis of the conduction pathways,
points of disruption can be identified and appropriate interventions prescribed (Figure 8.5 and Table 8.1).

Mechanisms of Arrhythmia Generation

Most experts agree that there are three generally understood substrates that set the stage for tachyarrhythmias. These are reentry, enhanced automaticity, and triggered automaticity. While these substrates

FIGURE 8.5

The His bundle electrogram. The diagram illustrates the different catheter positions and the respective electrograms. Position 1 measures the left bundle branch
(LBB) potential, position 2 presents a right bundle branch (RBB) potential, position 3 shows a His bundle (HB) potential, position 4 shows a potential in both
the atria and ventricle from the perspective of the coronary sinus (CS), and position 5 illustrates an atrial potential from the right atrium. MS = membranous septum, AVN = atrioventricular node, SN = sinus node, Ao = aorta, PA = pulmonary
artery.

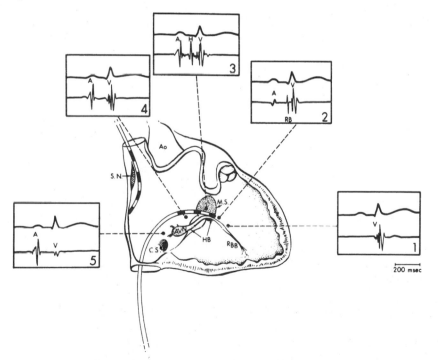

Adapted from: Gallagher JJ, Damato AN. Technique of recording His bundle activity in man. In: Grossman W, ed. *Cardiac Catheterization and Angiography*. 2nd
ed. Philadelphia: Lea and Febiger; 1980. Used with permission.

TABLE 8.1

Conduction System Intervals

Measured Area	Description	Normal Values
PA interval	Measures intra-atrial conduction	<45 ms
AH interval	Conduction time from the low right atrium through the AV node to the His bundle	50–150 ms
AV interval	Time from the earliest His deflection to the earliest ventricular activation	35–55 ms

can occur in a healthy heart, most often they result from abnormal conduction pathways, accessory pathways, or diseased myocardium. Scar tissue and drug toxicity can also contribute to the development of these mechanisms.

Reentry

The most common form of abnormal conduction resulting in tachyarrhythmias is the reentry phenomenon. Reentry is commonly found to be the culprit in malignant supraventricular and ventricular arrhythmias that are not responsive to drug therapies. Reentry can occur anywhere in the heart when certain conditions are present.[2] For a reentrant rhythm to occur there needs to exist:

1. A dual or bifurcated pathway somewhere within the conduction system,
2. A portion of the pathway that is blocked or depressed,
3. Delayed activation of tissue beyond the region of block, and
4. Reexcitation of tissue proximal to the block.[5]

Reentrant ventricular arrhythmias are generally the result of chronic ventricular disease resulting from coronary artery ischemia or infarct, or cardiomyopathy. Dual AV nodal pathways and accessory AV pathways can also be a substrate for reentry. The reentry pathway can include any part of the normal conduction system, atrial muscle, or ventricular muscle tissue. The reentrant mechanism is sustained when the refractory period in the region of block is short enough to allow the next impulse entering the depressed tissue to be conducted slowly once again. The major factors in the initiation and propagation of this circular reentry phenomenon are (1) conduction velocity and (2) relative refractoriness in both antegrade and retrograde pathways (Figure 8.6). Since the reentry pattern can produce both supraventricular and ventricular tachycardias and patients may have mild to severe symptoms in either case, the EP test is most useful in determining the type of tachycardia. Once

FIGURE 8.6

Mechanism of reentry. The impulse, blocked in limb A, is conducted slowly through limb B. By the time the impulse traverses limb B, limb A is recovered and as the block in limb A is unidirectional; the stimulus is retrogradely conducted through limb A as well as antegradely conducted through the distal common pathway of limbs A and B. Examples of dysrhythmias associated with reentry include AV nodal reentry tachycardia (AVNRT), certain atrial tachycardias, and the most common ventricular tachycardias.

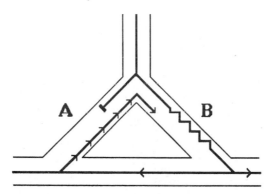

that has been established, treatment can be initiated and evaluated (Figure 8.7).

Preexcitation, a common substrate of reentry, occurs in the normal heart where there is an interruption in the ring of nonconducting tissue that separates the atria from the ventricles. This tissue, the annulus fibrosus, is usually only interrupted at the AV node and His junction. Abnormalities in this ring, usually congenitally formed, provide accessory pathways (APs) consisting of conductile tissue. These APs are a direct link between the atria and ventricles and can conduct much more rapidly than the AV node. An impulse originating in the atria can propagate down the AP and result in partial or full depolarization of the ventricles. There are many locations and variations in accessory pathways. The most common type of accessory pathway is the Kent bundle, which connects the atrium to the ventricle and is the most common pathway found in patients with Wolff-Parkinson-White syndrome. Patients with antegrade conduction over Kent's bundle can be identified on surface ECGs by a short PR interval plus a slurring of the beginning of the QRS complex (delta wave).

Another type of accessory pathway is the Mahaim fiber, which connects the AV node with the right ventricle or right bundle branch. On the surface ECG this phenomenon is shown as a normal PR interval with a prolonged QRS complex, typically with a delta wave (Figure 8.8).

Quite often, the patient with accessory pathways experiences a number of tachyarrhythmias.[6] These include atrial fibrillation or flutter as well as various forms of reentrant tachycardias. Occasionally these

FIGURE 8.7

Initiation of common AV nodal reentry. In (A) the premature stimulus is not able to propagate a tachycardia at an interval of 210 ms. However, in (B) the premature stimulus (S_2) at 380 ms causes an increase in the AV node conduction time and the tachycardia ensues. The retrograde conduction from the His bundle to the atria is 45 ms (HA interval).

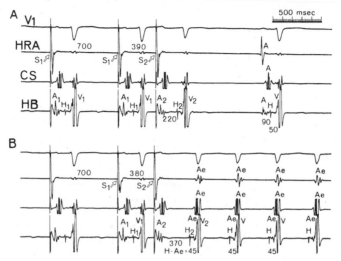

Adapted from: El-Sherif N, Samet P. *Cardiac Pacing and Electrophysiology*. 3rd ed. Philadelphia: WB Saunders; 1991:173. Used with permission.

tachycardias are so rapid that the patient has syncope or dizziness or other symptoms and may also be at risk for sudden death. EP testing is extremely helpful in this situation because it allows identification of the specific tachycardia and provides a mechanism for therapeutic intervention.

Enhanced Automaticity

Enhanced automaticity is another mechanism by which tachyarrhythmias may be generated. It results from a shift in threshold potential from a normal -60 mV to a -70 or -80 mV. When the threshold potential shifts closer to the resting membrane potential of -90 mV, a smaller stimulus is needed to initiate depolarization. It simply requires less energy to change the voltage from -90 mV to -80 mV than it does to change from -90 mV to -60 mV. This shift allows transient depolarizations to induce repetitive tachyarrhythmias, especially in patients being treated with digitalis glycosides or in whom catecholamine stimulation is occurring.[2] There are many factors that contribute to enhanced automaticity, including acute or chronic myocardial ischemia, certain antiarrhythmic drugs, electrolyte imbalance (especially hypokalemia), increased metabolism related to hyperthyroidism, and mechanical irrita-

FIGURE 8.8

Accessory pathways can connect almost any part of the conduction system to another part. Kent, Mahaim, James, and Lev bundles have been illustrated with their common connection sites. The Kent bundle typically connects atria to ventricle and is the substrate for Wolff-Parkinson-White syndrome. The Mahaim, James, and Lev bundles provide a conduit between either the AV node or bundle of His and the atria or ventricular muscle.

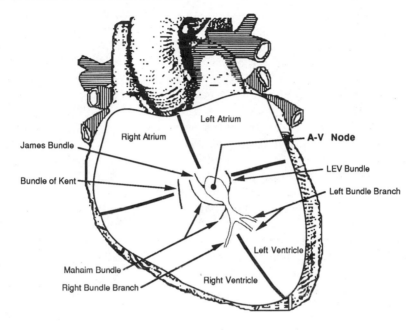

tion related to chronic stretching of the ventricle (as seen in congestive heart failure).[2]

Patients with enhanced automaticity often have a ventricular tachycardia that can produce symptoms ranging from palpitations to loss of consciousness. Often this VT is slower than that from a reentrant focus. For study purposes, an infusion of isoproterenol can be used to help reproduce the tachycardia in these patients.

Triggered Automaticity

Triggered automaticity is believed to be caused by small potentials that occur during the latter portion of the QRS depolarization. *Afterdepolarizations*, as they are called, are too small to be detected by the surface ECG. These late potentials are most commonly seen in patients with ischemic heart disease, cardiomyopathy, digitalis toxicity, multifocal atrial tachycardia (MAT), or long QT syndrome. Researchers believe that afterdepolarizations cause enough stimulation during the terminal portion of the QRS complex (relative refractory period) to initiate VT in these high-risk patients. The use of signal-averaged ECG may help detect patients with afterdepolarizations.

THE ELECTROPHYSIOLOGY STUDY

Indications

Sudden cardiac death affects approximately 400,000 people each year. Those surviving an episode of sudden cardiac arrest without signs of an acute myocardial infarction will benefit from EP testing to guide subsequent therapy. Likewise, patients with a history of syncope of unknown etiology can benefit from EP testing because the differential diagnosis of syncope is vague, and with EP a precise diagnosis can be established. In patients with sinus node or AV node disease, the EP evaluation helps determine the need for a permanent pacemaker. The EP test can also be used to test drug efficacy, to perform preoperative mapping, to directly terminate a tachycardia, and to evaluate the need for and the efficacy of an implantable device.[1] Direct destruction of the arrhythmia focus is also possible using catheter ablation or modification.

Electrophysiology (EP) tests are especially useful in the evaluation of preexcitation syndromes such as Wolff-Parkinson-White or paroxysmal tachycardia of unknown origin. One of the most valuable uses of EP tests is in the differentiation of supraventricular tachycardia (SVT) from ventricular tachycardia (VT), particularly when the patient is symptomatic and diagnosis by surface ECG is questionable. Patients who experience tachyarrhythmias, whether ventricular or supraventricular in origin, may undergo EP testing to enable the physician to select the most appropriate drug/intervention regimen.

Some physicians study patients who have short, documented episodes of VT, such as might occur during routine in-hospital monitoring. The purpose of the test in this case is to determine the patient's risk of having sustained ventricular tachycardia. In some instances, the patients with frequent, complex PVCs but without documented VT are evaluated. Patients without a history of sudden death who are noninducible for sustained ventricular tachycardia in the laboratory are generally considered to be low risk for a future sudden death episode. These patients are usually not treated with antiarrhythmic drugs because of the high incidence of intolerable drug side effects and the possibility of proarrhythmia.

Patient Preparation

To prepare for an electrophysiology study, the patient should take nothing by mouth for 6 to 8 hours prior to the procedure. In most cases, all antiarrhythmic agents will be held for at least 24 hours prior to the procedure in order to study the arrhythmia without the influence of any drugs. Because of the risk of a sudden onset of arrhythmias in the patient who is coming off antiarrhythmic therapy, the patient's rhythm should be constantly monitored. In most cases, the right groin will be shaved and prepped in the electrophysiology lab.

Patient education is very important (see Patient Education Box 8.1). The patient may have to have repeated studies and multiple drug trials; some patients will not achieve successful termination of their arrhythmias with drugs and will need device therapy. Although it is not possible to predict the outcome of the first study, if subsequent studies are needed then the length of stay in the hospital will extend an average of 2 days for each additional study.

Equipment

Electrophysiology tests are usually performed in the cardiac catheterization laboratory. The equipment needed to perform the procedure includes a stimulator, amplifier, oscilloscope, and recording device in addition to catheters and fluoroscopy equipment.

The stimulator is used to pace the heart as well as to introduce multiple (up to five) extrastimuli, of varying amplitudes and durations, at any desired interval. The stimuli are synchronized with cardiac depolarization during sinus rhythm or tachycardia. The amplifier filters the electrograms, which are displayed on an oscilloscope. The oscilloscope provides constant monitoring of the surface and intracardiac ECG as well as the arterial pressure tracing.

Catheter Insertion

A variety of electrode catheters can be used to perform an EP test. Multipolar catheters are positioned in the heart under fluoroscopy via the right or left femoral vein. They are placed routinely in the high right atrium, across the tricuspid valve to record His bundle activity, in the right ventricular apex, and right ventricular outflow tract or coronary sinus. If necessary, a catheter can also be placed in the left ventricle. Study of the left ventricle involves placement of an arterial catheter, which can increase risk of complications such as bleeding and loss of arterial pulse. Therefore, it is only done when the right heart study is inconclusive.[4] Since the induction of ventricular tachycardia may cause the patient to experience loss of consciousness and pulselessness, a defibrillator is on hand and connected to the patient at all times during the study. Usually, a small arterial catheter is inserted in patients with suspected ventricular tachycardia or fibrillation to monitor blood pressure.

Electrophysiology tests are performed with the patient awake. Occasionally, sedation will be used if the patient is unusually anxious, but since patient cooperation and verbal response to stimulation are ex-

PATIENT EDUCATION BOX 8.1

Electrophysiology Study

The purpose of the EPS is to study your heart's electrical system. This study will be done so that the best treatment for you can be prescribed. The study will last from 1 to 3 hours.

BEFORE THE TEST

Do not eat or drink anything after midnight the evening before the test unless instructed to do so by your doctor or nurse.

You may be taken off your usual medications in preparation for this test.

DURING THE PROCEDURE

The doctor will inject into your right or left groin a numbing medicine. Then a special tube will be placed into the vein in your groin. Through this tube catheters will be threaded into your heart. Occasionally an arm or neck vein is used instead of one in your groin.

The doctor will use a special wire to increase your heart rate and produce the irregular beats that cause your symptoms.

You will be awake during the procedure. It is very important to tell your doctor if you feel any chest pain, shortness of breath, or dizziness.

If symptoms occur, the doctor may ask you to cough. Do so forcefully and concentrate on the instructions you are given.

AFTERCARE

After the test you will feel some pressure in the groin site as the catheters are removed.

Pressure will be applied on your groin to stop the bleeding. After this, a dressing is applied and you will be instructed to stay flat in bed for a few hours. This helps prevent bleeding.

The nurse will check the dressing, along with your vital signs, at frequent intervals. The dressing can be removed 24 hours after the study.

Be sure to notify the nurse *immediately* of any symptoms you may feel including dizziness, palpitations, or warmth/wetness at the groin site.

The doctor will discuss the results of your study with you and suggest treatment alternatives.

You may resume your normal activities after you are allowed up from bed.

tremely helpful to the study, heavy sedation is undesirable. As with any invasive procedure, informed, written consent must be obtained. Surface ECG leads are placed on the chest so that simultaneous recordings can be made.

Intracardiac Recordings

Intracardiac ECG recordings help the investigator establish the origin and direction of electrical conduction. The His bundle recording is helpful in analyzing AV node function. Atrial recordings are used to distinguish between ventricular and atrial depolarizations during the arrhythmia. By observing the timing of His bundle activation during the tachycardia, the investigator can distinguish a ventricular tachycardia from a supraventricular tachycardia with bundle branch block or aberration.

Occasionally, recordings are simultaneously taken from the His bundle area, the coronary sinus, and the high right atrium. This method permits accessory paths to be localized.

Diagnostic Procedures

Programmed Electrical Stimulation of the Ventricle

The purpose of programmed electrical stimulation (PES) is to examine the tachyarrhythmia by reproducing it through an intracardiac catheter. Before the stimulation protocol is begun, a baseline recording is done. A single premature ventricular depolarization is delivered with a pacing catheter during sinus rhythm. After eight to ten sinus beats (identified by the designation V_1 or S_1), a premature ventricular depolarization (PVD) is applied (called V_2 or S_2). This stimulus is gradually moved toward V_1S_1 in 10-ms increments. Therefore each subsequent PVD is 10 ms more premature after each cycle. This process continues until the ventricle becomes refractory (no QRS complex or depolarization is noted on ECG), or a response is evoked (sustained or nonsustained ventricular tachycardia).

If a tachycardia is noninducible, that is, no response is seen after one extrastimulus (V_2), then two extrastimuli may be introduced. The two extrastimuli are usually delivered at differing cycle lengths (rates), beginning at 600 or 500 ms (100 or 120 bpm). PVDs are again introduced after every eight to ten beats. V_2, the first premature stimulus, is introduced and moved toward V_1 until the effective refractory period of the ventricle is found or a tachycardia is initiated. If no response is generated, V_2 is introduced 30 to 40 ms outside the refractory period and a second premature extrastimuli (V_3) is tried in the same fashion as V_2. If a second extrastimuli does not evoke a response then a third, or triple, extrastimulus may be used (Figure 8.9). V_3 is set 30 to 40 ms outside its refractory period and V_4 is introduced. All extrastimuli are synchronized to appear

FIGURE 8.9

Programmed electrical stimulation of ventricular tachycardia. Surface leads I, II, and III are illustrated, as are the distal and proximal His bundles and the right ventricle. Ventricular pacing at a rate of 100 bpm was interrupted by 3 premature paced extrastimuli (S_2, S_3, S_4), which resulted in a sustained monomorphic ventricular tachycardia.

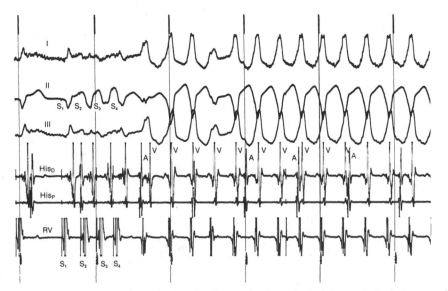

From Tilkian AG, Daily EK. *Cardiovascular Procedures, Diagnostic Techniques and Therapeutic Procedures.* St. Louis: CV Mosby; 1986:221.

late in diastole during ventricular pacing. Stimulation is usually first tried at the right ventricular apex, then at the right ventricular outflow tract.

It should be noted that use of triple extrastimuli more often results in ventricular fibrillation. In many cases ventricular fibrillation has not been documented clinically and may not actually be responsible for the patient's symptoms. The end point of the study is the induction of a reproducible, sustained (greater than 30 sec) ventricular tachycardia. Adjunctive use of isoproterenol sometimes helps to reproduce the clinical tachyarrhythmia. Isoproterenol may also help to provoke ventricular tachycardia when VT has not been induced after two or three extrastimuli. In some patients, isoproterenol increases the sinus rate to 125 to 150 bpm, and ventricular tachycardia then may occur spontaneously or can be initiated easily by programmed stimulation.

Programmed Electrical Stimulation of the Atria

Supraventricular tachycardia can originate in atrial or junctional tissue or can be caused by reentrant or accessory pathways. Stimulation of the atria through programmed premature depolarizations is used to provoke the tachycardia in the EP lab. Once the arrhythmia is reproduced, its focus, conduction pathways, and response to treatment can be analyzed.

Atrial stimulation is performed using a single test stimulus during basic atrial pacing. Premature stimuli are then introduced at various cycle lengths in 10-ms increments until a tachycardic response occurs. Once the tachycardia is produced, the patient is observed for symptoms and hemodynamic measurements are obtained.[4,7]

Endocardial Mapping

Intraventricular endocardial mapping is a procedure during which the precise location of an arrhythmic focus is identified. Mapping is essential when certain treatments such as surgical resection or catheter ablation are being considered. The actual point of origin is determined through recordings taken at many sites in the right and/or left ventricular endocardium. The earliest onset of electrical activation on the endocardial surface and the morphology of the QRS complex determine the origin of the arrhythmia circuit. Endocardial mapping involves the placement of an electrode catheter in multiple sites within the ventricles. The right ventricle is mapped first, followed by the left. Recordings are done while the patient is having the tachycardia. At least two radiographic/fluoroscopic views from different angles are needed for precise localization of the catheter site or zone. The patient must be hemodynamically stable in the tachycardia long enough to complete the mapping procedure. Some induced VTs may be too rapid to map. Therefore, the administration of antiarrhythmic drugs to slow the rate may be helpful to adequately map the site. Studies have shown that the use of drugs to slow the rate of VT does not alter the site of origin, although it may change the morphology of the complexes.

The mapping procedure usually takes between 15 and 45 minutes. This depends on the rate of the tachycardia, the patient's response to the arrhythmia, and the experience of the investigator. A 12-lead ECG is used to provide a guide to the general zone of the tachycardia. If the patient has complications such as a drop in blood pressure, loss of consciousness, or angina during the tachycardia, the arrhythmia must be terminated. The study is continued as soon as the patient is stabilized.

EVALUATION OF ANTIARRHYTHMIC THERAPY

Once a tachyarrhythmia has been identified through EP testing, the next step is to choose the most effective treatment regimen. *Electropharmacologic therapy* is the selection of an antiarrhythmic drug based on the results of the EP test. Studies have shown that arrhythmia induction via programmed stimulation and serial drug testing are highly effective in the selection of long-term drug therapy.[1]

Antiarrhythmic drug efficacy was historically assessed via ECG and Holter monitoring. Success was measured by a reduction in the number of complex premature ventricular beats and/or short runs of ventricular tachycardia after initiation of drug therapy. In some patients, however, there is frequent and unpredictable variability in the appearance of ectopic ventricular activity on the Holter monitor. A decrease in spontaneous ventricular ectopy may not be a highly sensitive indication that sudden death due to ventricular tachycardia or fibrillation will not occur.[6] EP testing gives a more reliable indication of drug efficacy by demonstrating whether or not tachycardic events occur during programmed electrical stimulation in the presence of the drug. Some studies have shown that although the number of PVCs may be reduced after the initiation of drug therapy, the arrhythmia may still be inducible in the EP laboratory or may occur spontaneously.[8]

Drugs that do not suppress sustained ventricular tachycardia would be dropped from the plan for long-term therapy. The end point to testing drug efficacy, according to some investigators, is to induce runs of ventricular ectopics of less than 5 beats during programmed stimulation, which demonstrates an appropriate and favorable response to a specific antiarrhythmic regimen.[9]

Serial antiarrhythmic testing begins with an antiarrhythmic-free baseline study, during which the patient's clinical arrhythmia is induced. An antiarrhythmic drug is then administered for a period of at least 48 hours. Another EP study is done to reproduce the tachycardia with programmed stimulation. If the tachycardia is not inducible after treatment with the antiarrhythmic drug—a positive response—the drug is considered successful. The patient is usually discharged on that drug and followed. Should adverse side effects occur, the process is repeated to find another effective drug.

If ventricular tachycardia is induced after drug therapy, the first drug is discontinued and a second drug is tried. Studies have demonstrated that a negative response to procainamide, quinidine, or both correlates strongly with unfavorable results of all class I antiarrhythmic agents.[8,9,10] Therefore, if a patient fails a trial of procainamide, often a class III antiarrhythmic agent such as amiodarone or sotalol may be tested.

Although serial drug testing and repeat EP studies are not without risk, they have been shown to be a safe, efficient, reliable method of diagnosing tachyarrhythmias and measuring responses to antiarrhythmic drug therapy. A successful response to the first antiarrhythmic drug may limit the hospital stay to 2 to 5 days. A significant benefit of EP testing is the security of knowing that the antiarrhythmic drug is effective.

It is important to stress these points when educating the patient on the need for electrophysiologic evaluation of antiarrhythmic drug therapy.

DISEASE OF THE CONDUCTION SYSTEM

The Patient with Sinoatrial Disease

Patients with sinoatrial disease may present with a wide range of symptoms. The patient may complain of occasional dizziness, fatigue, or weakness. These mild symptoms may be precursors to episodes of sudden loss of consciousness (Stokes-Adams attacks), which could be due to pronounced bradycardia or asystole. In the majority of patients who present with symptoms associated with bradyarrhythmias, documentation on surface ECG is indication enough for permanent pacemaker implantation and EP study is not necessary.[1] However, electrophysiology studies may be the only definitive diagnostic tool for those patients who have symptoms such as syncope or presyncope (weakness/faintness without actual loss of consciousness) but for whom repeated 24-hour Holter monitoring and other noninvasive tests have produced no explanation for the symptoms.[1]

Evaluating SA Node Function

The evaluation of sinus node function includes the assessment of sinus node automaticity, sinoatrial conduction time, and the effects of catecholamines and/or drugs. Sinus node function is tested in the EP lab using rapid atrial pacing.

Rapid atrial pacing is begun at a rate slightly faster than the patient's own sinus rate. Pacing is performed at cycle lengths down to 300 ms (200 bpm) for 30 to 60 seconds. To evaluate sinus node automaticity, measurements of the sinus node recovery time (SNRT) and the corrected sinus node recovery time (CSNRT) are taken. The SNRT is a measurement of the patient's sinus response to overdrive pacing. Pacing is abruptly terminated; the interval measured between the last paced atrial beat and the first spontaneous sinus beat is the SNRT. This cycle is repeated at atrial pacing rates of 60 to 150 bpm, increasing in 10-bpm increments. To allow for possible differences in the patient's intrinsic sinus rates, the investigator uses the corrected sinus node recovery time as the basis of the evaluation of sinus node function. This interval is gained by taking the longest SNRT found and subtracting the sinus cycle length prior to pacing. Normal values are usually less than 600 ms.[1]

Patients found to have a prolonged CSNRT may benefit from a pacemaker, especially if dizziness, lightheadedness, or syncope reappear during the postpacing pauses. The patient's response to atropine or iso-proterenol infusion is also assessed to determine whether the arrhythmia is due to abnormal increased autonomic tone. Abnormal autonomic response can be treated with beta-blockers, disopyramide, or other agents, while serious sinoatrial disease is treated with a permanent pacemaker.

THE PATIENT WITH ATRIOVENTRICULAR CONDUCTION DISEASE

Atrioventricular conduction refers to that area of the electrical pathway from the upper atrioventricular node through the His bundle to the bundle branches and Purkinje fibers. On the surface ECG the PR interval represents conduction through the atrium and AV node (AH interval) and the His-Purkinje system (HV interval). Thus, a prolonged PR interval on the surface ECG represents a conduction delay, that may occur at any point from the upper AV node through the Purkinje network. The His bundle electrogram provides a much more detailed assessment of conduction through the AV node and His-Purkinje system and can reveal the precise site of the atrioventricular conduction delay or block. On the His bundle recording, a prolonged AH interval indicates delayed conduction in the AV node, while delayed conduction through the His-Purkinje conduction system prolongs the HV interval.

The atrioventricular node effective refractory period (ERP) is measured to provide evidence for the existence of AV node disease, with atrial premature stimulation the technique most widely used. The right atrium is paced and a premature atrial depolarization (PAD) is introduced near or on the last paced beat in 10-ms increments. The interval at which the premature stimulus depolarizes the atrium but is blocked on its way to the ventricles is the ERP. If the site of block is in the AV node proximal to the His bundle, there is an absence of the His bundle deflection. If the site of block is distal to the His bundle, this usually indicates significant conduction disease in the terminal portion of the ventricular conduction network.

The presence of atrioventricular block is initially seen on a standard 12-lead ECG. Depending on the exact site of block, a permanent pacemaker may be necessary. The EPS is used to localize the block and validate the need for a pacemaker. For example, if the site of block occurs at the level of the AV node, it may be a benign block and a pacemaker may not be indicated, but if the level of block is in the His-Purkinje system, it is almost always necessary to implant a permanent pacemaker. Other factors, including the location and rate of the escape rhythm and the patient's response to exercise, carotid sinus massage, and atropine, are also considered in the pacemaker evaluation.[1]

Analysis of His bundle conduction is important in patients with loss or near loss of consciousness. Evaluation of both His bundle conduction and ventricular stimulation is usually performed to differentiate symptoms resulting from blocks occurring within the His-Purkinje network and those produced by episodic ventricular dysrhythmias.

THE PATIENT WITH SUPRAVENTRICULAR TACHYCARDIA

Supraventricular tachycardia can originate in atrial or junctional tissue or can be caused by automatic, reentrant, or accessory pathways. Stimulation of the atria through programmed premature depolarizations is used to provoke the tachycardia in the EP lab and determine the mechanism responsible for its initiation.

Accessory Pathways

The EP study can identify the presence and location of accessory pathways. The direction of conduction through the pathway is also determined (antegrade versus retrograde). Next, the role of the pathway in propagating the tachyarrhythmia is evaluated. Methods of terminating the tachycardia and responses to antiarrhythmic medications are assessed.

Treatment of SVT

Pharmacologic therapy for preexcitation syndromes and SVTs may be attempted with the following considerations:[6,11]

- Decreasing or preventing spontaneous atrial or ventricular premature beats that may initiate the tachycardia
- Increasing the retrograde refractory period of the accessory pathway with Type I antiarrhythmic drugs like procainamide, disopyramide, or quinidine
- Depressing AV nodal conduction, thereby lengthening the antegrade refractory period with calcium channel blockers, beta-blockers, or digitalis

Drug therapy is not suited for all patients, especially those with a rapid antegrade bypass conduction. Most of the Type I antiarrhythmic agents have been associated with multiple side effects including proarrhythmia, which can cause sudden death.

Pacemakers

Another treatment used in the EP lab is the termination of arrhythmias through specifically designed programmable pacemakers.

These can be useful in patients with certain reentrant forms of SVT. Patient-triggered pacemakers or automatic triggering rate-sensitive pacemakers have proven successful in treating these patients, but the efficacy must be established via electrophysiology study. They are especially helpful in the treatment of patients who are unable or unwilling to endure long-term antiarrhythmic therapy (Figure 8.10).

Intracardiac Transcatheter Interventions

Intracardiac transcatheter ablation is used to destroy accessory bypass tracts, reentrant pathways, or pathways within the AV node. A special catheter is used to produce an injury to the target site using radiofrequency energy. The injury destroys the cells in the area and prevents them from propagating the arrhythmia (Figure 8.11).

Transcatheter radiofrequency (RF) ablation has become the treatment of choice for ablating pathways within the AV node as well as accessory pathways in patients with preexcitation. Because the RF beam can be more precisely placed, the process is less destructive than direct current catheter ablation and carries less risk to the surrounding tissue. The minimal complication rate and the high degree of success incurred by this method have allowed many patients to enjoy a complete cure of their tachycardia.

In one recent study, 93% of patients with accessory pathways that were causing supraventricular tachycardias had complete cure after RF ablation of the pathways. A 92% success rate was reported in several studies where AV node ablation was performed for the treatment of AV nodal reentry tachycardia.[12] Complications following RF ablation were minimal

FIGURE 8.10

Example of antitachycardia burst pacing. A six-beat burst of rapid pacing is delivered during the tachycardia, which interrupts the cycle and allows the normal rhythm to resume.

Fixed Burst

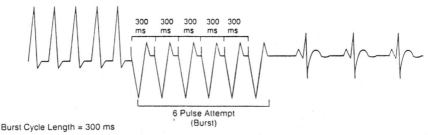

300 ms 300 ms 300 ms 300 ms 300 ms

6 Pulse Attempt (Burst)

Burst Cycle Length = 300 ms

Courtesy CPI, Minneapolis, Minn.

FIGURE 8.11

Radiofrequency catheter ablation. **(A)** The RF current is applied at 35 watts and the delta wave disappears almost immediately. This demonstrates successful destruction of the accessory pathway (AP). **(B)** The current is turned on and, after one last beat, the delta wave disappears, again indicating successful destruction of the AP.

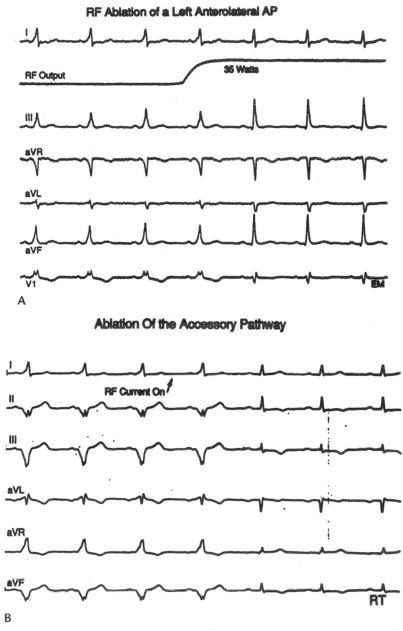

Courtesy Dr. S. Adam Strickberger, University of Michigan Hospitals, Ann Arbor, Mich.

and included a transient heart block and a mild burning sensation in the chest during the application of the RF current. Very few patients had heart block that was severe enough to warrant a permanent pacemaker after AV node ablation.[12]

THE PATIENT WITH VENTRICULAR TACHYCARDIA

Ventricular Tachyarhythmias

Electrophysiology testing is of great value in the diagnosis and treatment of life-threatening ventricular tachyarrhythmias. Ventricular tachycardia has a wide QRS complex and may be associated with AV dissociation. Activation of the His bundle during ventricular tachycardia usually occurs after the QRS complex due to retrograde conduction and is hidden in the QRS complex. EP study with programmed ventricular stimulation allows physicians to determine if the arrhythmia can be induced, which will allow for serial drug testing as needed.

Differentiating Wide Complex Tachycardias

Electrophysiologic testing can precisely differentiate a ventricular from a supraventricular mechanism. For example, VT can be differentiated from SVT with aberrant conduction by noting the relationship of the His bundle and atrial electrograms to the ventricular depolarization. During SVT, a His deflection comes before each QRS complex; with VT, the His deflection follows the QRS complex or is absent.[12] Since successful treatment of any wide complex tachycardia is dependent upon accurate diagnosis, the use of EP testing helps ensure that appropriate treatment will be employed.

Termination of Ventricular Tachycardia in the EP Laboratory

There are several techniques available in the EP lab to terminate ventricular tachycardia. One method is to use pacing. Precisely timed extrastimuli and burst pacing are often very effective in terminating a reentry circuit, while overdrive pacing is generally successful in terminating VT when the rate is slower (140–160 bpm).[4]

Synchronized cardioversion is used to terminate ventricular tachycardia in patients who develop hemodynamic instability. Most patients respond to external cardioversion. However, internal cardioversion with pacing wires may be used when external cardioversion fails and the tachyarrhythmia produces symptoms of cardiac ischemia, decreased cerebral perfusion, or hypotension. The patient may complain of chest pain or feel faint or confused. Should VT degenerate into ventricular fibrillation, electrical defibrillation is the only effective means to convert it.

Termination of Chronic VT on a Long-term Basis

Long-term treatment of ventricular tachycardia can be carried out with drugs (see above), devices, or ablation of the focus or pathway. Ablation of the focus is becoming more common as intracardiac techniques are improved. The most impressive success, however, has been seen in the use of implantable devices.

Implantable Cardioverter Defibrillators

Implantable cardioverter defibrillators (ICDs) are widely used to control ventricular tachycardia and fibrillation. The ICD can be implanted using either an epicardial lead system or a nonthoracotomy transvenous lead system. The transvenous lead system eliminates the need for open chest surgery, reduces the attendant risks associated with a thoracotomy and is the preferred method of device implantation. The basic device senses the intrinsic heart rate, analyzes the rate for an alarm violation, and delivers a shock if necessary. Up to five consecutive shocks are given in sequence to convert the lethal rhythm. This device has been implanted in tens of thousands of patients worldwide and has resulted in dramatic improvement in the survival rates of patients with ventricular tachycardias.[13,14]

The latest development in ICD devices is a three-tiered therapy that combines defibrillation with low energy cardioversion and antitachycardia pacing. The newer ICDs also have bradycardia pacing capability. These devices are programmable and allow for a combination of therapies (Figure 8.12). For example, patients with VT often respond to pacing or low-energy cardioversion. Low-energy cardioversion uses a small shock (0.1–5 joules) to terminate the VT. Most patients find these low energy shocks to be considerably less painful than the defibrillating shock. Successful antitachycardia pacing spares the patient the pain of any shock, and often converts the VT before the patient has any serious symptoms.[15] Patients who demonstrate reliable antitachycardia pacing to terminate ventricular tachycardia and who do not lose consciousness may be allowed to resume previously prohibited activities such as driving.[16]

POSTPROCEDURE CARE

One potential problem that can occur during an EP study is the development of a vasovagal reaction with either catheter insertion or withdrawal. Pallor, diaphoresis, nausea, vomiting, dizziness, bradycardia, or hypoten-

FIGURE 8.12

Third-generation implantable cardioverter defibrillators. In most of these devices, antitachycardia pacing, low-energy cardioversion, defibrillation, and bradycardia pacing are programmable features. The Medtronic Jewel and the Ventritex Cadence V = 110 are smaller devices. (A) Ventak Prx. (B) Ventak P2. (C) Medtronic Jewel. (D) Medtronic PCD. (E) Cadence V-110. (F) Cadence V-100. (G) Res-Q ACD.

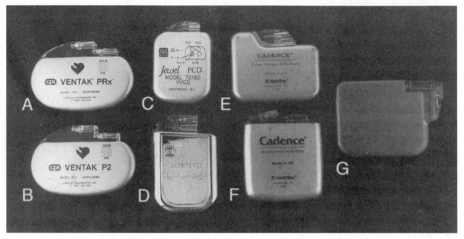

A, B. Courtesy CPI, Minneapolis, Minnesota. C,D. Courtesy Medtronic, Inc., Minneapolis, Minnesota. E,F. Courtesy Ventritex, Inc., Sunnyvale, California. G. Courtesy Intermedics, Inc., Freeport, Texas.

sion can result from vagal stimulation. Additionally, a rare complication is the development of a pericardial effusion resulting from a small ventricular puncture. Small leaks usually repair themselves without complication. However, a rapid leaking of blood into the pericardial sac can result in cardiac tamponade. Symptoms associated with this include pallor, hypotension, diaphoresis, loss of voltage on ECG, and chest pain. The pericardial sac must be decompressed to restore adequate cardiac output. In general, complications following EP testing are very rare.

Before being discharged from the lab, the patient's response to the procedure is noted and the physician may discuss the preliminary findings. The catheter insertion site is dressed. The procedural findings and any complications are documented. The patient's neurological status is checked after each cardioversion in the EP lab. If antiarrhythmic drug trials are performed, the patient's response to therapy is assessed by measuring vital signs, any ECG changes, side effects of the drug, and the efficacy of the drug in controlling the patient's rhythm.

Postprocedure nursing care involves a full cardiovascular assessment upon the patient's return. Vital signs, heart sounds, cardiac rhythm, and level of consciousness should be noted. Listen for a pericardial friction rub, which may indicate bleeding into the pericardial sac. Check the catheter site for bleeding, swelling, or diminished circulation to the distal extremity. If blood is seen on the dressing, place a new, firm pressure dressing on the site and check as indicated—but at least every 15 minutes—for a period of 1 hour. Placing a 5 to 10-pound sandbag over the site for 2 or 3 hours will help stop bleeding and may decrease the risk for hematoma formation. Remind the patient of the importance of keeping the affected extremity straight for the prescribed time. Encourage the patient's oral intake of fluids. While intravenous fluids may not be needed, IV access should be maintained since arrhythmias may occur. This is easily accomplished through the use of a heparin lock.

Following the first study to test drug efficacy, a new antiarrhythmic drug may be ordered if the patient is still inducible for VT. Over the next few days, the patient may be "loaded" with this other drug and returned to the lab for a follow-up study. Monitoring for tachyarrhythmias and/or side effects from the new drug is very important. Document any further episodes of arrhythmias on rhythm strips and be prepared to intervene for lethal arrhythmias. Allowing patients to verbalize fears and anxieties about future studies, impending surgery, or the need for long-term antiarrhythmic drug therapy promotes comfort and aids compliance with the treatment regimen. Slow, deep breathing and relaxation techniques may be helpful in reducing anxiety.

REFERENCES

1. Prystowsky EN, Noble RJ. Electrophysiological studies: Who to refer. *Heart Disease and Stroke.* 1992;1:188–194.
2. Braunwald E. *Heart Disease: A Textbook of Cardiovascular Medicine.* 4th ed. Philadelphia: Saunders; 1991.
3. Hurst JW. *The Heart, Arteries and Veins.* 7th ed. New York: McGraw-Hill; 1990.
4. Josephson M. *Clinical Cardiac Electrophysiology Technique.* 2nd ed. Philadelphia: Lea and Febiger; 1993.
5. Marriott HJ. *Practical electrocardiography.* 8th ed. Baltimore: Williams & Wilkins; 1988.
6. Prystowsky EN. Diagnosis and management of the preexcitation syndromes. *Curr Probl Cardiol.* 1988;13:227–310.
7. Warren J, Lewis R. *Diagnostic Procedures in Cardiology: A Clinician's Guide.* Chicago: Yearbook Medical Publishers; 1985.
8. Prystowsky EN. Electrophysiologic-electropharmacologic testing in patients with ventricular arrhythmias. *PACE.* 1988;11:225–251.
9. Prystowsky EN, Knilans TK, Evans JJ. Diagnostic evaluation and treatment strategies for patients at risk for serious cardiac arrhythmias, part 2: Ventricular tachyarrhythmias and Wolff-Parkinson-White syndrome. *Mod Concepts Cardiovasc Dis.* 1991;60:55–60.
10. Kienzle MG, Williams PD, Zygmont D, et al. Antiarrhythmic drug therapy for sustained ventricular tachycardia. *Heart Lung.* 1984;13:614.
11. Miles WM, Prystowsky EN. Supraventricular tachycardia in patients without overt preexcitation. *Clin Cardiol.* 1986;4:429–446.

12. Calkins H, Sousa J, el-Atassi R, et al. Diagnosis and care of the Wolff-Parkinson-White syndrome or paroxysmal supraventricular tachycardias during a single electrophysiology test. *N Engl J Med*. 1991;324:1612–1618.
13. Winkle RA, Mead RH, Ruder MA, et al. Long-term outcome with the automatic implantable cardioverter defibrillator. *J Am Coll Cardiol*. 1989; 13:1353–1361.
14. Akhtar M, Avitall B, Jazayeri M, et al. Role of implantable cardioverter defibrillator therapy in the management of high risk patients. *Circulation*. 1992;85(suppl 1):131–139.
15. Horwood L, VanRiper S, Davidson T. Antitachycardia pacing: An overview. *Am J Crit Care*. 1995;4:397–404.
16. Davidson T, VanRiper S, Harper P, Wenk A. Implantable cardioverter defibrillators: A guide for clinicians. *Heart Lung*. 1994;23:205–215.

INDEX

Note: Page numbers in *italics* refer to illustrations; page numbers followed by t refer to tables.